HERNIA
SURGICAL ANATOMY AND TECHNIQUE

HERNIA

SURGICAL ANATOMY AND TECHNIQUE

John E. Skandalakis, M.D., PH.D., F.A.C.S.

Chris Carlos Professor of Surgical Anatomy and Technique
Director of the Thalia and Michael Carlos Center for Surgical
* Anatomy and Technique*
Emory University School of Medicine
Senior Attending Surgeon
The Piedmont Hospital, Atlanta, Georgia

Stephen W. Gray, PH.D.

Professor Emeritus of Anatomy
Associate Director of the Thalia and Michael Carlos Center
* for Surgical Anatomy and Technique*
Emory University School of Medicine
Consultant to the Medical Staff for Congenital Anomalies
The Piedmont Hospital, Atlanta, Georgia

Arlie R. Mansberger, Jr., M.D., F.A.C.S.

Professor and Chairman
Department of Surgery, Medical College of Georgia
Augusta, Georgia

Gene L. Colborn, PH.D.

Professor of Anatomy
Director of the Center for Clinical Anatomy
Medical College of Georgia, Augusta, Georgia

Lee J. Skandalakis, M.D.

Former Assistant Professor of Surgery
Medical College of Georgia
Attending Surgeon
The Piedmont Hospital, Atlanta, Georgia

Contributions by

A. Cullen Richardson, M.D.   **Gerald T. Zwiren**, M.D., F.A.C.S.
(Gynecologic Surgery)   (Pediatric Surgery)

Editorial Assistant: Lynne McIntyre, M.A.L.S.

McGraw-Hill Information Services Company
Health Professions Division
New York St. Louis San Francisco Colorado Springs Auckland
Bogotá Caracas Hamburg Lisbon London Madrid Mexico Milan
Montreal New Delhi Panama Paris San Juan São Paulo
Singapore Sydney Tokyo Toronto

HERNIA: Surgical Anatomy and Technique

1234567890 KGPKGP 89321098

ISBN 0-07-057789-7

This book was set in Caslon by York Graphic Services, Inc.
The editors were Ray Moloney and Mariapaz Ramos-Englis; the
production supervisor was Elaine Gardenier; the cover was
designed by Edward R. Schultheis.
Arcata Graphics/Kingsport was printer and binder.

Library of Congress Cataloging-in-Publication Data

Hernia: surgical anatomy and technique/John E. Skandalakis . . . [et al.]; contributions
by Gerald T. Zwiren, A. Cullen Richardson.
  p. cm.
  ISBN 0-07-057789-7
  1. Hernia—Surgery—Atlases. I. Skandalakis, John Elias, date.
  [DNLM: 1. Hernia—surgery—atlases. WI 17 H557]
RD621.H48 1989
617′ .559—dc19
DNLM/DLC
for Library of Congress   88-13559
                          CIP

To our wives, who tolerated us for so many years . . .

Mimi   (J.E.S.)
Betty   (S.W.G.)
Ellen   (A.R.M., Jr.)
Sarah   (G.L.C.)
Vita   (L.J.S.)

Contents

vii

POSTERIOR (LUMBAR) BODY WALL

SECTION TWO   HERNIAS OF THE PELVIC WALL, PERINEUM, AND PELVIC FLOOR

SECTION THREE INTERNAL ABDOMINAL HERNIAS

SECTION FOUR HERNIAS OF THE DIAPHRAGM

THE SURGICAL TREATMENT OF HIATAL HERNIA

CONGENITAL DIAPHRAGMATIC HERNIAS

SECTION FIVE EPONYMOUS HERNIAS

Preface

We have made every sea the highway of our daring.

RICHARD HAKLUYT, 1587
Geographer

This Atlas was begun with the hope that we could present to residents in surgery and to practicing surgeons the surgical embryology, the anatomy and technique, and the anatomical complications of hernias in such a way that their study is easier, their presentation is simpler, and their importance is clearer.

We have presented the surgical repair of most of the hernias as a series of steps by means of which the surgeon can be assured of full control of the procedure.

This Atlas does not present every existing repair of hernias; only the most currently acceptable surgical techniques are described, with or without modifications. We apologize to those surgeons, friends as well as strangers, whose original work or modifications have been left out.

We also present unusual hernias, for the treatment of which we have relied upon the experience of those surgeons with the good fortune to have encountered such rare lesions. Many of these were reproduced on cadavers in the dissecting room in order to determine the anatomical entities involved or to follow the pathway of the hernial sac. Although we have exercised special care with regard to the anatomical details, there may be errors in our descriptions. For this we ask forgiveness. In the words of John Dusseau, then editor at Saunders, on the subject of another one of our books: "Do you want it to be perfect or do you want it published?"

Alas, Anatomy, once the queen of the basic sciences, has today become the neglected stepchild. The embryology and anatomy of the abnormal are no longer emphasized in our schools. With this in mind, we have described normal and abnormal anatomy at considerable length, lest the reader feel lost in the details of surgical procedure. We have described the known seas and indicated approaches to unknown seas, the "highway of our daring."

We are two old surgeons (JES, ARM) and one old anatomist (SWG) in the springtime of our senility. This period is also known as one of wisdom and experience. We have lightened our burden with a young surgeon (LJS) and a mature anatomist at the height of his powers (GLC).

Surgeons and anatomists, no matter how wise or experienced, do not produce an actual book to put on the bookshelf; they need professional help. We wish to praise the Department of Medical Illustration of Emory University Medical School, especially its director, Grover Hogan, and the artists, Charles Boyter, Patsy Bryan, and Michael Budowick, for their skillfully drawn illustrations and for their patience in dealing with the changes and corrections that are always a part of so large an enterprise.

A good clinical teacher is himself a medical school.
OLIVER WENDELL HOLMES

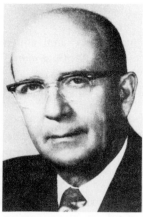

OLIVER H. BEAHRS, M.D.

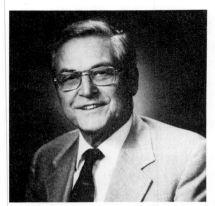

CHESTER B. McVAY, M.D., PH.D.

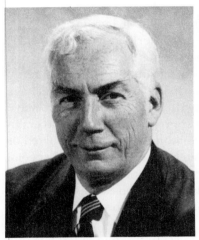

ROBERT E. CONDON, M.D.

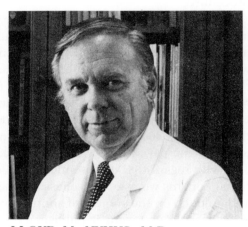

LLOYD M. NYHUS, M.D.

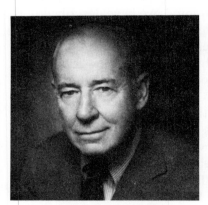

JOHN L. MADDEN, M.D.

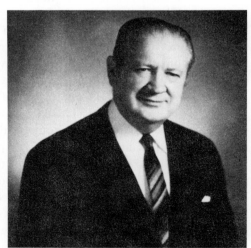

JOSEPH L. PONKA, M.D.

Because they teach the students to be good doctors,
and the doctors to be good surgeons,
and the surgeons to be good teachers.

The authors owe much to Kathy Magruder, our former editorial assistant, who rearranged our English, kept track of the myriad illustrations in their various stages, and reconciled the conflicting views of the authors. We also wish to thank Mariapaz R. Englis of McGraw-Hill Health Professions Division for her editorial and executive help.

Last but not least, our love, gratitude, and appreciation go to our great benefactors, Michael and Thalia Carlos, without whose help this Atlas would not have been published . . .

. . . and to a special group of authors who inspired the students of *Surgery of Hernia* with the biblical

Be ye doers of the word, and not the hearers only

James 1:22

and the Homeric

To be both a speaker of words and a doer of deeds

Homer, The Iliad IX, 443

How grateful, indeed, we are to these navigators of our ship.

Decalogue

Today's status quo was yesterday's new idea.

R.L. VARCO

General Principles

A decalogue of principles of hernia repair should be followed strictly, without deviation.

We do not claim that the decalogue presented here is complete, but we feel that if the surgeon follows these procedures, both surgeon and patient will reach the promised land.

A Decalogue on Herniorrhaphy

1. **Surgical embryology and congenital anomalies.**
   Example: The surgeon must understand the descent of the testes and understand that the testis is retroperitoneal and not intraabdominal.
   Example: The surgeon must understand diaphragmatic defects and their embryonic origin.

2. **Surgical anatomy and anatomical variations.**
   Example: The surgeon should know that collateral testicular circulation is from arteries outside the external inguinal ring. If the testis is not exteriorized, no swelling, inflammation, or gangrene will take place.
   Example: The "touch down" of the external oblique aponeurosis for participation of the anterior lamina of the rectus sheath must be known in order to make a good relaxing incision.

3. **Surgical anatomy and pathology.**
   Example: It is in extremely rare cases only that microscopic pathology will be needed.
   Example: Complete mobilization of the viscus involved in a sliding indirect inguinal hernia would be a catastrophe.

4. **Surgical procedures and modifications.**
   We agree with Nyhus that no one procedure is adequate for all patients with hernia. The surgeon should be flexible, knowledgeable about all of the techniques and their modifications, and able to select the one best for the patient. Recurrence is very unpleasant for both surgeon and patient.

5. **Position and incision.**
   It is essential that the patient be placed in a convenient position.
   The incision should fulfill the requirements of Maingot: accessibility, extensibility, and security.
   We do not advise dogmatically which incision to make. Some surgeons

like vertical incisions, others prefer transverse or oblique incisions with or without muscle splitting.

Much has been written about incision, most of it good. Knowing the anatomy of opening and of closing an incision is the mark of good technique.

6. **The operating room.**

It is not within the scope of this Atlas to give the details of operating room procedure, but we would like to emphasize the following:

   a. Do not break dress code; always wear a clean operating room suit. Go straight from the doctors' dressing room to the operating room.

   b. Do not break sterile technique.

   c. Obtain and keep good hemostasis.

   d. Use a drain when it is necessary. We prefer a Jackson-Pratt device, but a simple Penrose drain is acceptable.

   e. Select appropriate suture and prosthetic material. Table 1 shows a list of suture materials from Ponka (*Hernias of the Abdominal Wall,* 1980, p. 344), with some additions. The choice is up to the surgeon. The controversy over absorbable or nonabsorbable sutures continues. We thought the requiem of catgut had been played and the epitaph carved several years ago, but our old friend Dr. Oliver Beahrs has reopened the subject.

   Dr. Beahrs loves catgut; he has had remarkable success with catgut sutures. Others support silk, or synthetic or metallic material.

   Since we trained with, and thus prefer, nonabsorbable biomaterial, we nonetheless recognize that permeable or nonpermeable sutures may be used to close a defect without tension. There are surgeons who always use prosthesis (e.g., Bellis) for the repair of direct inguinal hernias. Again, we cite (Table 2) a list of such materials from Ponka (p. 538). The choice of whether to use stapling devices, absorbable or nonabsorbable, is up to the surgeon.

7. **The natural history of the disease.**

A hernia is usually first seen by the internist, who, in most cases, does not advise early operation. This is unfortunate because, over time, the protrusion will destroy more and more of the anatomical entities and their normal relationships. A small hernia can be repaired more easily than a large one. The patient will benefit more from early surgery despite the small but real recurrence rate. Remember, an untreated hernia is usually incapacitating and may lead to intestinal obstruction and death.

8. **Physical examination.**

This should include the detection of metabolic problems, collagen deficiency disease, and the possibility of allergic reaction. Such findings may influence the surgeon in his choice of a preperitoneal nonabsorbable prosthesis or the use of the "plug" technique of Lichtenstein. General anesthesia, spinal, epidural, or local anesthesia should each be evaluated in terms of the patient's welfare. Remember, the patient may have debilitating problems other than the hernia.

9. **Preoperative preparations.**

Polk, in Sabiston's *Textbook of Surgery* (1986), has proposed a simple preoperative checklist. We consider this to be one of the best of such lists available today.

1. Operative permit—appropriately signed and witnessed.
2. Dietary considerations.
   a. For abdominal operation, liquid diet and laxatives to ensure clean collapsed bowel.
   b. NPO (nothing by mouth) at least 6 h before operation.
3. Review of life support systems.
   a. Vital signs recorded often enough to establish "normal."
   b. Pulmonary system—chest x-rays; other studies as indicated.
   c. Cardiac function—ECG; other studies as indicated.
   d. Renal function—urinalysis; BUN (blood urea nitrogen) and creatinine determinations.
4. Adequate hydration up to time of operation—especially to compensate for laxatives and fasting.
5. Area of operation washed with appropriate germicidal detergent and shaved, clipped, or cleansed with depilatory agent.
6. Blood transfusions prepared as anticipated.
7. Order that patient should void on call to operating room.
8. Preoperative medications—vagolytic and sedative drugs.
9. Special medications—digitalis, insulin.

10. Postoperative care.

Observation for a few hours for uncomplicated procedures, or observation and hospitalization for several days after complicated procedures or celiotomy (internal hernia). The following is the postoperative checklist:
1. Vital signs
2. I & O (intake and output)
3. Wound care
   a. Dressing change
   b. Seroma
   c. Infection
   d. Dehiscence
4. Pulmonary complications: atelectasis
5. Cardiovascular complications
   a. Arrhythmia
   b. Myocardial infarction
6. Gastrointestinal complications
   a. Bleeding (hematemesis—melena)
   b. Intestinal obstruction
7. Antibiotics PRN (as necessary)
8. NPO if indicated
9. IV fluids

TABLE 1
A Classification of Suture Materials*

Nonabsorbable	Absorbable
A. Natural	A. Natural
1. Cotton	1. Catgut
2. Silk	*a.* Plain
B. Synthetic	*b.* Chromicized
1. Polyamide	*c.* Iodized
a. Nylon	2. Reconstructed collagen
b. Nylon-braided (Nurolon, Surgilon)	B. Synthetic
2. Polyester	1. Polyglycolic acid (Dexon)
a. Multifilament (Dacron, Mersilene)	2. Polyglactin (Vicryl)
b. Teflon-coated (Ethiflex, Deknatel, Tevdek, Polydek)	3. Polyparadioxanone (PDS)
c. Silicone-treated (Tycron)	4. Clips
3. Polyolefins	5. Staples
a. Polypropylene (Prolene)	
b. Polyethylene	
4. Metallic	
a. Steel: Monofilament / Braided	
b. Tantalum	
c. Clips	
d. Staples	

*Adapted from Ponka, *Hernias of the Abdominal Wall,* 1980, p. 344, with modifications.

TABLE 2
**A Classification of Reinforcing Materials
for Hernia Repair***

I. Autografts	IV. Metallic
A. Fascia lata	A. Stainless steel
1. Free	B. Tantalum
2. Pedicle	C. Silver
B. Tendon	V. Synthetic-plastic
C. Cutis graft	A. Marlex mesh (high-density polyethylene)
D. Whole skin	B. Mersilene (Dacron polyester)
II. Homograft	C. Nylon (Polyamide)
A. Fascia lata	D. Others
B. Aorta	1. Teflon (polytetrafluoroethylene)
III. Heterografts	2. Ivalon sponge (formalized polyvinyl)
A. Fascia	
B. Tendon	
C. Pericardium	

*From Ponka, *Hernias of the Abdominal Wall,* 1980, p. 538.

HERNIA
SURGICAL ANATOMY AND TECHNIQUE

SECTION ONE
HERNIAS OF THE ABDOMINAL WALL

ANTERIOR BODY WALL

Embryogenesis of the Upper Anterior Body Wall

The anterior body wall forms as a result of the rapid growth of the embryonic body and a simultaneous decrease in the growth of the body stalk.

The primitive wall is a layer of ectoderm and mesoderm (somatopleure)— at first without muscle, vessels, or nerves. In the sixth week, mesoderm from the myotomes on each side of the vertebral column invades the somatopleure. The segmental pattern is lost, and the mesoderm grows laterally and ventrally as a sheet. The leading edges of the sheet will differentiate into right and left rectus abdominis muscles, at first widely separated. The remainder of the mesodermal sheet splits into an external layer, which will differentiate into the external oblique muscle (ventral) and the serratus muscles (dorsal); a middle layer, which will form the internal oblique muscle; and an inner layer, which will become the transversus abdominis muscle. All of these muscles are distinguishable by the middle of the seventh week.

As these muscles differentiate, the rapidly growing intestine, with a portion of coelom, herniates into the umbilical cord. Normally, the intestines return to the growing abdominal cavity in the tenth week. Following this return, the recti approximate, and their sheaths form the linea alba in the midline, leaving a fibrous ring about 1 cm in diameter surrounding the attachment of the umbilical cord. Anteriorly the skin attaches directly to the ring, and after birth it covers the whole ring with no intervening subcutaneous fat. Inferiorly the transversalis fascia and peritoneum form the floor of the ring.

Surgical Anatomy of the Upper Anterior Abdominal Wall

For practical purposes, the anterior abdominal wall may be divided into two portions, lateral and medial. Laterally the wall is composed of the external and internal oblique muscles and the transversus abdominis muscle. Medially the wall is formed by the rectus abdominis and pyramidalis muscles.

The three muscles of the lateral portion are arranged so that their fibers are roughly parallel at their insertion on the rectus sheath. Muscle-splitting incisions will not encounter markedly different directions between fibers of the three muscles. Laterally, toward the flank, the direction of the fibers becomes divergent, and muscle transection may be necessary during urologic procedures performed through flank incisions.

The Rectus Abdominis Muscle and the Rectus Sheath
The rectus abdominis muscle arises from the pubic crest and pubic symphysis and inserts on the fifth, sixth, and seventh costal cartilages; occasionally fibers insert on the xiphoid process.

The pyramidalis muscle arises from the anterior surface of the pubis and inserts on the linea alba midway or less between the umbilicus and the pubis. It is inconstant, being absent on one or both sides in from 10 to 20 percent of subjects.

The rectus and pyramidalis muscles are contained in a stout sheath formed by the aponeuroses of the three muscles of the lateral abdominal wall. These aponeuroses fuse, then split to enclose the rectus abdominis and rejoin as the linea alba in the midline (Plate 1A,B). In the inferior one-fourth of the abdominal wall, the aponeuroses pass only anterior to the rectus (Plate 1A,C). The linea semicircularis (of Douglas) marks the level at which the posterior aponeurotic layer of the sheath disappears (Plate 1A). The differences in the wall above and below this line may be summarized as follows:

Upper Midline	Lower Midline
Linea alba well developed	Linea alba poorly developed
Right and left recti well separated	Right and left recti close together
Anterior and posterior layers of sheath present	Only anterior layer of sheath present
Aponeurosis of external oblique weak or absent	Aponeurosis of external oblique strong and well developed

Blood Supply to the Anterior Abdominal Wall

Three superficial branches of the femoral artery help supply the abdominal wall below the umbilicus, giving off rami that pass upward in the subcutaneous connective tissue. From lateral to medial, they are the superficial circumflex iliac artery, the superficial epigastric artery, and the superficial external pudendal artery. The superficial epigastric artery anastomoses with the contralateral artery, and all have anastomoses with the deep arteries.

Deep arteries lie between the internal oblique and the transversus abdominis muscles. They are the tenth and eleventh posterior intercostal arteries, the anterior branch of the subcostal artery, the anterior branches of the four lumbar arteries, and the deep circumflex iliac artery.

The blood supply to the rectus sheath is from the superior and inferior epigastric arteries. They frequently anastomose.

The superior epigastric artery enters the upper end of the sheath deep to the rectus muscle. Cutaneous branches pierce the anterior lamina of the sheath close to the lateral border of the rectus, to supply the skin. Too lateral an incision may cut these perforating arteries as well as musculocutaneous nerves.

The inferior epigastric artery enters the rectus sheath at or about the semilunar line, between the rectus muscle and the posterior lamina of the sheath.

Nerve Supply to the Anterior Abdominal Wall

Both the lateral abdominal wall and the recti are supplied by the anterior rami of the VIIth to the XIIth thoracic (Plate 1D) and the Ist lumbar nerves (Plate 1E). Each ramus gives off a lateral branch which pierces the transversus abdominis and internal oblique muscles to innervate the external oblique muscle and form the lateral cutaneous nerve. The anterior branches of the VIIth to XIIth thoracic nerves enter the rectus sheath, innervating the rectus muscle and piercing the anterior lamina of the sheath to form the anterior cutaneous nerves. The subcostal nerve (T_{12}) supplies the pyramidalis muscle (Plate 1D). The first lumbar nerve forms anterior cutaneous nerves (iliohypogastric and ilioinguinal) without entering the rectus sheath (Plate 1E). There is little if any communication between the segmental nerves to the rectus muscle, so that section of more than one nerve results in rectus paralysis with a weakened abdominal wall.

Formation of the Linea Alba

The linea alba is formed by interdigitation and fusion of the aponeurotic fibers of the anterior and posterior laminae of the rectus sheath between the medial borders of the rectus muscles. The rectus sheath is composed of the fascial layers and aponeuroses of the external oblique, internal oblique, and transversus abdominis muscles.

As they approach the midline, the aponeuroses form a three-layered system of interlacing fibers, described in detail by Askar (1984) (Plate 2). Fibers of the external oblique aponeurosis cross the midline to become continuous with fibers of the contralateral internal oblique aponeurosis and the contralateral anterior rectus sheath lamina. Similarly, the posterior lamina of the internal oblique aponeurosis and that of the transversus abdominis form the posterior lamina of the rectus sheath. Fibers of the transversus abdominis also cross the midline.

The number of crossings of fibers (decussation) at the linea alba varies. In 30 percent of Askar's subjects there was a single anterior and single posterior crossing. In 10 percent there was a single anterior and a triple posterior crossing. In 60 percent both anterior and posterior crossings were triple. One can only speculate that subjects with single fibrous crossings may be more susceptible to linea alba hernia than those with triple crossings.

Surgical Anatomy of the Umbilical Region

In a study of the umbilical region, Orda and Nathan (1973) found that in most individuals (74 percent), the round ligament of the liver passed over the superior margin of the umbilical ring and crossed the ring to attach to the inferior margin (Plate 3A). In about one-fourth of subjects, the round ligament bifurcated and attached to the superior margin of the ring (Plate 3B). In such cases, the floor of the ring was formed by transversalis fascia and peritoneum only.

The floor of the umbilical ring may be further strengthened by a thickening of the transversalis fascia in this area, the fascia umbilicalis. This thickened fascia may cover the umbilical ring entirely (Plate 3C) or partially (Plate 3D,E). It may fail to cover the ring (Plate 3F), and it was completely absent in 16 percent of specimens.

There are thus two structures, the round ligament and the fascia umbilicalis, that protect the umbilical area. If both are absent (Plate 3B,F), the floor of the umbilical ring is relatively unsupported. Herniation through such a ring has been called *direct* umbilical hernia by Orda and Nathan (1973).

Where the umbilical fascia partly covers the ring (Plate 3D,E), the superior or inferior edge may form a fold or recess through which a hernia may occur. Such an "indirect" umbilical hernia descends into the umbilical ring from a superior fascial fold, or ascends into the ring from an inferior fold. A combination of the variations shown in Plates 3B, and D or E would appear to predispose to herniation through the umbilical ring. Far from supporting the ring in such cases, the umbilical fascia may predispose to hernia.

Anatomy of the Umbilical Cord

The covering of the umbilical cord at its junction with the body is a simple epithelium continuous distally with the amnion and proximally with the skin. At term, the cord contains the stroma of the embryonic connective tissue (Wharton's jelly) as well as the following structures (Plate 4, Table 1):

1. Two umbilical arteries
2. One left umbilical vein
3. Vestige of the allantoic duct (urachus)

These structures pass through the abdominal wall at the umbilical ring, an opening in the linea alba about 1 cm in diameter.

TABLE 1
Structures Associated with the Umbilical Cord and Umbilicus

In the Primitive Body Stalk	At the Umbilicus at Term	In the Neonatal Abdomen	Pathology
Yolk stalk (vitelline duct)	Absent or vestigial	Absent	Meckel's diverticulum or umbilical sinus or fistula
Extraembryonic coelom	Absent	None	
Herniated intestine	Returned to abdomen	Returned to abdomen	Failure of return: omphalocele
Vitelline arteries	Absent	Celiac, superior, and inferior mesenteric arteries	
Vitelline veins	Absent	Part of portal vein	
Allantois	Absent or vestigial	Urachus (median umbilical ligament)	Patent urachus; undescended bladder
Umbilical arteries	Both present	Medial umbilical ligaments	Single umbilical artery (1%)
Umbilical veins	Only left vein present	Round ligament in falciform ligament	
Undifferentiated mesenchyme	Embryonic connective tissue at cord	None	

PLATE 1

Anatomy of the Anterior Abdominal Wall

A. The anterior body wall and some landmarks.

B. Section through the anterior abdominal wall at level 1 showing the rectus abdominis muscle, the rectus sheath, and the layers of the lateral abdominal wall.

C. Section through the abdominal wall at level 2. The posterior aponeurotic lamina of the sheath is absent. The posterior lamina is formed only by the transversalis fascia.

D. The course of the anterior rami of the VIIth to XIIth thoracic segmental nerves in the anterior body wall.

E. The course of the anterior ramus of the first lumbar nerve.

Source: Orda R, Nathan H: Surgical anatomy of the umbilical structures. *Int Surg* 58(7): 454–464, 1973.

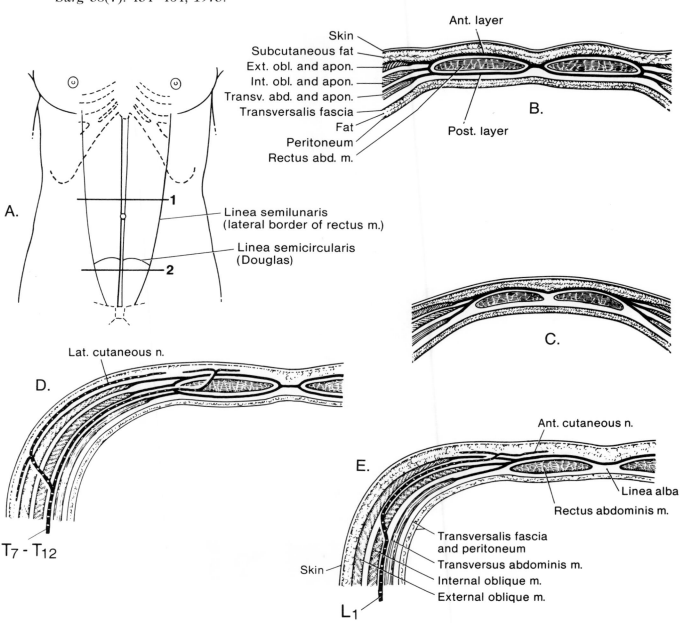

PLATE 2
Muscles of the Anterior Abdominal Wall

A. Aponeurotic fibers of the external oblique muscle cross the midline to form the anterior lamina of the contralateral internal oblique aponeurosis.

B. Aponeurotic fibers of the transversus abdominis muscle cross the midline to form the posterior lamina of the contralateral internal oblique aponeurosis.

C. Aponeurotic fibers of the transversus abdominis muscle cross the midline to form the contralateral aponeurosis.

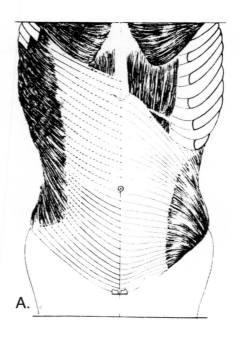

A.

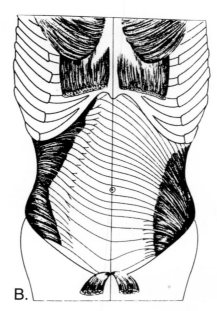

B.

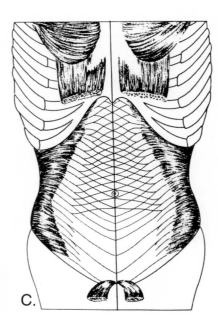

C.

D. Askar's concept of the linea alba formed by decussating aponeurotic fibers of the rectus sheath:

1. Single decussation of fibers of the anterior and posterior rectus sheaths (30 percent of specimens).
2. Single decussation of anterior and triple decussation of posterior rectus sheath (10 percent of specimens).
3. Triple decussation of aponeurotic fibers of both anterior and posterior rectus sheaths (60 percent of specimens).

Source: Askar OM: Aponeurotic hernias, recent observations upon paraumbilical and epigastric hernias. *Surg Clin North Am* 64:315–333, 1984 (Fig 3; Fig 8B).

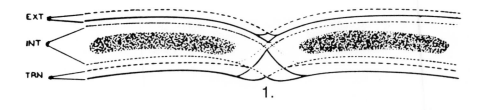

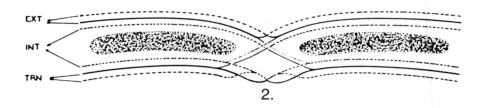

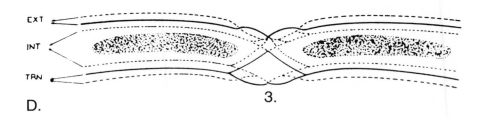

D.

PLATE 3

Variations in the Umbilical Ring and the Umbilical Fascia

Variations in the umbilical ring and the umbilical fascia as seen from the posterior (peritoneal) surface of the body wall. Arrows indicate:

A. Usual relations (74 percent) of the umbilical ring (UR), the round ligament (RL), the urachus (U), and the medial umbilical ligaments (MUL). The round ligament crosses the umbilical ring to insert on its inferior margin.

B. Less-common configuration (24 percent). The round ligament splits and is attached to the superior margin of the umbilical ring.

C. The thickened transversalis fascia which forms the umbilical fascia covers the umbilical ring (36 percent).

D. The umbilical fascia covers only the superior portion of the umbilical ring (38 percent).

E. The umbilical fascia covers only the inferior portion of the umbilical ring (6 percent).

F. Though present, the umbilical fascia does not underlie the umbilical ring (4 percent).
   The fascia is entirely absent in 16 percent.

Source: Orda R, Nathan H: Surgical anatomy of the umbilical structures. *Int Surg* 58(7): 454–464, 1973.

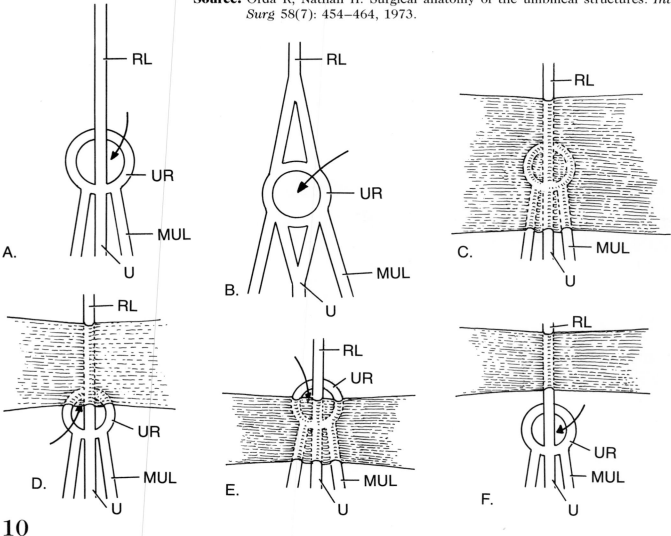

PLATE 4
Surgical Anatomy of the Umbilical Region

A. The posterior surface of the anterior abdominal wall of a newborn infant is seen from inside the abdomen. The umbilical cord is still attached. The medial umbilical ligaments (obliterated umbilical arteries) and the urachus (obliterated allantoic duct) participate in the formation of the fibrous umbilical ring. The round ligament (obliterated umbilical vein) arises from the inferior margin of the ring and passes superiorly in the falciform ligament.

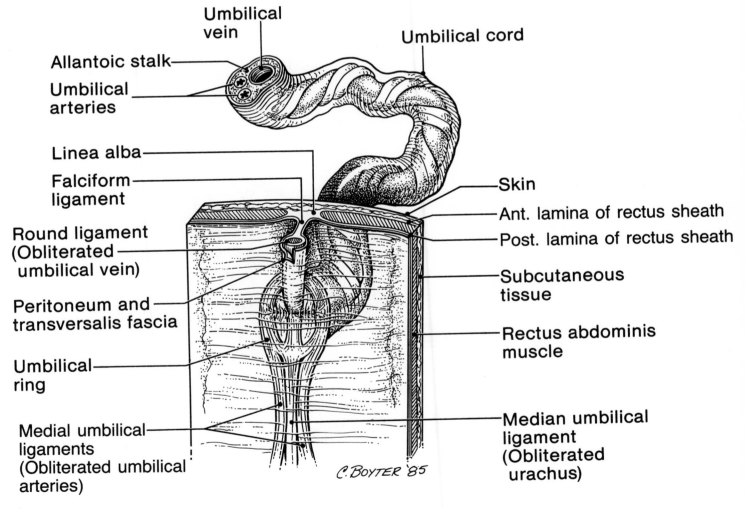

Umbilical vein

Umbilical cord

Allantoic stalk

Umbilical arteries

Linea alba

Falciform ligament

Skin

Ant. lamina of rectus sheath

Round ligament (Obliterated umbilical vein)

Post. lamina of rectus sheath

Subcutaneous tissue

Peritoneum and transversalis fascia

Rectus abdominis muscle

Umbilical ring

Medial umbilical ligaments (Obliterated umbilical arteries)

Median umbilical ligament (Obliterated urachus)

C. BOYTER '85

A.

11

PLATE 4 (*Continued*)
Surgical Anatomy of the Umbilical Region

B. Diagrammatic sagittal section through a normal umbilicus showing the relation of the umbilical ring to the linea alba, the round ligament, the urachus, and the umbilical and transversalis fasciae. Note the absence of subcutaneous fat over the umbilical ring.

C. Diagrammatic sagittal section through a small umbilical hernia. The hernial sac is covered by skin only.

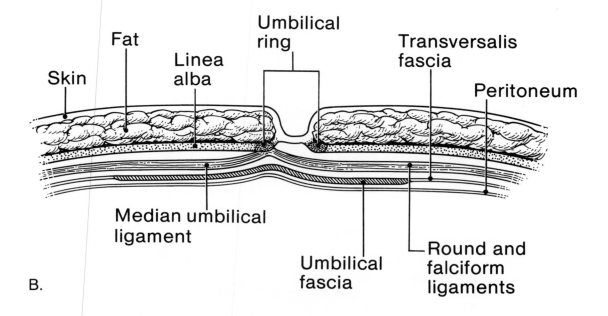

B.

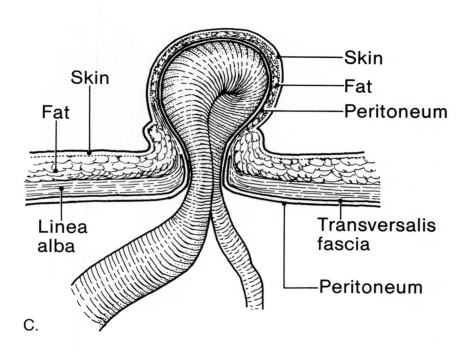

C.

Incisional Hernia

Pray before surgery,
but remember God will not
alter a faulty incision.

ARTHUR H. KEENEY

Definition

Incisional hernia is the abnormal protrusion of peritoneum through a separation of the edges of a musculoaponeurotic wound. The wound may be fresh, recent, or even old. The peritoneal sac may or may not contain a viscus.

Predisposing Pathogenic Factors

1. Obesity (the most important single factor)
2. Wound infection
3. Wound dehiscence
4. Postoperative hematoma or seroma
5. Type of incision
6. Poor technique of wound closure
7. Inadequate available abdominal wall (resulting from surgery or trauma)
8. Postoperative distension
9. Ascites secondary to liver cirrhosis
10. Concomitant steroid therapy
11. Malnutrition (hypoproteinemia scurvy)
12. Pulmonary complications

There are many types of abdominal incisions; some have descriptive names, and others are eponymous. Few surgeons can deny a secret wish to have a procedure, or at least a modification of a procedure, named for them. Here we will, however, describe only major types of incision commonly used without discussing their variations (Plate 6).

In any given case the choice of operation should be governed by the three requirements of Maingot[1]: *accessibility, extensibility,* and *security.* Although transverse incisions take more time and cause more bleeding than do longitudinal incisions, they result in slightly fewer incisional hernias. Statistically, the difference is not highly significant. Postoperative herniation occurs more often in vertical incisions due to contractions of muscles pulling on the edge of the wound.

Abdominal muscle returns to its preoperative strength in about 8 weeks after operation. In the absence of complicating factors, dehiscence and herniation will occur soon after the operation, if they occur at all.

Good healing without incisional hernia or a disfiguring scar results from the absence of tension on sutures; from little or no pressure or dead space; and from the presence of good debridement, hemostasis, irrigation, and good skin approximation.

[1]Maingot R: *Abdominal Operations,* 5th ed. Appleton-Century-Crofts, New York, 1969.

13

Treatment

The role of preoperative care in preventing incisional hernia must not be overlooked. We recommend the following regimen:

1. Wash abdomen with Hibiclens or PhisoHex 12 h and 1 h prior to surgery.
2. Shave abdomen 1 h prior to surgery.
3. Insert Foley catheter.
4. Insert nasogastric tube.
5. Provide intravenous antibiotics prior to surgery and for the first 24 h after surgery.
6. Bowel preparation:

   Cathartics
   Erythromycin base 500 mg qid for 1 day prior to surgery.
   Neomycin 1 g qid for 1 day prior to surgery.
   Barium enema.
   Gastrointestinal and small bowel series.

PLATE 5
Basic Types of Abdominal Incision

The choice of incision must be based on Maingot's principles:
1. The incision must provide *access* to the viscus or lesion to be treated.
2. The incision must permit *extension* should it be necessary.
3. The incision must permit *secure* closure.

A. Midline (linea alba) incision

B. Paramedian (rectus) incision with muscle retraction

C. Subcostal incision

D. Two transverse abdominal incisions

E. McBurney incision

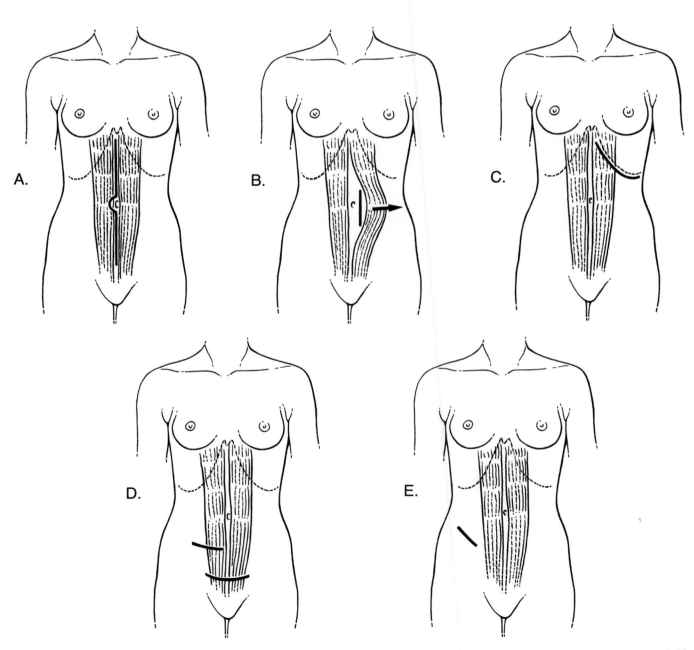

PLATE 5 (*Continued*)

Basic Types of Abdominal Incision

F,G. Two thoracoabdominal incisions

H. Pararectus incision[1]

I. Paramedian (rectus) incisions with muscle splitting[1]

[1]Incisions H and I are not recommended.

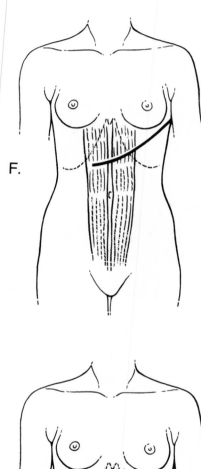

F.

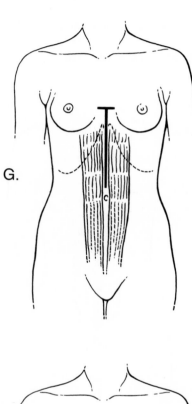

G.

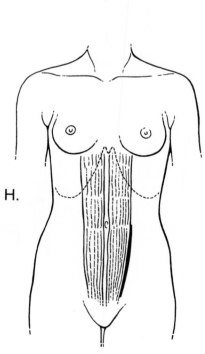

H.

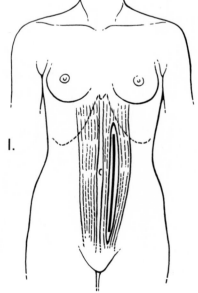

I.

PLATE 6
Abdominal Incisions—Sectional View

A. Vertical midline incision through the linea alba.

B. Paramedian (rectus) muscle-splitting incision.

C. Pararectus incision. Dashed line indicates the course of thoracic segmental nerve.

D. Paramedian (rectus) muscle-retracting incision. Opening the sheath and retracting the muscle laterally will avoid the muscle splitting shown in part B.

E. As above, with release of retraction allowing the rectus to bridge the incision through the sheath (compare with part B above). Muscle retraction is preferred over muscle splitting.

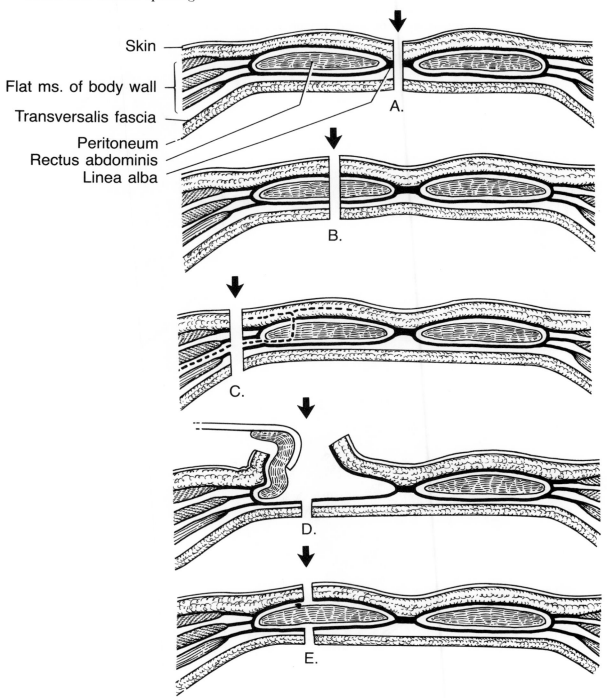

Skin

Flat ms. of body wall

Transversalis fascia

Peritoneum
Rectus abdominis
Linea alba

A.

B.

C.

D.

E.

PLATE 7
Repair of Incisional Hernia

For obvious reasons, it is impossible to describe the technique for every incisional hernia. A good knowledge of the anatomy of the anterior and lateral abdominal wall is a must for a good repair.

A. Herniation at the site of a left rectus incision.

B. *Step 1*. Make an elliptical incision over the hernia and around the scar. Apply clamps to the skin over the hernial sac and to the subcutaneous tissue peripherally.

Step 2. Dissect skin flaps and subcutaneous tissue on both sides of the defect to the aponeurotic level. This facilitates exact identification of the defect and the hernia sac.

C. *Step 3*. Expose the hernia sac and open it. The hernia ring may be round or ovoid, large or small. Peripheral dissection of the ring may be necessary to reach a strong "white" musculoaponeurotic tissue. Remove old sutures if encountered.

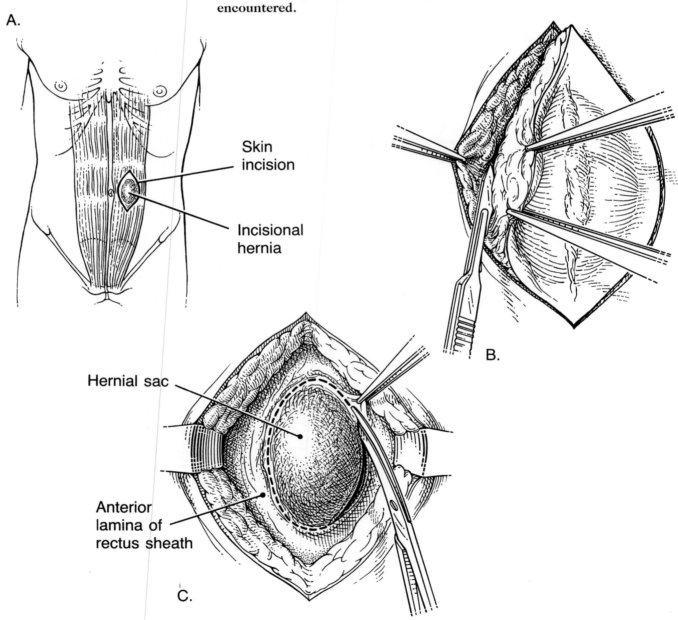

A.

Skin
incision

Incisional
hernia

B.

Hernial sac

Anterior
lamina of
rectus sheath

C.

18

D. *Step 4.* Elevate the opened hernial sac. Dissect any adhesions between the sac and its contents.

Step 5. Remove the sac and scar tissue. The hernial ring has been trimmed. In the patient shown here, the posterior and anterior laminae of the rectus sheath were obvious after removal of scar tissue.

Step 6. They were separated, and the decision was made to close the incision in two layers. Both sheaths were prepared accordingly.

E. *Step 7.* Dissect for about 3 cm around the ring. Digital examination around the ring may reveal more small defects of the abdominal wall.

Step 8. The operator may choose to close the small defect if it is some distance from the principal defect or to convert several defects into one large defect. In the latter case, peripheral dissection around the ring should be generous.

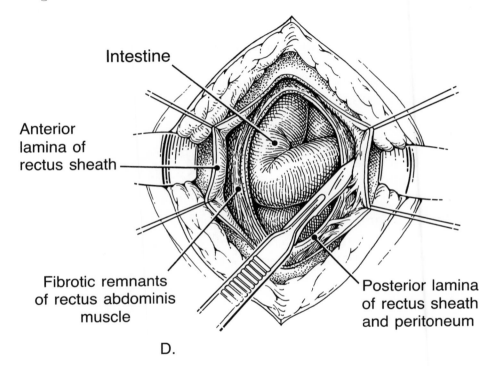

Intestine

Anterior lamina of rectus sheath

Fibrotic remnants of rectus abdominis muscle

Posterior lamina of rectus sheath and peritoneum

D.

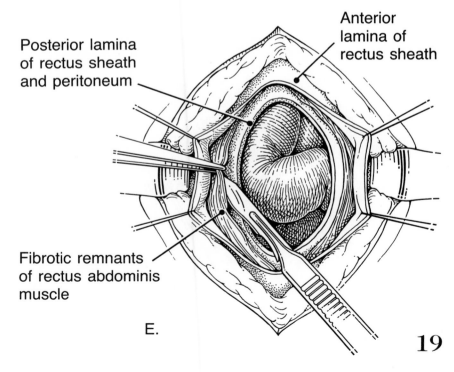

Posterior lamina of rectus sheath and peritoneum

Anterior lamina of rectus sheath

Fibrotic remnants of rectus abdominis muscle

E.

19

PLATE 7 (*Continued*)

Repair of Incisional Hernia

F. *Step 9.* Closure of the posterior lamina may be accomplished in several ways. In this illustration closure is by continuous no. 1 Prolene with interrupted no. 0 Dexon every three bites.

G. *Step 10.* Close the anterior rectus lamina in the same manner.

Step 11. Close the subcutaneous tissues with a few interrupted 00 plain catgut sutures.

H. The defect has been closed transversely in one layer with continuous Prolene no. 1 sutures with interrupted Dexon no. 0 incorporating the peritoneum, the transversalis fascia, and the aponeuroses. We prefer this closure. Damage to underlying intestine must be avoided.

I. *Step 12.* Close the skin with interrupted sutures.

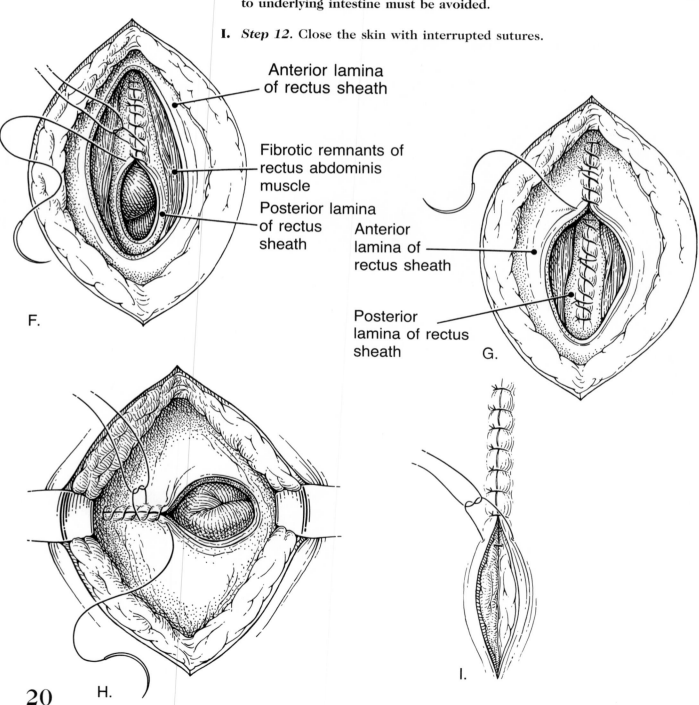

Anterior lamina of rectus sheath

Fibrotic remnants of rectus abdominis muscle

Posterior lamina of rectus sheath

Anterior lamina of rectus sheath

Posterior lamina of rectus sheath

F.

G.

H.

I.

PLATE 8
Alternative Closures for Incisional Hernia Repair

Remember: The defect may be closed by any of several methods:

A. Imbrication with side-to-side closure.

B. Appositional interrupted sutures with edge-to-edge closure.

C. Continuous suture with edge-to-edge closure. Interrupted sutures every third bite may or may not be considered necessary. Insert sutures not less than 2 to 2.5 cm from the ring. Keep in mind the three Bs: Big-Bites-Better. Strategically located relaxing incisions occasionally help to close a defect without tension.

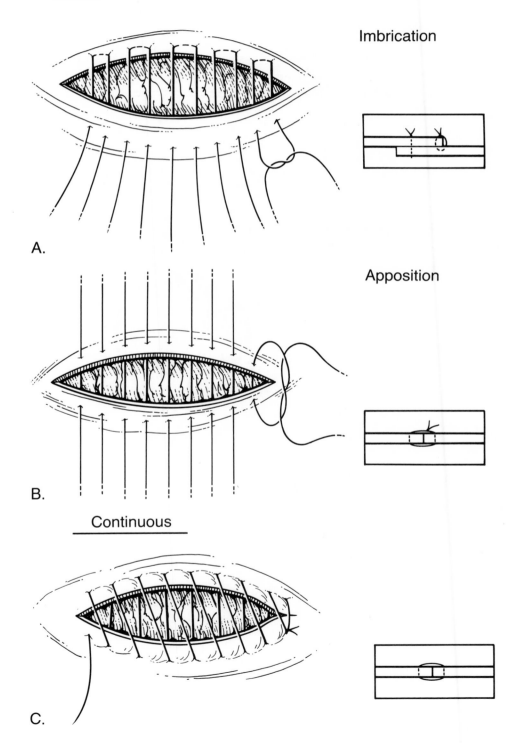

Imbrication

A.

Apposition

B.

Continuous

C.

PLATE 8 (*Continued*)

Alternative Closures for Incisional Hernia Repair

D. If the defect is large, use the Usher repair with two layers of Marlex or Prolene mesh. Fix the deep layer to the posterior surface of the transversalis fascia.

E. Fix a second layer to the anterior surface of the fascia with interrupted 0 or 00 polypropylene monofilament sutures. Our preference is Prolene mesh.

F. Use drains in large hernias. The J-P or Snyder apparatus is the best. Use separate stab wounds, and secure the catheter with skin sutures.

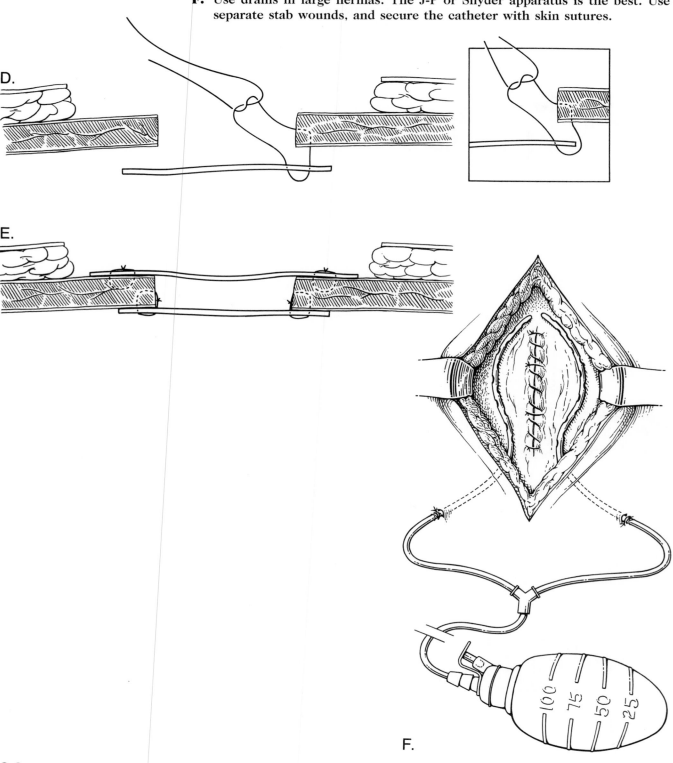

TABLE 2
Summary of Anatomical Complications of Abdominal Incisions

Procedure	Vascular Injury	Nerve Injury	Organ Injury	Inadequate Procedure
All abdominal incisions	Hemorrhage; hematoma; ischemia	Muscle paralysis; neuroma formation	Perforation of abdominal viscus	Evisceration; dehiscence; incisional hernia
Upper midline incision	None	None	Perforation of abdominal viscus	Too short an incision may be extended upward and downward
Lower midline incision	None	None	Perforation of bladder	Too short an incision may be extended upward
Rectus incision	None, with lateral retraction	None, with lateral retraction	Perforation of abdominal viscus	Too short an incision may be extended upward and downward
Pararectus incision	Ischemia of medial portion of rectus	Injury to nerve supply to rectus muscle	Perforation of abdominal viscus	Too short an incision may be extended
Upper transverse incision	Superior epigastric artery	Injury to more than one nerve	Perforation of abdominal viscus	Too short an incision may be extended
Lower transverse incision	Inferior epigastric artery	Iliohypogastric nerve; ilioinguinal nerve	Perforation of bladder	Limited lateral extension possible
Subcostal incision	Hemorrhage	VIII and IX intercostal nerves	Perforation of abdominal viscus	May be extended in abdominal midline or chest wall
McBurney incision	Hemorrhage	Iliohypogastric nerve	Perforation of abdominal viscus	May be too small
Thoracoabdominal incision	Hemorrhage; ischemia of skin flap with T incisions	Intercostal nerves	Perforation of abdominal or thoracic viscus	

Source: Skandalakis JE, Gray SW, Rowe JS Jr.: *Anatomical Complications in General Surgery.* McGraw-Hill, New York, 1983, p. 301, Table 15-1. Used with permission.

23

Epigastric Hernia
(Hernia through the Linea Alba)

Definition

Epigastric hernia, or hernia through the linea alba, is a protrusion of preperitoneal fat or a peritoneal sac with or without an incarcerated viscus. It occurs in the midline between the xiphoid process and the umbilicus. The linea alba is wider above the umbilicus and more prone to penetration.

In the usual epigastric hernia, preperitoneal fat bulges through a small defect in the linea alba. Less commonly, the defect enlarges and a peritoneal sac is present. The sac may be empty or contain omentum or small or large intestine. Such a hernia is covered by skin, subcutaneous fat, and peritoneum.

PLATE 9

Diagram of Epigastric Hernia

A. Diagrammatic transverse section through the rectus abdominis muscles and the linea alba above the umbilicus.

B. Herniation of preperitoneal fat through the rectus sheath and the linea alba. In this illustration a peritoneal sac containing omentum has formed through a defect in the rectus sheath. The sac is covered only with skin and fat.

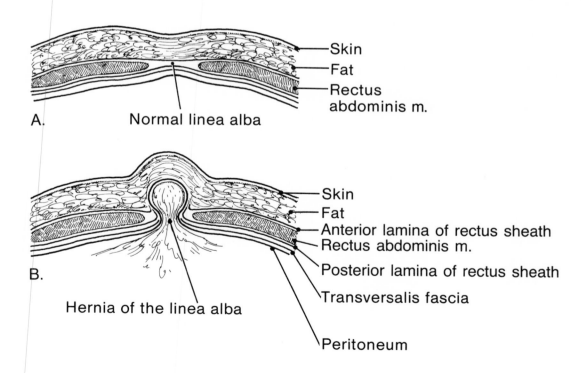

A. Normal linea alba

Skin
Fat
Rectus abdominis m.

B. Hernia of the linea alba

Skin
Fat
Anterior lamina of rectus sheath
Rectus abdominis m.
Posterior lamina of rectus sheath
Transversalis fascia
Peritoneum

PLATE 10
Repair of Epigastric Hernia

A. *Step 1.* Make a vertical or transverse incision over the mass.

B. *Step 2.* Dissect the fat down to the linea alba superiorly and inferiorly and to the anterior lamina of the rectus sheath laterally.

C. *Step 3.* Separate the preperitoneal tissues from the subcutaneous fat and the anterior lamina of the rectus sheath.

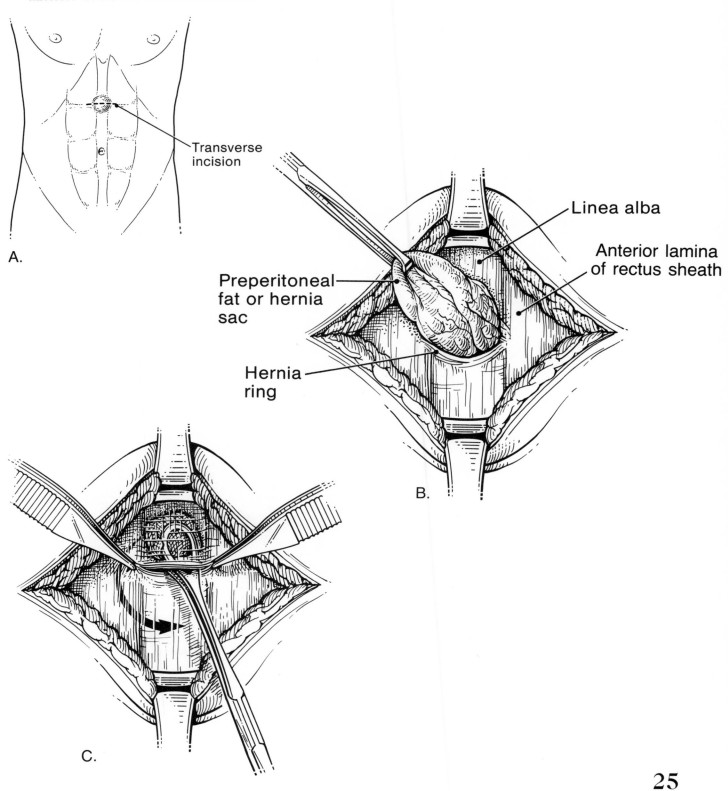

A.

Transverse
incision

Linea alba

Anterior lamina
of rectus sheath

Preperitoneal
fat or hernia
sac

Hernia
ring

B.

C.

PLATE 10 (*Continued*)
Repair of Epigastric Hernia

D. *Step 4.* Expose the hernial ring. If the defect is small, push the protruding fat inside. Rarely is there a hernial sac. If one is present, open it; ligate with 00 or 000 silk and invert. With incarceration, the ring can be enlarged by incising the linea alba upward or downward sufficiently to release the tissue or viscus.

E. *Step 5.* Close the small defect in the linea alba transversely with interrupted 0 Surgilon suture or with continuous 0 Prolene and interrupted 0 Dexon if the defect is large.

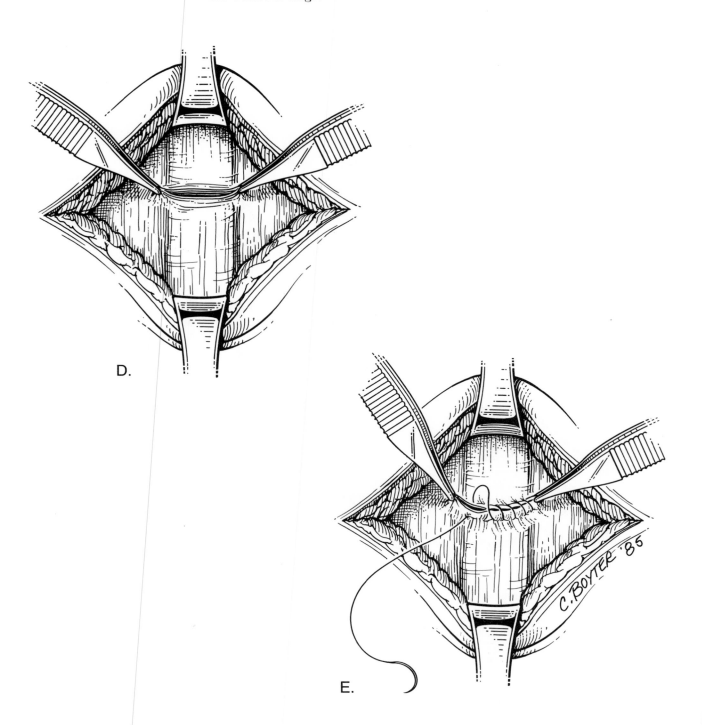

D.

E.

F. *Step 6.* Imbrication may be used, but not at the risk of overstretching the aponeurosis.

G. *Step 7.* Close large defects vertically. Closure may be achieved in a single layer with continuous 0 Prolene and interrupted 0 Dexon every three bites. Closure in two layers is done by suturing the posterior and anterior laminae of the rectus sheath separately. In extreme cases, a prosthetic mesh may be needed.

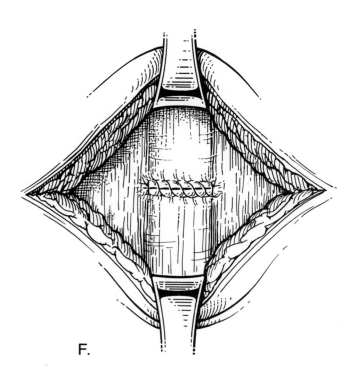

F.

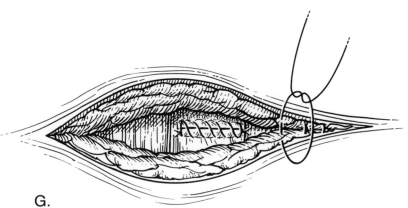

G.

Umbilical Hernia

I have resolved to restore this science [surgery] to life,
and to consecrate this treatise to that purpose. I will
proceed by way of explanation and demonstration, in
curtailing that which is superfluous. I will give drawings
of surgical instruments and cauteries; I will describe them
and indicate the use of them.

ALBUCASIS (11TH CENTURY)
Introduction to Altasrif (Collection)

In Infants

Definition

Infantile umbilical hernia is a result of an abnormally large or abnormally weak umbilical ring in an otherwise normal abdominal wall. The defect is covered by skin.

The hernia is usually readily reduced and tends to close spontaneously. Strangulation is very rare. An enlarged ring is more frequent in premature infants, and closure continues at a reduced rate into postnatal life. A ring over 1.5 cm in diameter after the first year of postnatal life will probably not close spontaneously.

The herniation is typically at the umbilicus, but it may be above (supraumbilical) or below (infraumbilical) that level.

The umbilical ring is not covered by fat.

PLATE 11
Repair of Umbilical Hernia in Infants

A,B,C. *Step 1.* Make the incision in the inferior umbilical crease from 3 to 9 o'clock. Always preserve the umbilicus in children and young adults.

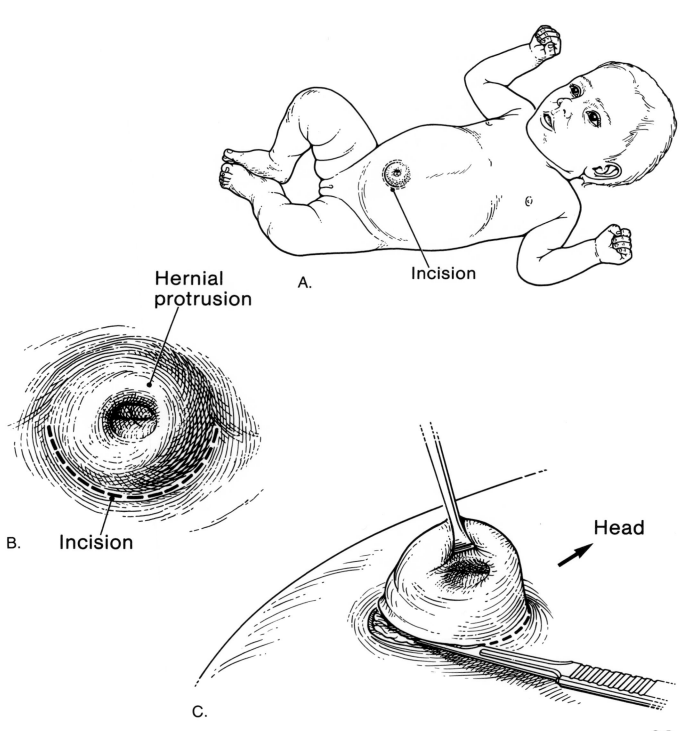

Incision

A.

Hernial protrusion

B.   Incision

Head

C.

PLATE 11 (*Continued*)
Repair of Umbilical Hernia in Infants

D.   *Step 2.* Elevate the umbilical skin gently and reflect it upward with Allis forceps fixed at the inside surface. (Do not clamp the skin.)

E.   *Step 3.* By careful dissection, separate the subcutaneous tissue from the anterior lamina of the rectus sheath and the umbilical stalk. The umbilical arteries may bleed immediately postpartum; they usually close a few days later. Closure may be incomplete, so the arteries must be ligated with 000 silk.

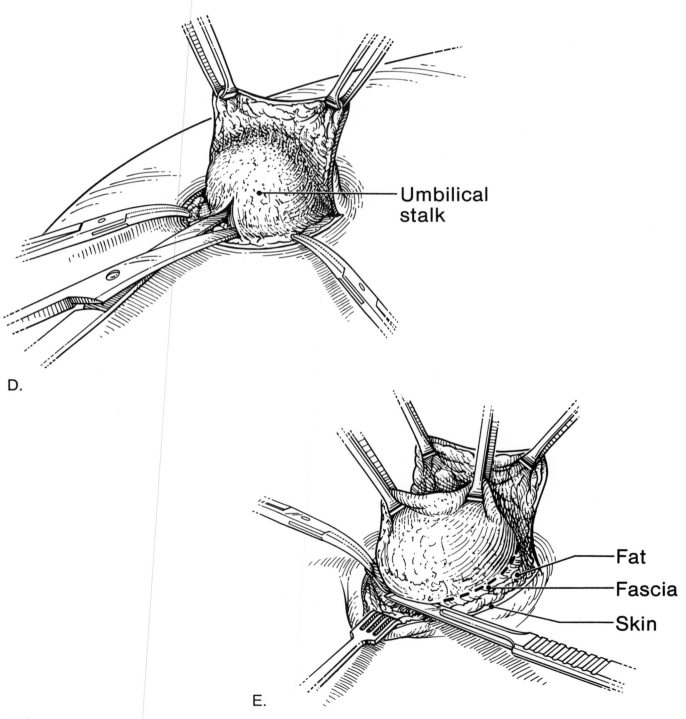

Umbilical stalk

D.

Fat

Fascia

Skin

E.

F.   *Step 4.* Isolate the sac and excise with scissors. The surgeon must decide whether or not to ligate the sac.

    Step 5. Ligate all bleeding points, especially in the area of the four tubular structures: round ligament (left umbilical vein); medial umbilical ligaments (umbilical arteries); median umbilical ligament (urachus). Be sure to ligate the falciform ligament.

G,H.   *Step 6.* Close the incision. We prefer a transverse closure of the ring. Whether to employ imbrication, interrupted apposition, or continuous suture technique is up to the surgeon.

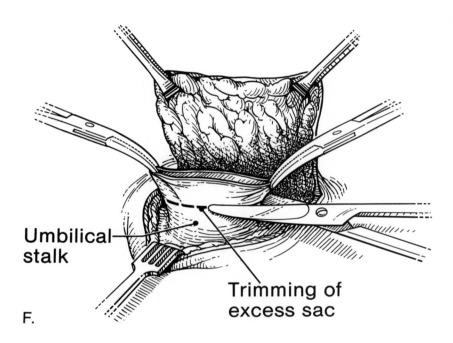

Umbilical stalk

Trimming of excess sac

F.

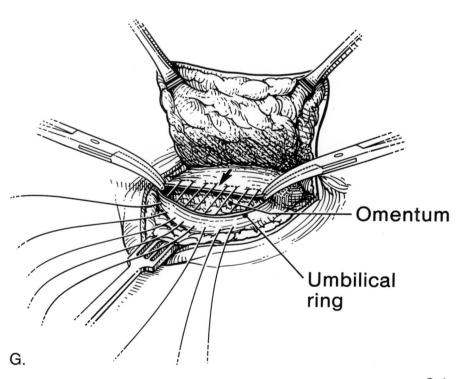

Omentum

Umbilical ring

G.

I,J. *Step 7.* Avoid dead spaces by suturing the inside of the umbilicus to the external lamina of the sheath of rectus abdominis. Use 0000 Dexon subcuticular continuous sutures for skin closure. Sterile strips are applied to the skin.

H.

I.

J.

Subcuticular
suture

In Adults

Definition

Umbilical hernias in adults may be the result of large, untreated infantile hernias that failed to close spontaneously. They are exacerbated in middle life by repeated pregnancies and by obesity or cirrhosis. Slow enlargement of the defect over a period of years is usual; umbilical hernias in the adult do not close spontaneously. It is probable that some conformations of the umbilical ring are more susceptible to herniation than are others.

PLATE 12
Repair of Umbilical Hernia in Adults

A. *Step 1.* If the skin is degenerated and if the patient is old, the umbilicus need not be preserved. However, try to save the umbilicus in all other cases, if possible, making an incision from 9 to 3 o'clock above or below the umbilicus.

B. *Step 2.* Separate the sac from the fat with knife or scissors and, after satisfactory isolation and elevation, open it. Gently push the abdominal contents into the abdomen, cutting any adhesions encountered.

Remember: In incarcerated hernia the fibers of the rectus sheath and posterior and anterior lamina run in a transverse way into the umbilical ring and linea alba. Therefore, with incarceration the ring should be incised laterally and the incision should be extended into both anterior and posterior laminae of the rectus abdominis with retraction of the muscle if necessary.

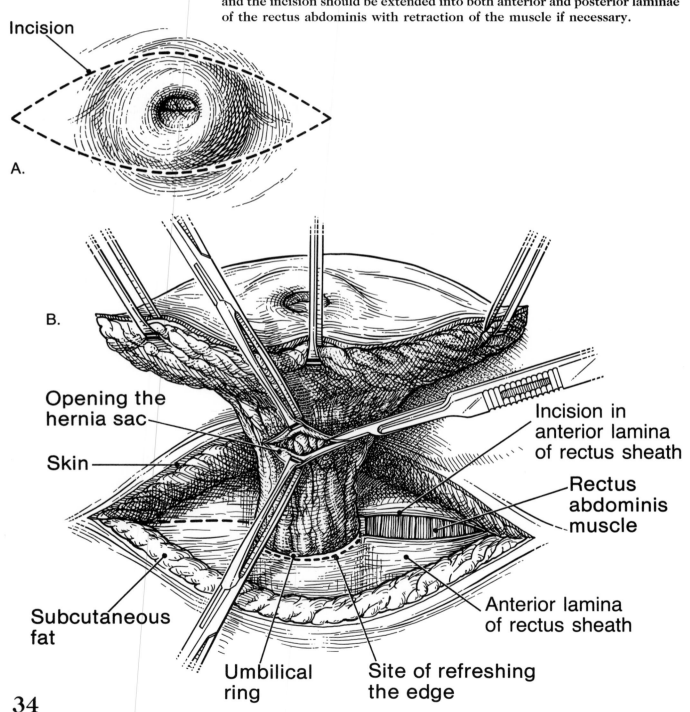

Incision

A.

B.

Opening the hernia sac

Skin

Subcutaneous fat

Incision in anterior lamina of rectus sheath

Rectus abdominis muscle

Anterior lamina of rectus sheath

Umbilical ring

Site of refreshing the edge

C. *Step 3.* Trim the sac down to the ring or just above the ring if the sac is to be closed separately. Ligate all bleeding points. We ligate all of the tubular structures with 000 silk.

D. *Step 4.* Close the sac and posterior lamina of the rectus sheath with interrupted 0 chromic or 00 Dexon suture. Prepare the anterior lamina of the rectus sheath for a distance of 1 to 2 cm all around the defect.

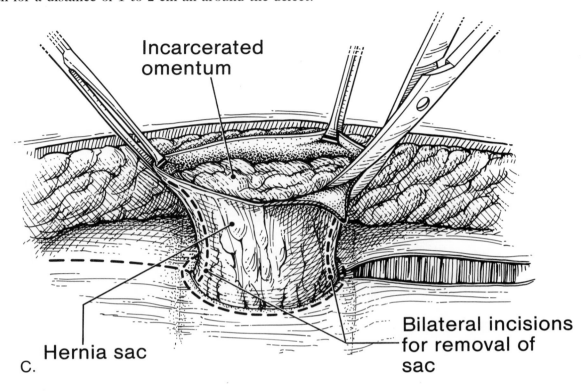

Incarcerated omentum

Hernia sac

Bilateral incisions for removal of sac

C.

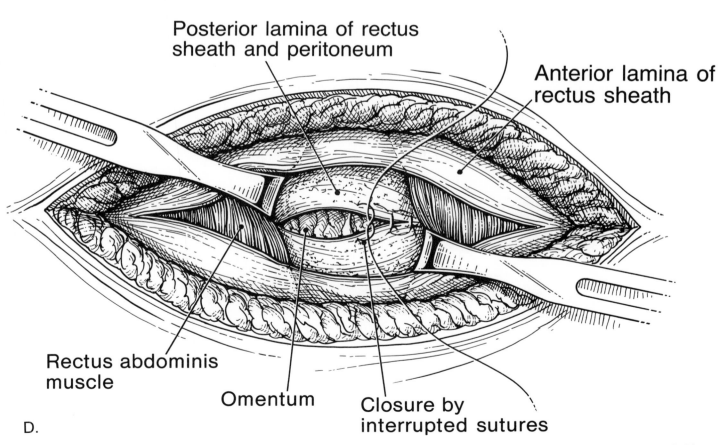

Posterior lamina of rectus sheath and peritoneum

Anterior lamina of rectus sheath

Rectus abdominis muscle

Omentum

Closure by interrupted sutures

D.

PLATE 12 (*Continued*)

Repair of Umbilical Hernia in Adults
Alternate Procedure

E. *Step 5.* Gently separate the posterior lamina of the rectus sheath from the peritoneum. Close the defect transversely, with or without imbrication or with continuous Prolene and interrupted 0 Dexon every three bites.

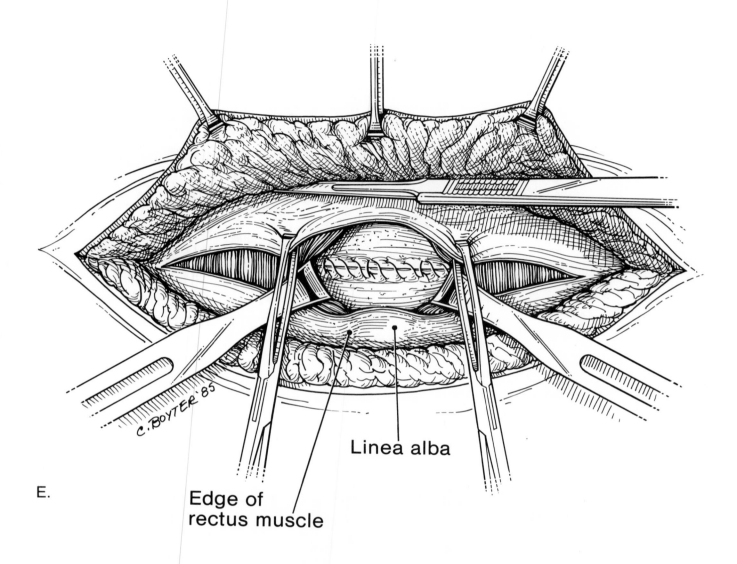

Linea alba

E.

Edge of
rectus muscle

F. *Step 6.* Undermine the linea alba.

G. *Step 7.* Close the linea alba with interrupted sutures.

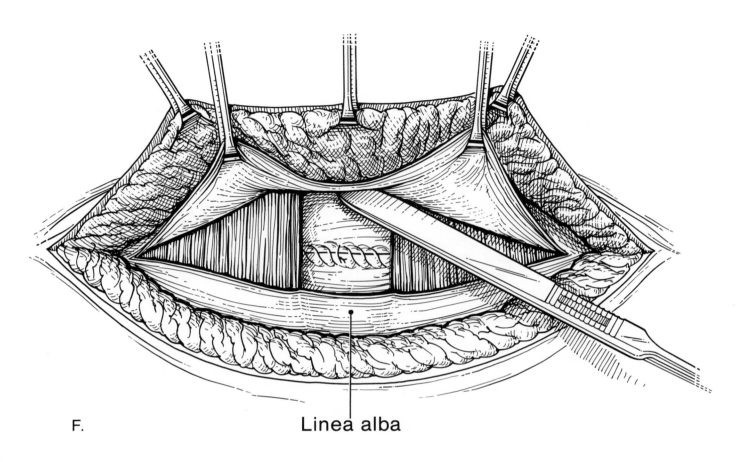

F.

Linea alba

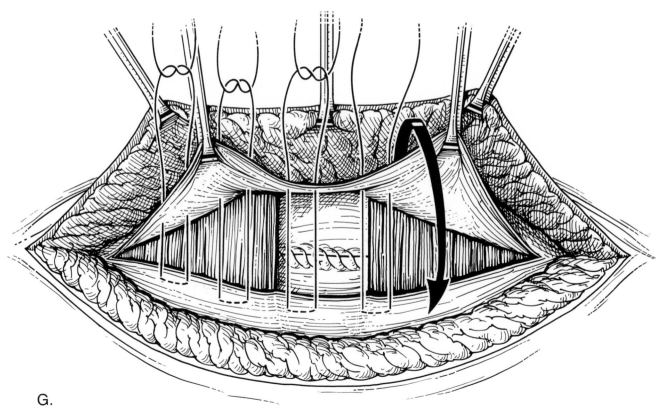

G.

PLATE 12 (*Continued*)

Repair of Umbilical Hernia in Adults

H. *Step 8.* Close the skin with interrupted sutures.

Many surgeons close the defect longitudinally in the same way that they close a midline incision. Also, many surgeons incorporate the peritoneum and fascia in one layer.

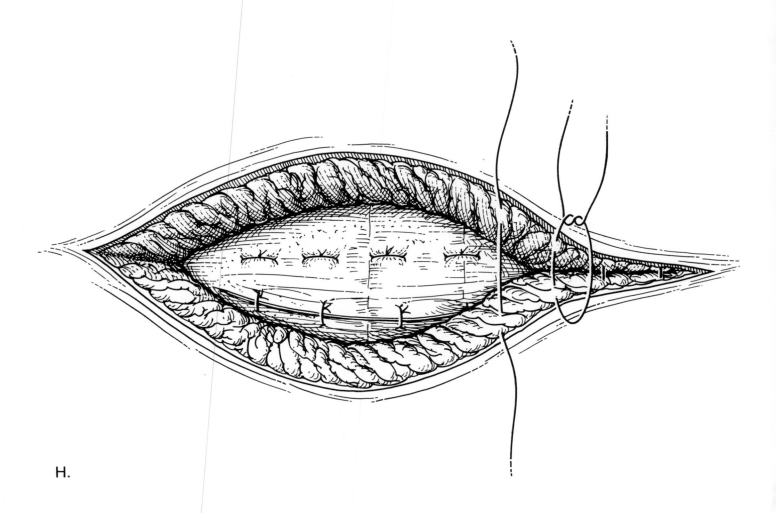

H.

Omphalocele (Exomphalos)

Definition

An omphalocele is a herniation of abdominal contents into the base of the umbilical cord. There is no skin overlying the defect, but there is a double layer of membrane consisting of amnion outside and peritoneum inside. There is a high incidence of associated anomalies.

Embryogenesis

Omphalocele represents a failure of the midgut to return to the abdominal cavity in the tenth prenatal week. As a result, the lateral folds are unable to meet and form the normal umbilical ring. In the absence of the normal intestinal mass, the abdominal cavity fails to reach its normal capacity.

Treatment and Repair

Omphalocele is a pediatric surgical emergency. The following procedures should be employed prior to surgery:

1. Avoid rupture of the avascular membrane. Do not manipulate the sac.
2. Cover the omphalocele with moist sterile gauze.
3. Keep the infant warm.
4. Insert a nasogastric tube.
5. Laboratory work must include blood glucose to rule out possible hypoglycemia.
6. Give intravenous (IV) fluids, e.g., dextrose in 0.25 normal saline.
7. Give antibiotics and vitamin K_1 (Aquamephyton).

At this point a decision must be made for either conservative treatment or surgery.

Conservative Treatment of the Nonruptured Omphalocele
Coat with Silvadene cream and allow skin ingrowth. Correct the hernia surgically at 6 to 24 months of age. The infant may be fed by hyperalimentation if necessary. Note: Avoid Mercurochrome; it causes mercury poisoning.

Surgical Repair
Omphaloceles may be divided into three groups by the size of the herniated mass and by the treatment required:

A *small* omphalocele, 2 to 4 cm in diameter, can be treated by reduction and a one-stage repair of the fascia and skin.

A *medium* omphalocele, 4 to 6 cm in diameter, can be treated by skin closure without repair of the fascial defect, leaving a ventral hernia to be closed six months to two years later.

A *massive* omphalocele, 7 to 10 cm in diameter, can contain parts of the liver, stomach, pancreas, spleen, transverse colon, or urinary bladder, in addition to small intestine. These organs cannot be placed into the inadequate abdominal cavity. A prosthetic "chimney" or "silo" must be constructed to contain them, and gentle, continuing pressure must be applied to stimulate enlargement of the space within the abdominal cavity.

Remember: The abdominal cavity is usually too small to receive the herniated mass all at once. Forcible attempts to reduce the hernia may result in fatal respiratory embarrassment from pressure on the diaphragm or reduced venous return to the heart due to compression of the inferior vena cava.

PLATE 13

Diagram of a Sagittal Section through a Small Omphalocele

The herniated viscera are covered with avascular amnion continuous with the skin of the abdominal wall. Care must be taken to avoid rupture of the sac.

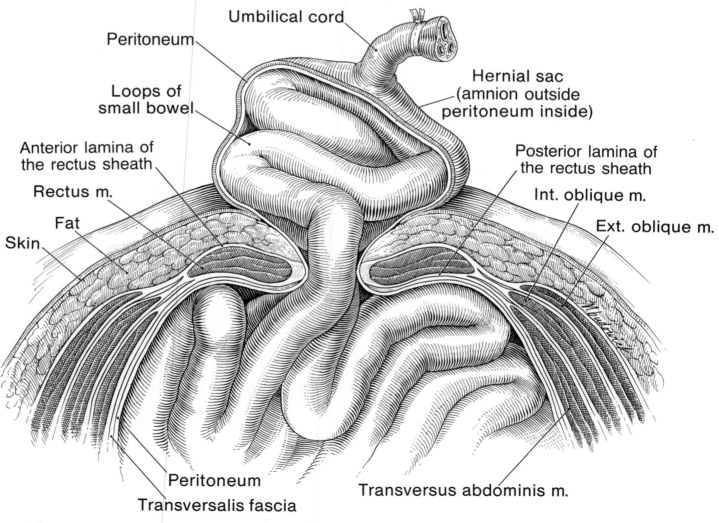

Umbilical cord

Peritoneum

Loops of small bowel

Hernial sac (amnion outside peritoneum inside)

Anterior lamina of the rectus sheath

Posterior lamina of the rectus sheath

Rectus m.

Int. oblique m.

Fat

Ext. oblique m.

Skin

Peritoneum

Transversalis fascia

Transversus abdominis m.

40

PLATE 14

Repair of Small Omphalocele

A. A small omphalocele: the herniated mass is 2 to 4 cm in diameter. If contents of the sac can be reduced within the peritoneum, a primary repair should be attempted.

B. *Step 1.* Make a circular incision with a scalpel at the junction of the true skin and the amnion forming the omphalocele sac.

C. *Step 2.* Carefully elevate the skin and subcutaneous tissue using scissors to undermine the flap down to the anterior lamina of the rectus sheath.

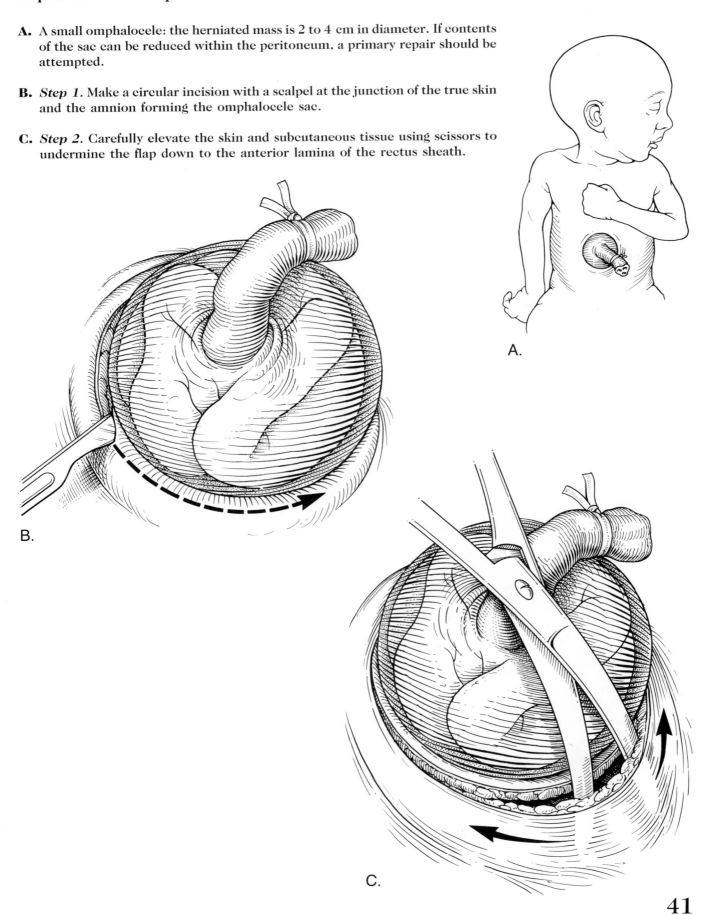

A.

B.

C.

41

PLATE 14 (*Continued*)

Repair of Small Omphalocele

D. *Step 3.* Clamp, ligate, and amputate the remnant of the umbilical cord.

E. Step 4. Trim skin from the base of the sac and gently push the sac into the abdomen. Close the hernial ring with interrupted 00 silk in one or two layers. In the example illustrated, closure is in one layer. Use subcutaneous 0000 Dexon and SteriStrips to close the skin.

Note: Some pediatric surgeons like to remove the sac and explore the abdomen to rule out other midgut anomalies.

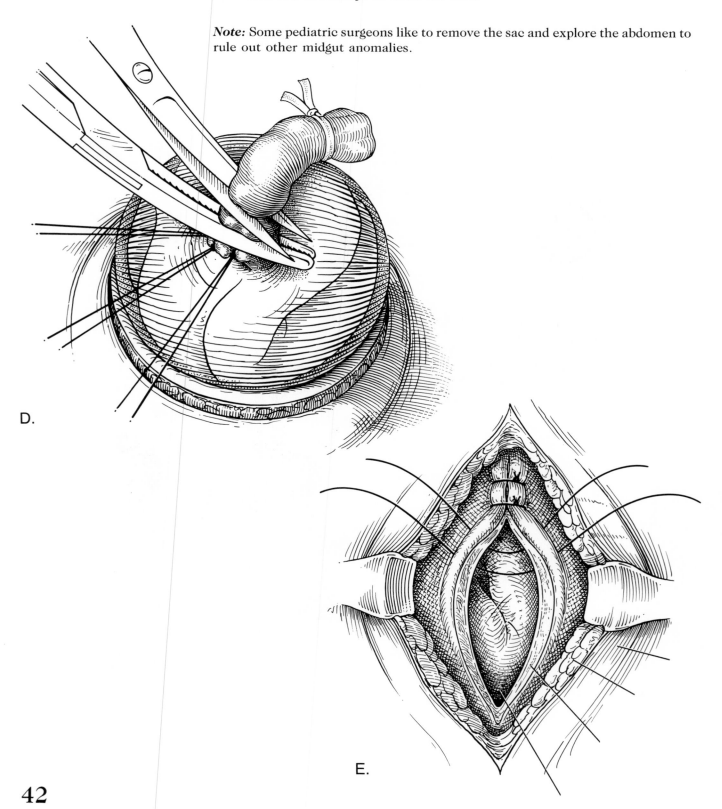

D.

E.

PLATE 15
Repair of Medium-Sized Omphalocele

A. A medium-sized omphalocele is 4 to 6 cm in diameter.

B. *Step 1.* Make a circular incision at the junction of the skin and amnion.

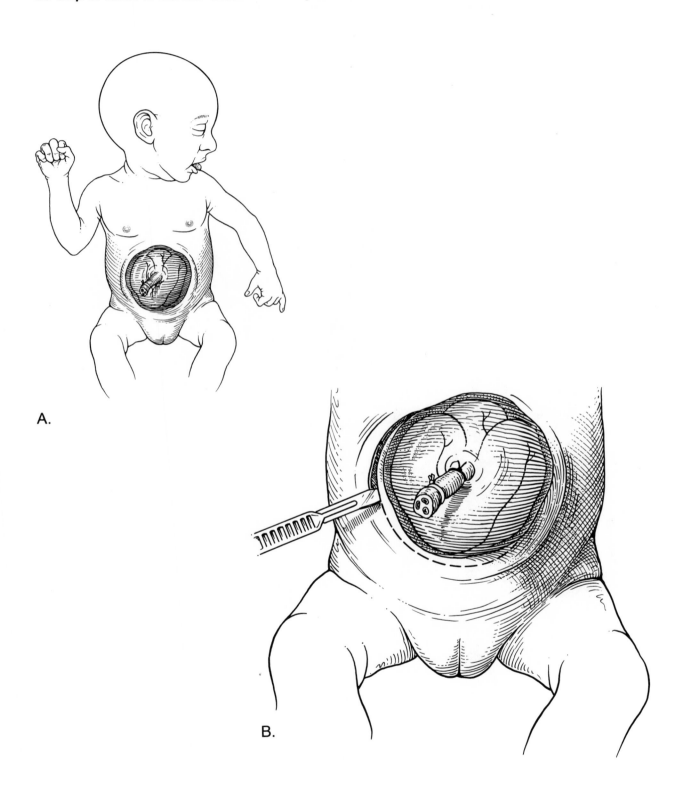

A.

B.

PLATE 15 (*Continued*)

Repair of Medium-Sized Omphalocele

C. *Step 2.* Elevate the skin and subcutaneous tissue using scissors to undermine the skin over the abdomen only, not over the ribs.

D. *Step 3.* Do not attempt to close the rectus fascia in one stage. Close only the skin over the hernia. If there is not enough skin, prepare flaps up to the costal margin. This converts the omphalocele into a ventral hernia to be repaired 6 to 24 months later.

Note: Gradual stretching of the abdominal wall with pneumoperitoneum will facilitate ventral hernia repair at a later date.

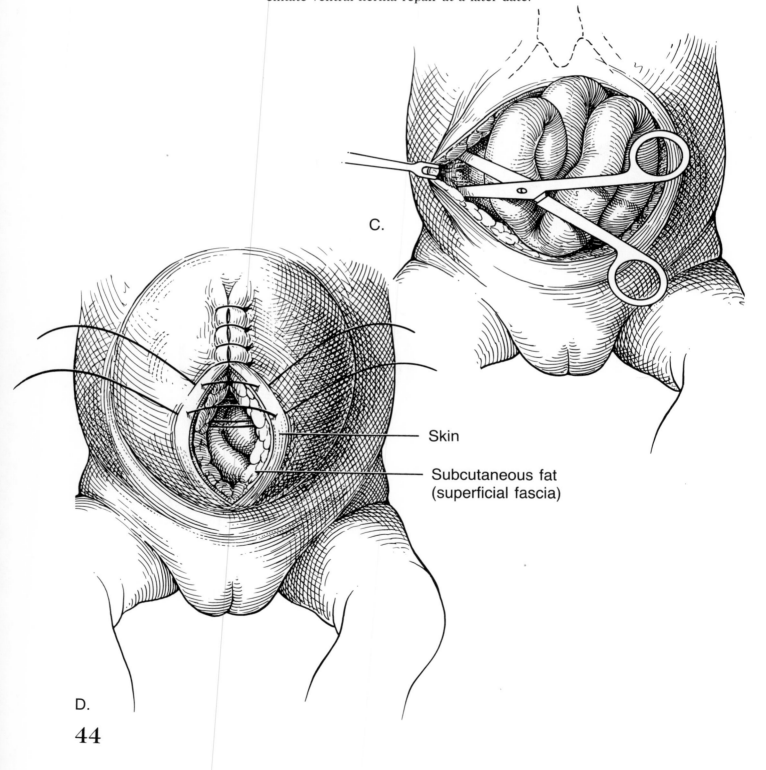

C.

Skin

Subcutaneous fat
(superficial fascia)

D.

PLATE 16
Repair of Massive Omphalocele

A. A massive omphalocele is 7 to 10 cm or more in diameter.

B. *Step 1.* Make a circular incision close to the edge of the skin, deep enough to expose the fascial ring and the edges of the right and left anterior rectus sheath lamina. Ligate all bleeding points with 0000 plain catgut. Try not to open the sac.

Step 2. Ligate the round and falciform ligaments, both umbilical arteries, and the urachus with 000 or 0000 silk.

C. *Step 3.* Suture two sheets of Silon or Teflon with a cuff of Dacron to the anterior rectus sheath on each side with interrupted 00 Dacron sutures. The Dacron cuff welcomes fibrous connective tissue and forms a solid foundation.

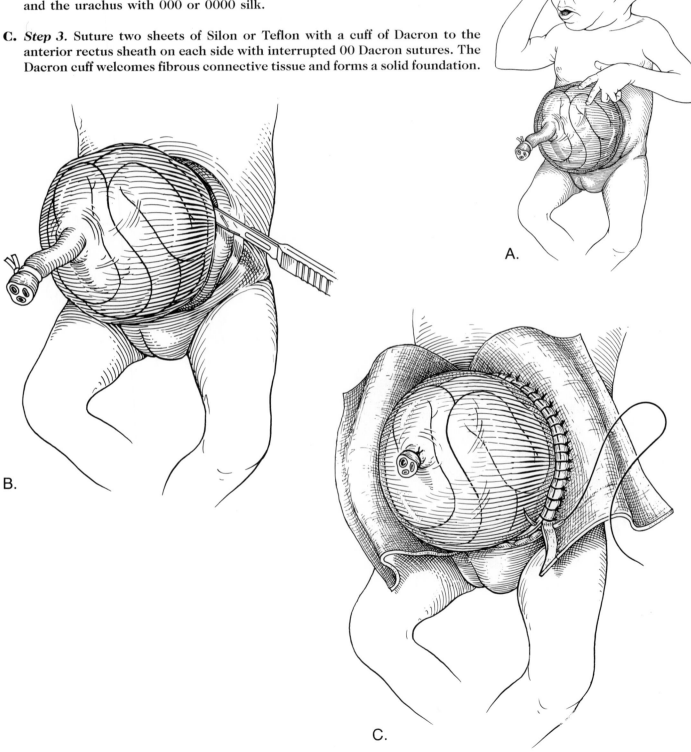

A.

B.

C.

45

PLATE 16 (*Continued*)

Repair of Massive Omphalocele

D. *Step 4.* Suture the right and left prosthetic sheets together superiorly and inferiorly; then close the top to create a "chimney" or "silo." A GIA stapling device may be used.

Step 5. Cut off the excess material and apply a sterile dressing.

E. *Step 6.* Two to three days after the operation, place a second row of interrupted sutures through the prosthesis 1 to 1.5 cm closer to the abdomen.

F. *Step 7.* Repeat this tucking procedure every 2 or 3 days until the intestines are placed entirely in the abdomen without pressure on the diaphragm.

G. *Step 8.* Remove the residual synthetic material in about 10 days, and close the abdomen fascia to fascia.

H. *Step 9.* Close the skin without tension with 00000 nylon or Prolene interrupted sutures. Apply Silvadene cream.

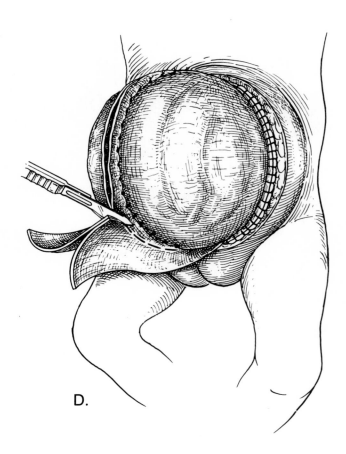

D.

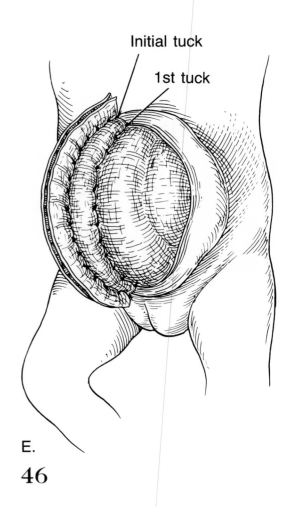

Initial tuck

1st tuck

E.

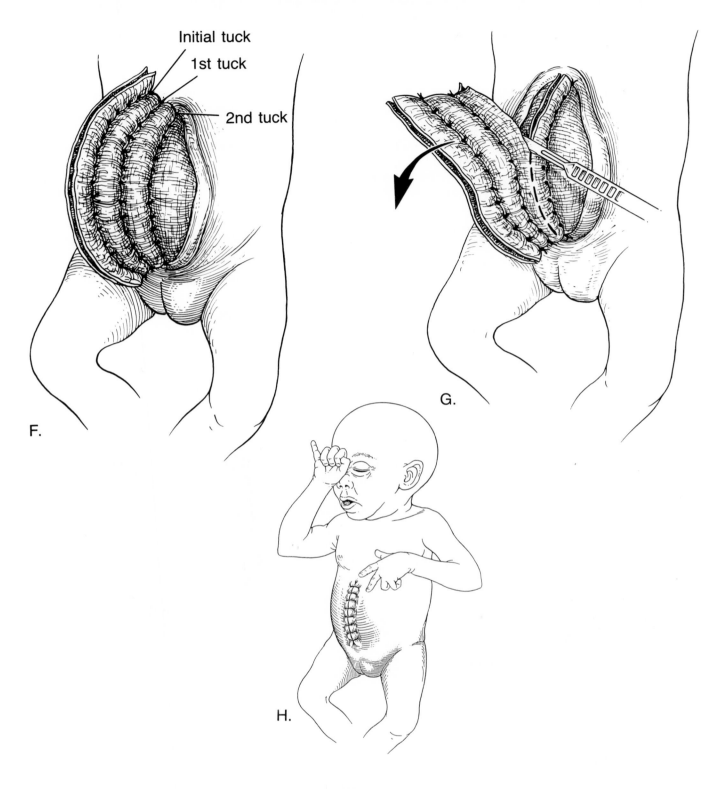

Initial tuck
1st tuck
2nd tuck

F.

G.

H.

Complications of Omphalocele, Umbilical Hernia, and Gastroschisis

1. Removal of the umbilicus.
2. Delay of operation on omphalocele or gastroschisis. (Note: Numbers 1 and 2 are iatrogenic complications.)
3. Seroma—hematoma.
4. Infection:
   Localized.
   Peritonitis due to perforated viscus.

Gastroschisis

Definition

Gastroschisis is a defect or cleft in the abdominal wall to the right of a normal umbilicus. There is no hernial sac. The liver is in the abdomen.

Anatomy

This defect is small, less than 3 to 4 cm, but the herniated mass is large. The abdominal cavity is fairly well developed. The infant is usually 500 g below normal weight.

The herniated intestines are not within a hernial sac as in an omphalocele, but they may be coated with a thick peel due to inflammation secondary to antenatal exposure to amniotic fluid. The midgut is nonrotated. In contrast to an omphalocele, there are few associated malformations.

Embryogenesis

Gastroschisis may arise from mesenchymal failure, usually to the right of the umbilicus, resulting in no sac or skin. It may occur secondary to resorption of somatic ectoderm.

The present concept of gastroschisis is that it is the result of prenatal rupture through the umbilical ring at the base of the umbilical cord. The hernia lies medial to the rectus abdominis muscle, without muscle fibers between it and the cord. A bridge of skin between the hernia and the cord may be a secondary development. Why the rupture occurs on the right side has not been explained.

Treatment

This is a pediatric surgical emergency. Care prior to surgery consists of the following:

1. Keep patient warm and keep bowel covered with sterile moist gauzes (Betadine-soaked).
2. Insert a nasogastric tube.
3. Give antibiotics, IV fluids, and vitamin K_1.

Use general endotracheal anesthesia; avoid nitrous oxide. Advance the nasogastric tube into the intestine and insert a rectal tube for decompression. If the herniated intestines are soft and pliable as in evisceration, the hernia may be reduced and the defect closed as in a small or medium-sized omphalocele (Plates 15 and 16).

If the intestinal wall is thickened with a firm peel or if reduction results in an unacceptably high abdominal pressure, the formation of a prosthetic silo or chimney must be undertaken. The procedure is that used for a massive omphalocele (Plate 17).

1. Close fascia and skin separately.
2. Manually stretch the abdominal wall.
3. Excise the umbilical vessels at skin level.

PLATE 17

Diagram of Gastroschisis—Parasagittal Section

Diagram of a parasagittal section through a patient with gastroschisis. The defect lies to the right of the insertion of the umbilical cord. The herniated mass is usually composed of small intestine only. There is no sac.

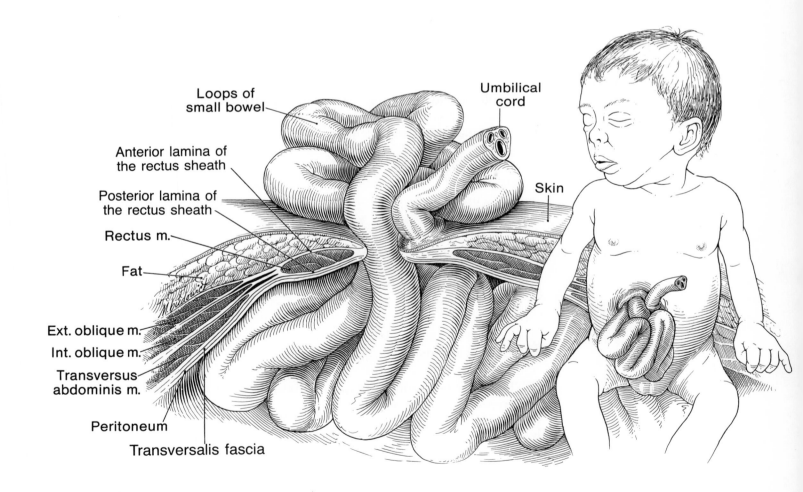

Spigelian (Lateral Ventral) Hernia

Definition

A Spigelian hernia is a spontaneous protrusion of preperitoneal fat, a peritoneal sac, or, less commonly, a sac containing a viscus, through the Spigelian zone (fascia) at any point along its length. The zone is bounded medially by the lateral margin of the anterior lamina of the rectus sheath and laterally by the muscular fibers of the internal oblique muscle.

Surgical Anatomy

The surgeon should be familiar with three entities in this area:

1. The semilunar line (of Spieghel), which marks the lateral border of the rectus sheath and extends from the pubic tubercle to the tip of the costal cartilage of the ninth rib.
2. The semicircular line (arcuate line, fold or line of Douglas) marks the caudal end of the posterior lamina of the aponeurotic rectus sheath, below the umbilicus and above the pubis. Unfortunately, the semilunar and semicircular lines are not easily seen in the operating room.
3. The Spigelian fascia (zone, aponeurosis) is composed of the aponeuroses of the external oblique, internal oblique, and transversus abdominis muscles. The region between these muscles and the lateral border of the rectus muscle defines the Spigelian fascia. For all practical purposes, the Spigelian fascia is formed by the approximation and fusion of the internal oblique and transversus abdominis aponeuroses. If the fusion of these aponeuroses is loose, a "zone" rather than a fascia is formed. The external oblique aponeurosis remains intact over the hernia.

The Spigelian fascia is widest between the umbilical plane above and the interspinous (ilium) plane below. The majority of Spigelian hernias occur here. For no obvious reason they occur more frequently on the right. Bilateral cases are known.

A fully developed Spigelian hernia is covered by peritoneum, transversalis fascia, aponeurosis of the external oblique muscle, and skin. In some cases, the hernia passes through the transversus abdominis aponeurosis only. It may then dissect between planes of the body wall.

Complications

There may be minimal complications of incisions of the abdominal wall. Recurrence is not reported.

PLATE 18
Anatomy of Spigelian Hernia

A. Diagram of cross sections of the anterior abdominal wall, above and below the semicircular line. The extent of the Spigelian fascia or zone is indicated.

B. Herniation usually begins with preperitoneal fat passing through defects in the transversus abdominis (A_1) and internal oblique (A_2) aponeuroses. Notice that the aponeurosis of the external oblique muscle remains intact and, with the skin, forms the covering of the hernia.

A_1 Transversus abdominis broken
A_2 Transversus abdominis and internal oblique broken
B_1 Transversus abdominis and internal oblique broken

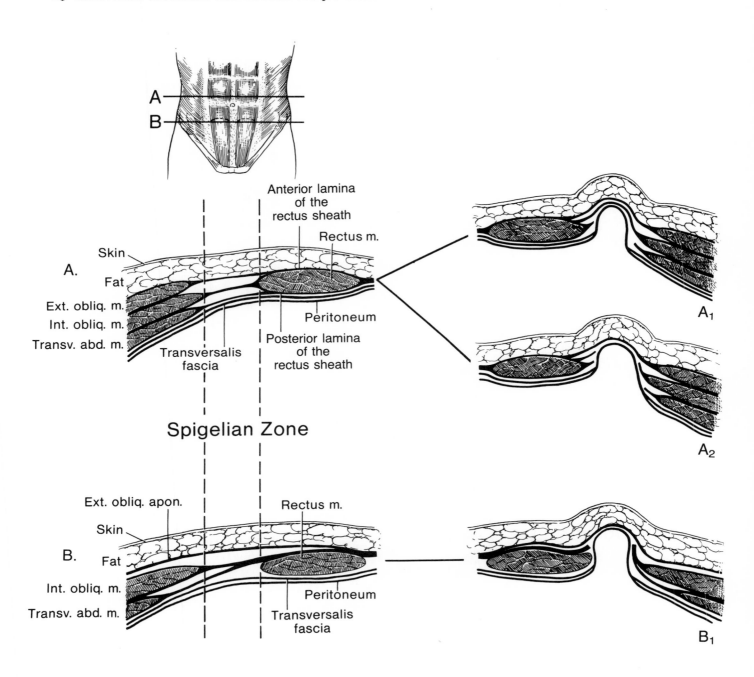

PLATE 19
Repair of Spigelian Hernia

A. *Step 1.* Make a transverse or vertical incision through the aponeurosis of the external oblique muscle over the palpable mass. If the mass is not palpable at examination, make a midline or vertical rectus incision. If the hernia is incarcerated, the ring should be incised medially toward the rectus abdominis muscle.

B. *Step 2.* Retract the aponeurosis of the external oblique muscle revealing the internal oblique muscle and the hernial sac.

Step 3. Open the sac; inspect its contents, ligate, and push the sac into the abdomen.

Step 4. Free the ring of Spigelian fascia from preperitoneal fat and peritoneal adhesions.

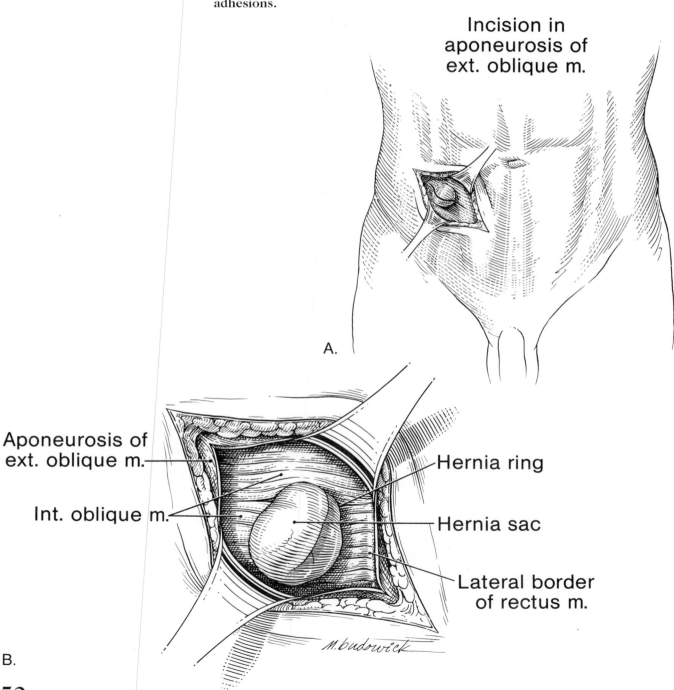

Incision in aponeurosis of ext. oblique m.

A.

Aponeurosis of ext. oblique m.

Int. oblique m.

Hernia ring

Hernia sac

Lateral border of rectus m.

M.budowick

B.

C. *Step 5.* Close the defect in the transversus abdominis and the internal oblique muscle with 0 or 00 Surgilon interrupted sutures.

D. *Step 6.* Close the defect in the aponeurosis of the external oblique muscle with interrupted sutures.

E. *Step 7.* Close the skin with interrupted sutures or clips.

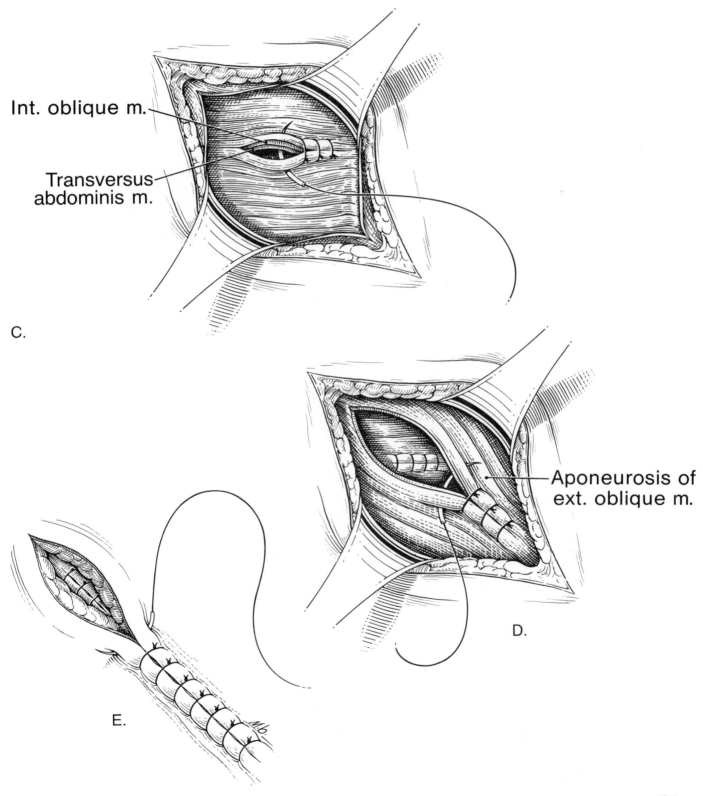

Int. oblique m.

Transversus abdominis m.

C.

Aponeurosis of ext. oblique m.

D.

E.

Inguinal (Groin) Hernias

Definition

The groin has been succinctly defined by Condon[1] as "that portion of the anterior abdominal wall below the level of the anterior superior iliac spines." In this area, a viscus may protrude, forming a visible and usually palpable swelling. Three types of hernia—direct inguinal, indirect inguinal, and external supravesical—may emerge through the abdominal wall by way of the external inguinal ring above the inguinal ligament; a fourth type, femoral hernia, emerges beneath the inguinal ligament by way of the femoral canal. These four hernias make up 90 percent of all hernias.

Other inguinal hernias, although not common, are important to the surgeon. In this chapter we also discuss female and pediatric inguinal hernias, undescended testis, and hydrocele.

Surgical Anatomy of Groin Hernias

Within the groin area are the inguinal and femoral canals. The inguinal canal is an oblique cleft about 4 cm long in the adult, lying about 4 to 5 cm above the inguinal ligament. The femoral canal below the inguinal ligament is 1.25 to 2 cm long and occupies the most medial compartment of the femoral sheath. The canal is conical with the apex of the cone at the fossa ovalis. This is the opening in the fascia lata of the thigh, through which the great saphenous vein passes to join the femoral vein.

The Layers of the Lower Anterior Body Wall
In the inguinal region, the layers of the abdominal wall are

1. Skin.
2. Subcutaneous or superficial fasciae (Camper's and Scarpa's) containing fat.
3. Innominate fascia (of Gallaudet). This is the superficial or external layer of fascia of the external oblique muscle. It is not always recognizable. Its absence is of no surgical importance.

---

[1]Condon RE: The anatomy of the inguinal region and its relationship to groin hernia, in *Hernia,* 2d ed. Nyhus LM, Condon RE (eds). Lippincott, Philadelphia, 1978, p. 14.

4. External oblique aponeurosis, including the inguinal (Poupart's), lacunar (Gimbernat's), and reflected inguinal (Colles') ligaments.
5. Spermatic cord in the male; round ligament of the uterus in the female.
6. Transversus abdominis muscle and aponeurosis, internal oblique muscle, falx inguinalis (Henle), and the conjoined tendon (when present).
7. Transversalis fascia and aponeurosis associated with the pectineal ligament (Cooper's), the iliopubic tract, falx inguinalis, and transversalis fascia sling.
8. Preperitoneal connective tissue with fat.
9. Peritoneum.
10. Superficial and deep inguinal rings.

Boundaries of the Inguinal Canal

Anterior: The aponeurosis of the external oblique muscle and, laterally, by the internal oblique muscle. Remember, there are no external oblique muscle fibers in the inguinal area, only aponeurotic fibers.

Posterior: (floor)   In about three-fourths of subjects, the posterior wall is formed laterally by the aponeurosis of the transversus abdominis muscle and the transversalis fascia; in the remainder, the posterior wall is transversalis fascia only. Medially the posterior wall is reinforced by the internal oblique aponeurosis.

Superior: (roof)   The roof of the canal is formed by the arched fibers of the lower edge of the internal oblique muscle and by the transversus abdominis muscle and aponeurosis.

Inferior: The wall of the canal is formed by the inguinal ligament (Poupart's) and the lacunar ligament (Gimbernat's).

The upper end of the inguinal canal is the internal or deep inguinal ring, which is a normal defect of the transversalis fascia. Its superior margin is formed by the transversus abdominis arch; its inferior margins by aponeurotic fibers from the iliopubic tract, the inferior epigastric vessels, and the interfoveolar ligament (Hesselbach's). The inferior epigastric vessels penetrate the transversalis fascia.

The external or superficial inguinal ring is a triangular opening in the aponeurosis of the external oblique muscle. The superior and inferior crura, which form the margins of the ring, are held together and reinforced by intercrural fibers.

Contents of the Inguinal Canal

MALE
The spermatic cord in the male contains a matrix of connective tissue continuous with the preperitoneal connective tissue (see no. 8 in the list above).
The cord consists of
   The ductus deferens
   Three arteries:
      Internal spermatic (testicular) artery
      Deferential artery
      External spermatic (cremasteric) artery
   One venous plexus (pampiniform)

Three nerves:
Genital branch of genitofemoral nerve
Ilioinguinal nerve
Sympathetic fibers from hypogastric plexus
Three layers of fascia:
The external spermatic fascia, a continuation of the innominate fascia
The middle, cremasteric layer, continuous with the internal oblique muscle fibers and muscle fascia
The internal spermatic fascia, an extension of the transversalis fascia

FEMALE
The round ligament of the uterus
Genital branch of the genitofemoral nerve
Cremasteric vessels
Ilioinguinal nerve
Coverings as described for the male, although usually less distinct

Fossae of the Anterior Abdominal Wall

The inner (posterior) surface of the anterior body wall above the inguinal ligament and below the umbilicus is divided into three shallow fossae on either side of a low ridge formed in the midline by the median umbilical ligament, the obliterated urachus. Each of these fossae is a potential site for a hernia. From lateral to medial, these fossae are

- The lateral fossa, bounded medially by the inferior epigastric arteries. It contains the internal inguinal ring, the site of indirect inguinal hernia.
- The medial fossa, between the inferior epigastric artery and the medial umbilical ligament (remnant of the umbilical artery). It is the site of direct inguinal hernia.
- The supravesical fossa, between the medial and median umbilical ligaments. It is the site of external supravesical hernia.

A hernia through either the supravesical or the medial fossa is, for all practical purposes, a direct inguinal hernia. A direct hernia may thus be inguinal, in the medial fossa, or supravesical, in the supravesical fossa.

The Femoral Sheath and the Femoral Canal

The femoral sheath is formed anteriorly and medially by the transversalis fascia and some transversus aponeurotic fibers, posteriorly by pectineus and psoas fasciae, and laterally by iliacus fascia. The sheath forms three compartments, the most medial of which is the femoral canal, through which a femoral hernia may pass. The femoral ring is relatively rigid. McVay[2] found the transverse diameter to be from 10 to 19 mm and the anteroposterior diameter to be from 12 to 16 mm in 70 percent of subjects. The boundaries are

Lateral: A connective tissue septum and the femoral vein
Posterior: The pectineal ligament (Cooper's)
Anterior: The iliopubic tract *or* the inguinal ligament *or* both
Medial: The aponeurotic insertion of the transversus abdominis muscle and transversalis fascia *or,* rarely, the lacunar ligament

[2]McVay CB, Anson BJ: Aponeurotic and fascial continuities in the abdomen, pelvis, and thigh. *Anat Rec* 76:213–231, 1940.

The Anatomical Entities of the Groin Defined

Superficial Fascia

This fascia is divided into a superficial part (Camper's) and a deep part (Scarpa's). The superficial part extends upward on the abdominal wall and downward over the penis, scrotum, perineum, thigh, and buttocks. The deep part extends from the abdominal wall to the penis (Buck's fascia), the scrotum (dartos), and perineum (Colles' fascia). Buck's fascia is attached to the pubic arch, the ischiopubic rami, and, posteriorly, to the posterior aspect of the urogenital diaphragm forming the superficial perineal pouch.

Another school of thought is that Buck's fascia is a downward continuation of the deep fascia of the anterior abdominal wall (innominate or Gallaudet). In the perineum it is represented as the muscle fascia of the superficial perineal pouch.

According to this theory, two spaces are formed: the superficial perineal cleft and the superficial perineal pouch. The cleft is situated between Colles' fascia and the muscle fascia that covers the muscles of the superficial perineal pouch.

The boundaries of the superficial perineal pouch are

Anterior: Perineal membrane
Inferior: External perineal fascia (Gallaudet)
Lateral: Ischiopubic rami

Inguinal Ligament (Poupart's)

This is the thickened lower part of the external oblique aponeurosis. It passes from the anterosuperior iliac spine laterally to the superior ramus of the pubis. The middle one-third has a free edge. The lateral two-thirds is attached strongly to the underlying iliopsoas fascia.

Aponeurosis of the External Oblique Muscle

Below the arcuate line (Douglas), this aponeurosis joins with the aponeuroses of the internal oblique and transverse abdominis muscles to form the anterior layer of the rectus sheath. This aponeurosis forms or contributes to three anatomical entities in the inguinal canal:

Inguinal ligament (Poupart's).
Lacunar ligament (Gimbernat's).
Reflected inguinal ligament (Colles').
[The pectineal ligament (Cooper's)—also formed from tendinous fibers of the internal oblique, transversus, and pectineus muscles—is sometimes included.]

Lacunar Ligament (Gimbernat's)

This is the most inferior portion of the inguinal ligament and is formed from external oblique tendon fibers arising at the anterior superior iliac spine. Its fibers recurve through an angle of less than 45° before attaching to the pectineal ligament. Occasionally it forms the medial border of the femoral canal.

Pectineal Ligament (Cooper's)

This is a thick, strong tendinous band formed principally by tendinous fibers of the lacunar ligament and aponeurotic fibers of the internal oblique, transversus abdominis, and pectineus muscles, and, with variation, the inguinal falx. It is fixed to the periosteum of the superior pubic ramus and, laterally, the periosteum of the ilium. The tendinous fibers are lined internally by transversalis fascia.

Conjoined Area

By definition, this is the fusion of fibers of the internal oblique aponeurosis with similar fibers from the aponeurosis of the transversus abdominis muscle just as they insert on the pubic tubercle, the pectineal ligament, and the superior ramus of the pubis.

The above configuration is rarely encountered; published data suggest that it will be found in 5 percent of individuals or fewer. We have proposed the term *conjoined area*. This has obvious practical application to the region containing the falx inguinalis (ligament of Henle), the transversus abdominis aponeurosis, the inferomedial fibers of the internal oblique muscle or aponeurosis, the reflected inguinal ligament, and the lateral border of the rectus sheath.

Arch of the Transversus Abdominis

The inferior portion of the transversus abdominis, the transversus arch, becomes increasingly less muscular and more aponeurotic as it approaches the rectus sheath. Close to the internal ring, it is covered by the much more muscular arch of the internal oblique muscle. Remember, in the vicinity of the internal ring, the internal oblique is muscular and the transversus abdominis is aponeurotic.

Falx Inguinalis (Ligament of Henle)

The ligament of Henle is the lateral, vertical expansion of the rectus sheath that inserts on the pecten of the pubis. It is present in from 30 to 50 percent of individuals and is fused with the transversus abdominis aponeurosis and transversalis fascia.

Interfoveolar Ligament (Hesselbach's)

This is not a true ligament. It is a thickening of the transversalis fascia at the medial side of the internal ring. It lies anterior to the inferior epigastric vessels.

Reflected Inguinal Ligament (Colles')

This is formed by aponeurotic fibers from the inferior crus of the external ring which pass superomedially to the linea alba.

Iliopubic Tract

This is an aponeurotic band extending from the iliopectineal arch to the superior ramus of the pubis. It forms part of the deep musculoaponeurotic layer together with the transversus abdominis muscle and aponeurosis and transversalis fascia.

The tract passes medially, contributing to the inferior border of the internal ring. It crosses the femoral vessels to form the anterior margin of the femoral sheath, together with the transversalis fascia. The tract curves around the medial surface of the femoral sheath to attach to the pectineal ligament. It can be confused with the inguinal ligament.

Transversalis Fascia

Although the name transversalis fascia may be restricted to the internal fascia lining the transversus abdominis muscle, it is often applied to the entire connective tissue sheet lining the abdominal cavity. In the latter sense, it is a fascial layer covering muscles, aponeuroses, ligaments, and bones. Fasciae such as this have little tensile strength and must not be confused with aponeuroses, which are flattened tendons. Aponeuroses are strong enough to transmit muscle force; fasciae are not.

Iliopectineal Arch

This is a medial thickening of the iliopsoas fascia deep to the inguinal ligament. The surgeon does not directly use this arch, but it is important as the junction of a number of structures of the groin. These are

1. Insertions of fibers of the external oblique aponeurosis and fibers of the inguinal ligament
2. The origin of part of the internal oblique muscle and a part of the transversus abdominis muscle
3. The lateral attachment of the iliopubic tract

Hesselbach's Triangle

As described by Hesselbach in 1814, the base of the triangle was formed by the pubic pecten and the pectineal ligament. The boundaries of this triangle as usually described today are

Superolateral: The inferior (deep) epigastric vessels
Medial: The rectus sheath (lateral border)
Inferior (or, the base): The inguinal ligament

This is smaller than that described by Hesselbach in 1814. Most direct inguinal hernias occur in this area. Most surgeons would prefer to use the iliopubic tract or the pectineal ligament rather than the inguinal ligament.

PLATE 20
Anatomy of the Inguinal Region

A. The skin of the lower abdominal wall has been removed to show superficial branches of the femoral artery.

B. The supericial fascia (Camper's and Scarpa's) and aponeurosis of the external oblique muscle have been removed to show the internal oblique muscle.

Source: Plate 20A and B from Gray SW, Skandalakis JE: *Atlas of Surgical Anatomy for General Surgeons.* Williams & Wilkins, Baltimore, 1985, p. 299, Plate 14-1.

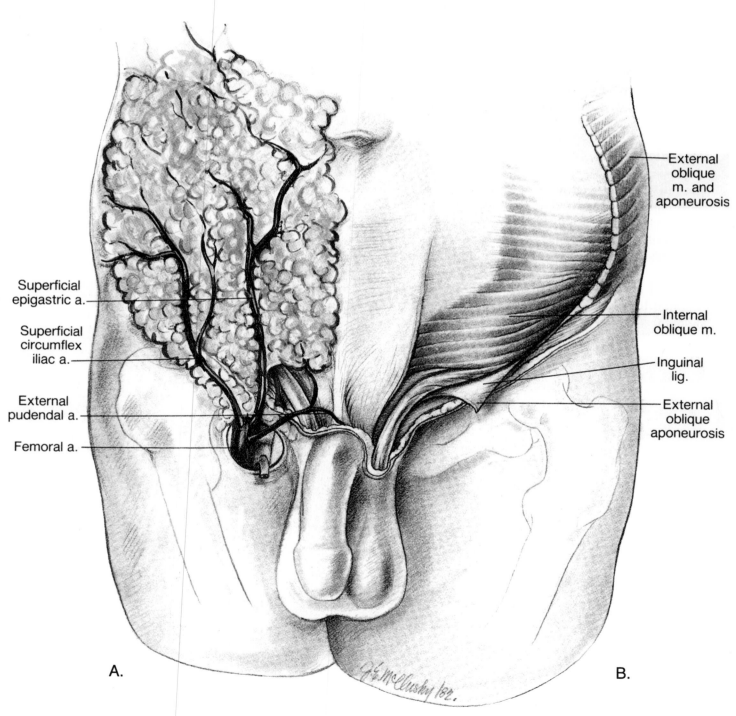

Superficial epigastric a.

Superficial circumflex iliac a.

External pudendal a.

Femoral a.

External oblique m. and aponeurosis

Internal oblique m.

Inguinal lig.

External oblique aponeurosis

A.

B.

C. Diagram of the relations of the superficial fasciae of the inguinal area showing the formation of the superficial perineal pouch.

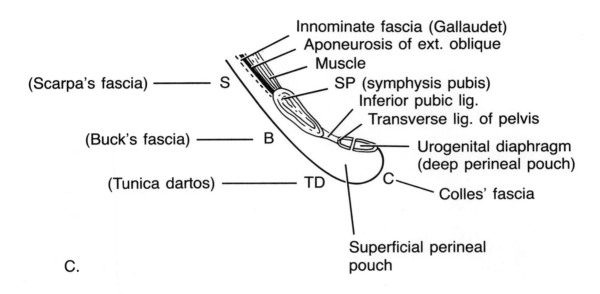

(Scarpa's fascia) ——— S

(Buck's fascia) ——— B

(Tunica dartos) ——— TD

Innominate fascia (Gallaudet)
Aponeurosis of ext. oblique
Muscle
SP (symphysis pubis)
Inferior pubic lig.
Transverse lig. of pelvis
Urogenital diaphragm
(deep perineal pouch)
C
Colles' fascia

Superficial perineal pouch

C.

PLATE 20 (*Continued*)
Anatomy of the Inguinal Region

D. The relations of the external inguinal ring and the spermatic cord are shown.

E. The external oblique aponeurosis is cut and reflected to show the inferior border of the internal oblique muscle and the ilioinguinal nerve. The ligament is retracted laterally and the external oblique aponeurosis is retracted medially.

Source: Plate 20D and E from Gray SW, Skandalakis JE: *Atlas of Surgical Anatomy for General Surgeons.* Williams & Wilkins, Baltimore, 1985, p. 301, Plate 14-2.

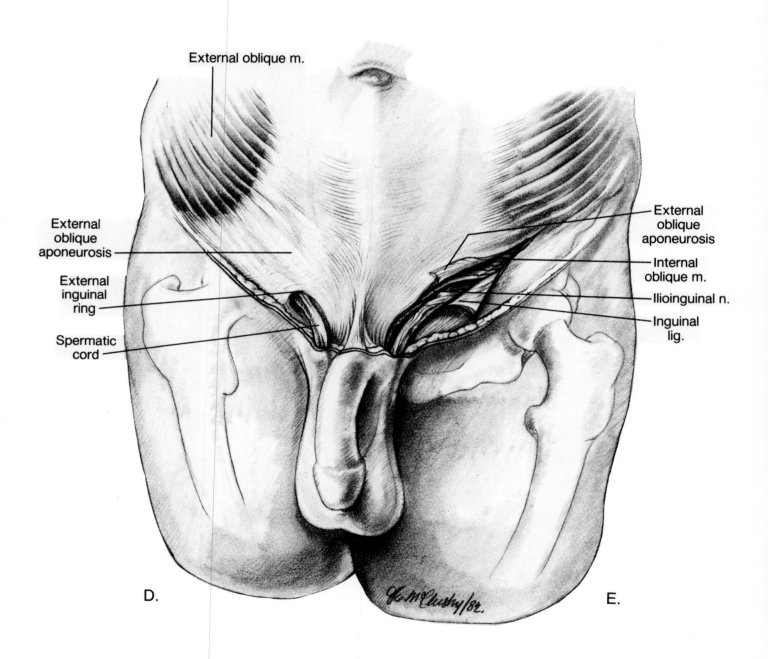

D.

E.

F. Some landmarks of the inguinal region.

G. The inguinal canal. The external oblique aponeurosis is cut and retracted upward and medially. The spermatic cord has been mobilized and retracted laterally.

Source: Plate 20F, G, H, and I from Skandalakis JE, Gray SW, Row JS: *Anatomical Complications in General Surgery.* McGraw-Hill, New York, 1983, p. 255, Figs. 13-2B, 13-3, 13-4; p. 256, Fig. 13-5.

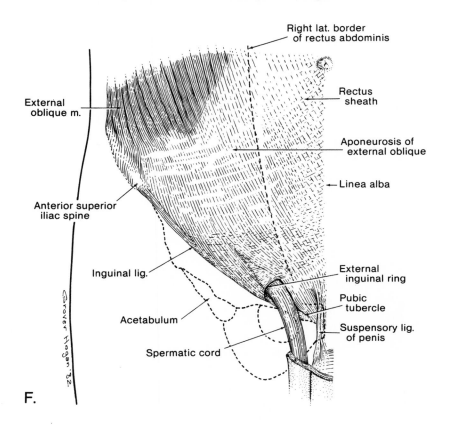

F.

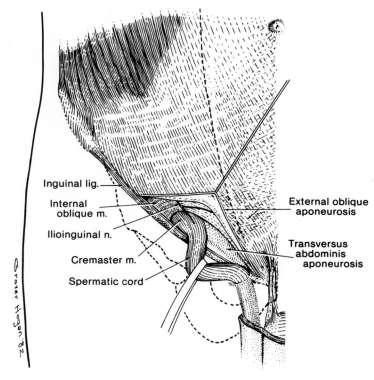

G.

PLATE 20 (*Continued*)

Anatomy of the Inguinal Region

H. The external oblique aponeurosis is removed to show the internal oblique muscle and arch. The spermatic cord is in situ.

I. Both oblique muscles and their aponeuroses have been removed to show the transversus abdominis muscle and aponeurosis.

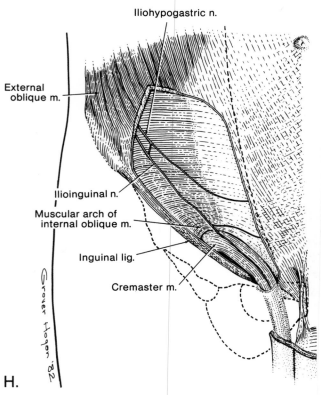

Iliohypogastric n.

External oblique m.

Ilioinguinal n.

Muscular arch of internal oblique m.

Inguinal lig.

Cremaster m.

H.

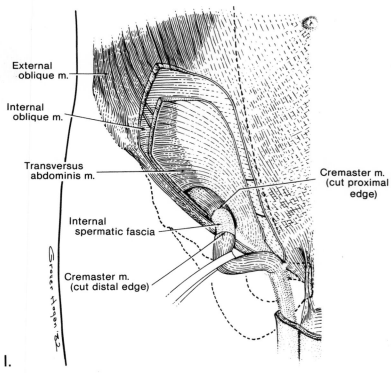

External oblique m.

Internal oblique m.

Transversus abdominis m.

Internal spermatic fascia

Cremaster m. (cut distal edge)

Cremaster m. (cut proximal edge)

I.

J. *Left:* The triangle described by Hesselbach in 1814.
   Right: The slightly smaller triangle accepted today.

Source: Skandalakis JE, Gray SW, Rowe JS: *Anatomical Complications in General Surgery.* McGraw-Hill, New York, 1983, p. 260, Fig. 13-8.

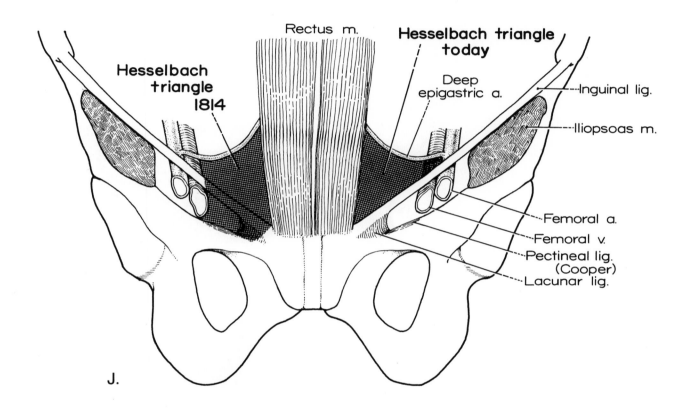

PLATE 20 (*Continued*)

Anatomy of the Inguinal Region

K. The "conjoined area" of the inguinal region.

Inset: The structures of the conjoined area. The concept of the "conjoined area" must replace that of the "conjoined tendon" of older anatomists and surgeons. The tendon was described as the fusion of lower fibers of the internal oblique aponeurosis with similar fibers of the aponeurosis of the transversus abdominis as they insert on the tubercle and superior ramus of the pubis. This tendon is present in only about 5 percent of individuals. For practical purposes, the "conjoined tendon" does not exist.

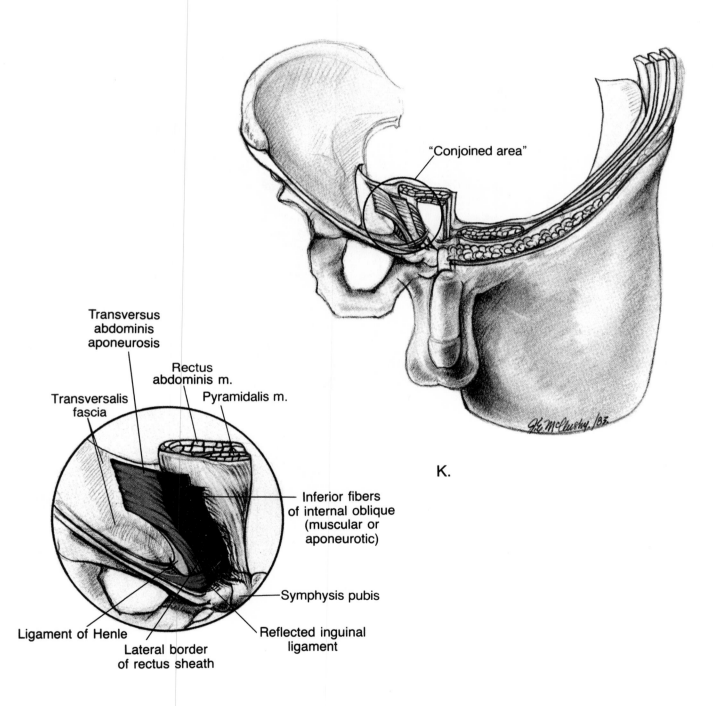

"Conjoined area"

Transversus
abdominis
aponeurosis

Rectus
abdominis m.

Pyramidalis m.

Transversalis
fascia

Inferior fibers
of internal oblique
(muscular or
aponeurotic)

Symphysis pubis

Ligament of Henle

Reflected inguinal
ligament

Lateral border
of rectus sheath

K.

L. Hesselbach's triangle is the site of direct inguinal hernia. The medial border of the triangle is the lateral border of the rectus abdominis muscle, the site of supravesical hernia.

Source: Plate 20K and L from Gray SW, Skandalakis JE: *Atlas of Surgical Anatomy for General Surgeons.* Williams & Wilkins, Baltimore, 1985, p. 302, Fig. 14-3A, B.

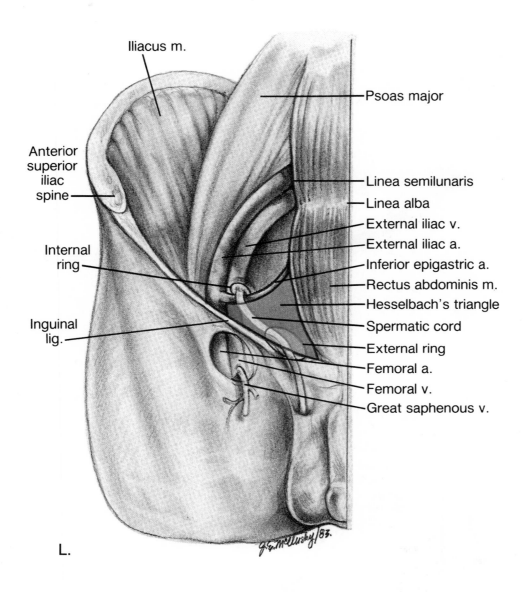

Iliacus m.

Psoas major

Anterior superior iliac spine

Linea semilunaris

Linea alba

External iliac v.

External iliac a.

Internal ring

Inferior epigastric a.

Rectus abdominis m.

Hesselbach's triangle

Spermatic cord

Inguinal lig.

External ring

Femoral a.

Femoral v.

Great saphenous v.

L.

PLATE 20 (*Continued*)

Anatomy of the Inguinal Region

M. The *left half* of the figure illustrates the arrangement of structures seen when the external oblique muscle and aponeurosis are removed. The *right half* of the figure shows an atypical arrangement of the same structure.

Inset: The inguinal canal and its contents

Source: Gray SW, Skandalakis JE: *Atlas of Surgical Anatomy for General Surgeons.* Williams & Wilkins, Baltimore, 1985, p. 305, Plate 14-4.

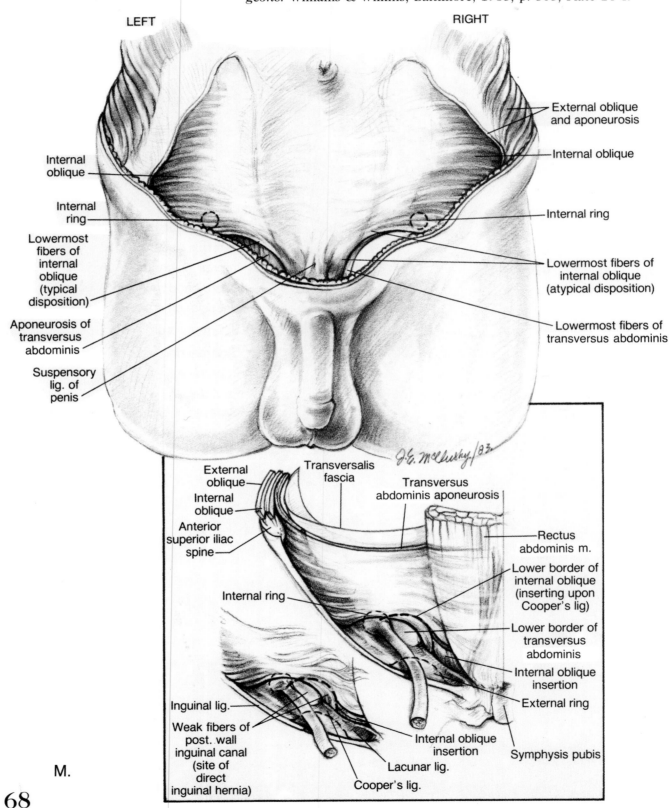

LEFT

RIGHT

External oblique and aponeurosis

Internal oblique

Internal oblique

Internal ring

Internal ring

Lowermost fibers of internal oblique (typical disposition)

Lowermost fibers of internal oblique (atypical disposition)

Aponeurosis of transversus abdominis

Lowermost fibers of transversus abdominis

Suspensory lig. of penis

J.E. McClusky/83

External oblique

Transversalis fascia

Transversus abdominis aponeurosis

Internal oblique

Anterior superior iliac spine

Rectus abdominis m.

Lower border of internal oblique (inserting upon Cooper's lig)

Internal ring

Lower border of transversus abdominis

Internal oblique insertion

External ring

Inguinal lig.

Weak fibers of post. wall inguinal canal (site of direct inguinal hernia)

Internal oblique insertion

Symphysis pubis

Lacunar lig.

Cooper's lig.

M.

68

N. A diagrammatic parasagittal section through the right midinguinal region illustrating the separation of the musculoaponeurotic lamina into the anterior and posterior inguinal canal.

Source: Plate 20N from Nyhus LM: The preperitoneal approach and iliopubic tract repair of inguinal hernia, in *Hernia,* 2d ed. Nyhus LM, Condon, RE (eds). Lippincott, Philadelphia, 1978, p. 216, Fig. 9-1.

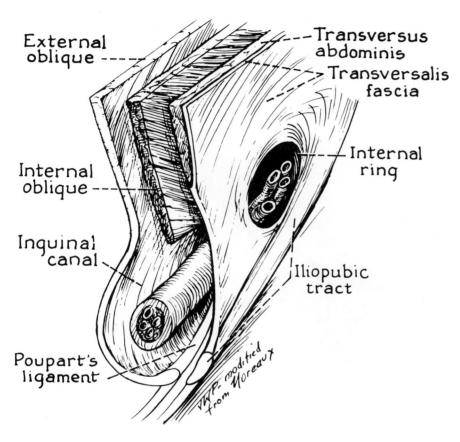

N.

TABLE 3
The Spermatic Cord and Its Coverings

Three fasciae:
   External spermatic (from external oblique fascia)
   Cremasteric (from internal oblique muscle and fascia)
   Internal spermatic (from transversalis fascia)
Three arteries:
   Testicular artery
   Cremasteric artery
   Deferential artery
Three veins:
   Pampiniform plexus and testicular vein
   Cremasteric vein
   Deferential vein
Three nerves:
   Genital branch of genitofemoral nerve
   Ilioniguinal nerve
   Sympathetic nerves (testicular plexus)
Lymphatics

PLATE 20 (*Continued*)
Anatomy of the Inguinal Region

O. The structures of the posterior wall of the inguinal canal.

    Inset: The vessels of the femoral sheath.

P. Direct inguinal hernia. Note the internal inguinal ring and the iliopubic tract.

Source: Gray SW, Skandalakis JE: *Atlas of Surgical Anatomy for General Surgeons.* Williams & Wilkins, Baltimore, 1985, p. 306, Plate 14-5A, B.

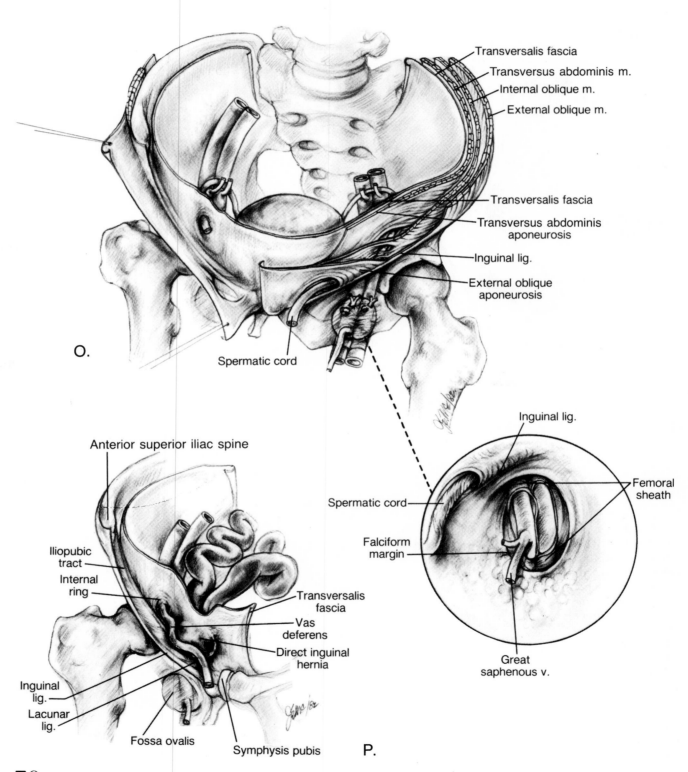

Q. Nerves of the inguinal region with which the surgeon should be familiar.

Source: Gray SW, Skandalakis JE: *Atlas of Surgical Anatomy for General Surgeons.* Williams & Wilkins, Baltimore, 1985, p. 311, Plate 14-7.

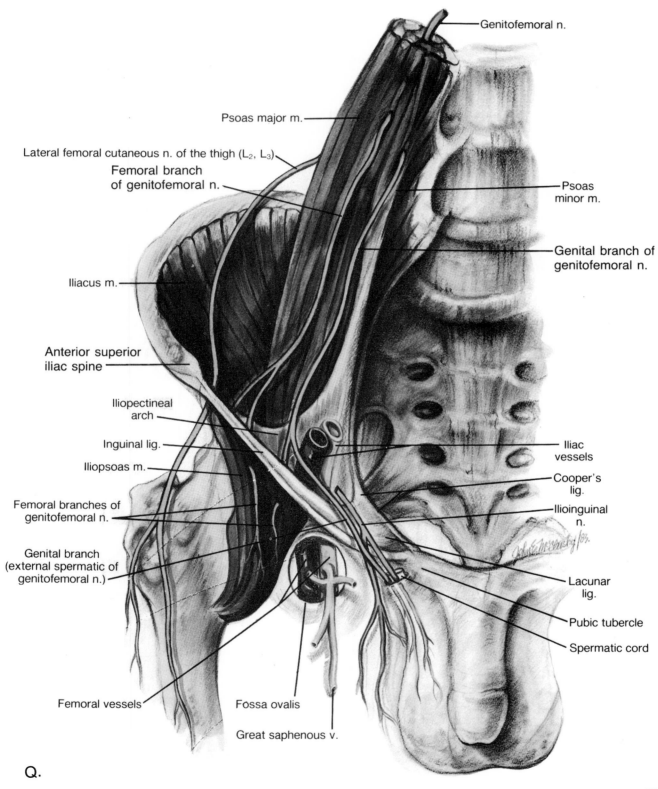

Genitofemoral n.

Psoas major m.

Lateral femoral cutaneous n. of the thigh (L$_2$, L$_3$)

Femoral branch of genitofemoral n.

Psoas minor m.

Genital branch of genitofemoral n.

Iliacus m.

Anterior superior iliac spine

Iliopectineal arch

Inguinal lig.

Iliopsoas m.

Femoral branches of genitofemoral n.

Genital branch (external spermatic of genitofemoral n.)

Iliac vessels

Cooper's lig.

Ilioinguinal n.

Lacunar lig.

Pubic tubercle

Spermatic cord

Femoral vessels

Fossa ovalis

Great saphenous v.

Q.

PLATE 20 (*Continued*)
Anatomy of the Inguinal Region

R. Diagram of the normal relations of the transversalis fascia in the lateral and lower parts of the abdominal cavity.

S. Diagrammatic cross section of a "strong" posterior inguinal canal wall. Notice the thickness and extent of the aponeurosis of the transversus abdominis muscle.

T. Diagrammatic cross section of a "weak" posterior inguinal canal wall. Compare with part B above.

Source: Plate 20R, S, and T from Lampe, EM: Transversalis fascia, in *Hernia,* 2d ed. Nyhus LM, Condon RE (eds). Lippincott, Philadelphia, 1978, pp. 61, 62, 63, Figs. 2-21, 2-23, 2-24.

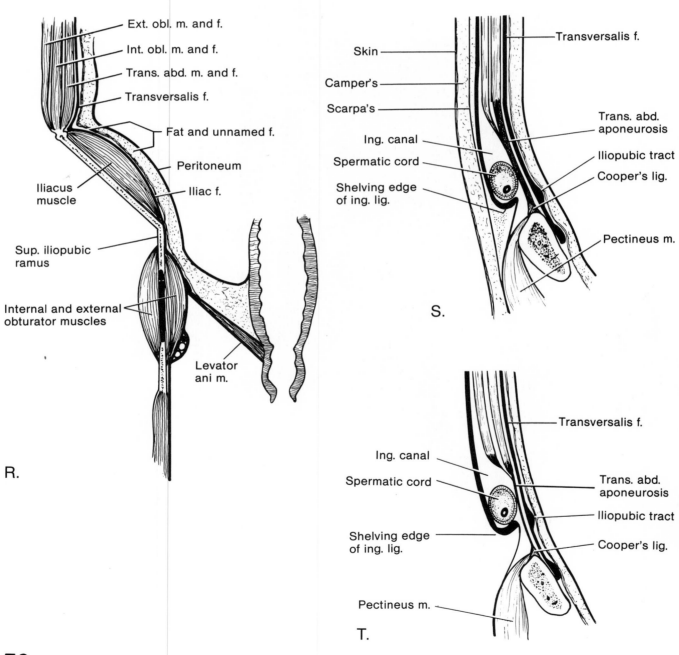

PLATE 21
The Surgical Ellipse

With the patient in the supine position, the surgeon is dealing with the following anatomical areas and entities of the inguinal region which are incorporated into an elliptical area:

The floor of the inguinal canal
A superior medial edge (above)
An inferior lateral edge (below)
A medial apex
A lateral apex

1. The floor (posterior wall) of the ellipse is formed by the transversus abdominis aponeurosis and transversalis fascia.

Remember: The transversalis fascia alone is not of adequate strength for satisfactory repair. It is not "good stuff." The transversalis fascia and transversus abdominis aponeurosis together are good stuff.

In a direct hernia, both the transversalis fascia and transversus abdominis aponeurosis are attenuated to some degree, contributing to a small or large defect. If the posterior wall is intact, none of the four types of inguinal hernia (indirect, direct, external supravesical, femoral) will develop.

The transversus abdominis layer is the most important of the three strata, according to McVay. Its integrity prevents herniation (see Plate 20S, T).

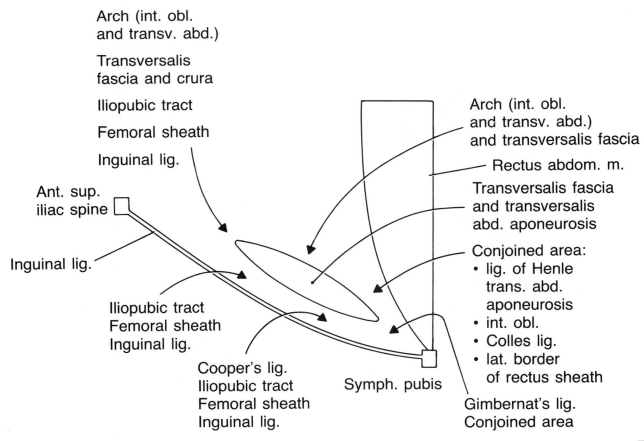

73

PLATE 21 (*Continued*)
The Surgical Ellipse

2. The superior medial (above) edge of the ellipse is formed by the
   Conjoined area
   Arch (internal oblique muscle and transversus abdominis muscle with their aponeuroses)

3. The inferior lateral edge (below) is formed by the
   Inguinal ligament
   Iliopubic tract
   Femoral sheath
   Cooper's ligament
   The iliopubic tract, femoral sheath, Cooper's ligament, and occasionally the inguinal ligament are used for repair

4. The medial apex, close to the symphysis pubis, is formed by
   Gimbernat's ligament below, and
   the conjoined area above

5. The lateral apex, at the internal ring, is formed by the
   Arch (internal oblique and transversus abdominis muscles and aponeuroses)
   Transversalis fascia and crura
   Iliopubic tract
   Femoral sheath
   Inguinal ligament

PLATE 22

Locations of Groin Hernias

A. Diagram of the relations of four groin hernias existing in the same patient. An indirect hernia with an interparietal diverticulum, as well as a direct hernia and an external supravesical hernia, was present.

1. Lateral umbilical ligament
2. Medial umbilical ligament

This illustrates the different sites of origin of each hernia.

B. Diagram of the fossae of the anterior abdominal wall and their relation to the sites of groin hernias: A, umbilicus; B, median umbilical ligament (obliterated urachus); C, medial umbilical ligament (obliterated umbilical arteries); D, lateral umbilical ligament containing inferior (deep) epigastric arteries; and E, falciform ligament. Sites of possible hernias: (1) lateral fossa (indirect inguinal hernia); (2) medial fossa (direct inguinal hernia); (3) supravesical fossa (supravesical hernia); and (4) femoral ring (femoral hernia).

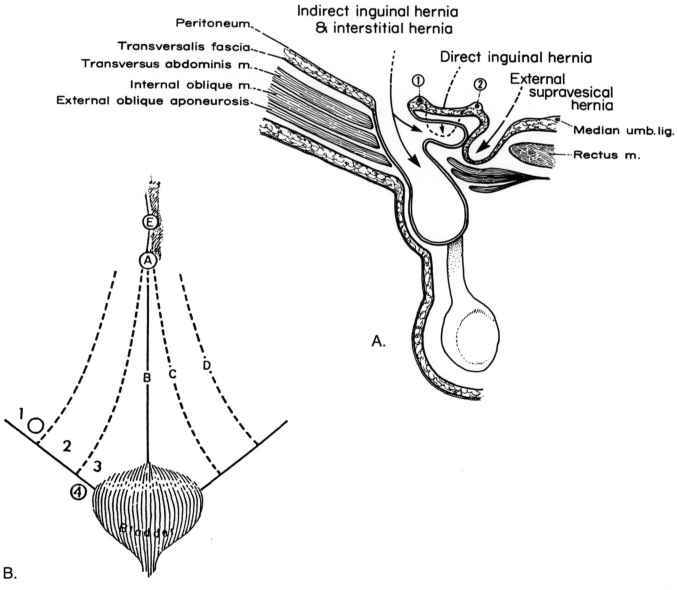

75

PLATE 22 (*Continued*)

Locations of Groin Hernias

C. Diagram of interparietal hernia. The sac, entering at the internal ring, may pass into any one or more spaces between layers of the abdominal wall: (1) properitoneal; (2), (3) interstitial; and (4) superficial. An indirect hernia also may be present.

Source: Plate 22A from Skandalakis JE: Internal and external supravesical hernia. *Am Surg* 42(2):142–146, 1976, Fig. 1. Plate 22B from Rowe JS Jr., Skandalakis JE, Gray SW: Multiple bilateral inguinal hernias. *Am Surg* 39(5):269–270, 1973, Fig. 2. Plate 22C from Skandalakis JE, Gray SW, Akin JT Jr: The surgical anatomy of hernial rings. *Surg Clin North Am* 54(6):1227–1246, 1974, Fig. 2.

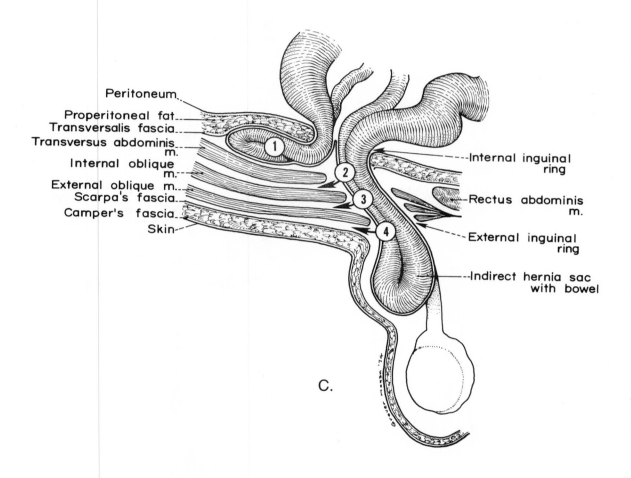

C.

76

Present Approaches to Groin Hernias

LLOYD M. NYHUS
Personal Communication, 1988

In the 1980s, the operative treatment of groin hernia continues to be based on an accurate knowledge of anatomy. Understanding the endoabdominal (transversalis) fascia and its analogues (iliopubic tract—anterior femoral sheath) is the key to our knowledge base relative to etiology, development, diagnosis, and cure of these common problems.

Although the Bassini repair continues to be popular (because of common usage), an overall recurrence rate of 10 percent has necessitated a search for other techniques. Experience has demonstrated that no one operative approach is superior. The surgeon today must have the ability to modify the approach according to individual operative findings.

The various anatomical defects of inguinal hernia and the specific best operative care for each are as follows:

1. Small indirect
   * Excision of hernial sac and high ligation (in all except direct)
   a. Transversalis fascia repair of internal ring

2. Large indirect
   a. Iliopubic tract repair of posterior inguinal wall
   b. Cooper ligament repair and modum McVay

3. Small direct
   a. Iliopubic tract repair of posterior inguinal wall

4. Large direct
   a. Cooper ligament repair of posterior inguinal wall
   b. Iliopubic tract repair with Marlex mesh buttress

5. Pantaloon hernia
   a. Iliopubic tract repair of posterior inguinal wall plus transversalis fascia closure of internal ring

6. Femoral
   a. Preperitoneal approach and iliopubic tract repair

7. Sliding indirect
   a. Preperitoneal approach and iliopubic tract repair
   b. Iliopubic tract repair (anterior approach)
   c. Cooper ligament repair

8. Strangulated indirect or femoral
   a. Preperitoneal approach, bowel resection and anastomosis, iliopubic tract repair

9. Recurrent hernia
   a. Preperitoneal approach and iliopubic tract repair with Marlex mesh buttress

10. Massive hernia (loss of "right of domain")
   a. 10 day pneumoperitoneum
   b. Iliopubic tract repair of posterior inguinal wall with Marlex mesh buttress
   c. Cooper ligament repair and modum McVay

Since a great number of surgeons in the United States and Canada use the Shouldice procedure for the repair of inguinal hernia, the authors have chosen to add this procedure for the benefit of surgeons who wish to use it. We have not described procedures of older surgeons such as Bassini, Halstead, and Marcy. Their contributions are so fundamental that modern surgery owes much to these great teachers of the past; without them, present methods of hernia repair would never have developed.

Indirect Inguinal Hernia

Definition

An indirect inguinal hernia leaves the abdomen through the internal inguinal ring and passes down the inguinal canal a variable distance with the spermatic cord or round ligament.

Occasionally the sac may not reach the scrotum or labia majora but may enter the abdominal wall through any cleavage plane between muscles. This is an interparietal hernia.

PLATE 23

Repair of Indirect Inguinal Hernia

A. *Step 1.* Incise the skin approximately 2 to 3 cm above and parallel to the inguinal ligament. (A transverse, gently curved incision following the lines of Langer is another option.) It is our practice to mark the location and length of the incision prior to covering the patient with sterile towels. The patient, male or female, will appreciate a symmetrical incision, especially on bilateral herniorrhaphy.

Incise the subcutaneous fascia (Camper's) and the fascia of Scarpa by sharp dissection. Open the aponeurosis of the external oblique muscle in the direction of its fibers. The external ring can be found with ease.

Remember:
- Ligate the large veins (superficial epigastric, superficial circumflex, and external pudendal) with plain catgut. Other small vessels may be treated by electrocoagulation.
- Protect the ilioinguinal nerve.
- If the hernia is recurrent, it is necessary to excise the preexisting scar, both for cosmetic reasons and for good healing.
- Do not dissect too much medially and laterally to the incision of the aponeurosis of the external oblique muscle. Avoid dead spaces.

B. *Step 2.* Elevate the spermatic cord carefully. Retract with a Penrose drain. We prefer significant skeletonization of the cord by careful partial dissection of the cremasteric muscles or any associated "cord lipoma." Proximal and distal ligation of the cremaster and the lipomatous structures is necessary. We use 000 or 0000 silk.

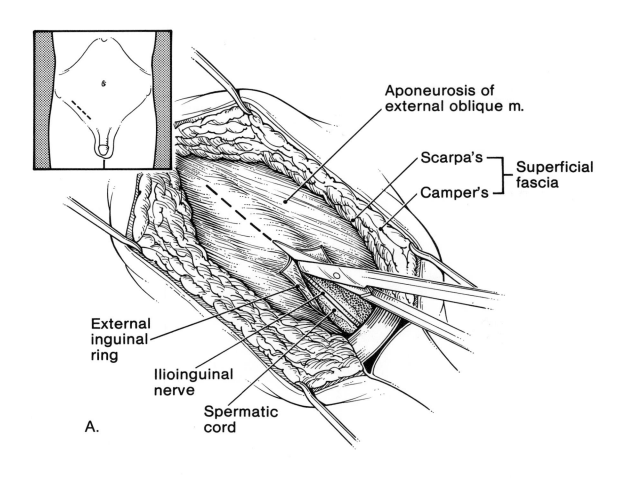

Aponeurosis of
external oblique m.

Scarpa's ⎤
Camper's ⎦ Superficial
fascia

External
inguinal
ring

Ilioinguinal
nerve

Spermatic
cord

A.

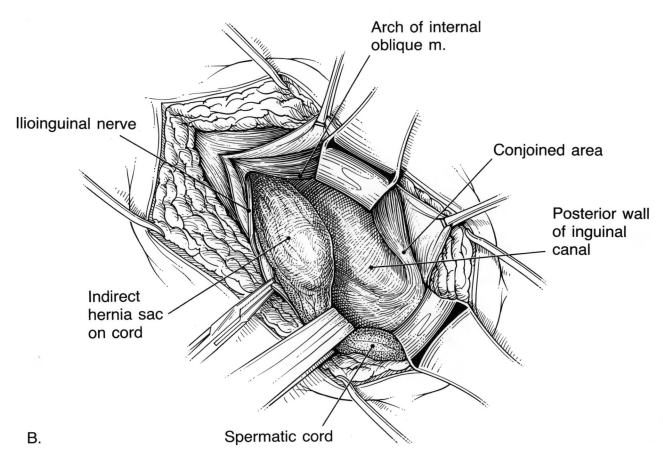

Arch of internal
oblique m.

Ilioinguinal nerve

Conjoined area

Posterior wall
of inguinal
canal

Indirect
hernia sac
on cord

Spermatic cord

B.

79

PLATE 23 (*Continued*)
Repair of Indirect Inguinal Hernia

C. *Step 3.* Identify the sac located anterior to the spermatic cord. Separate the sac using scissors and a wet sponge. Dissect it upward toward the internal ring and laterally to the deep epigastric vessels.

D. *Step 4.* Palpate the sac and open it.

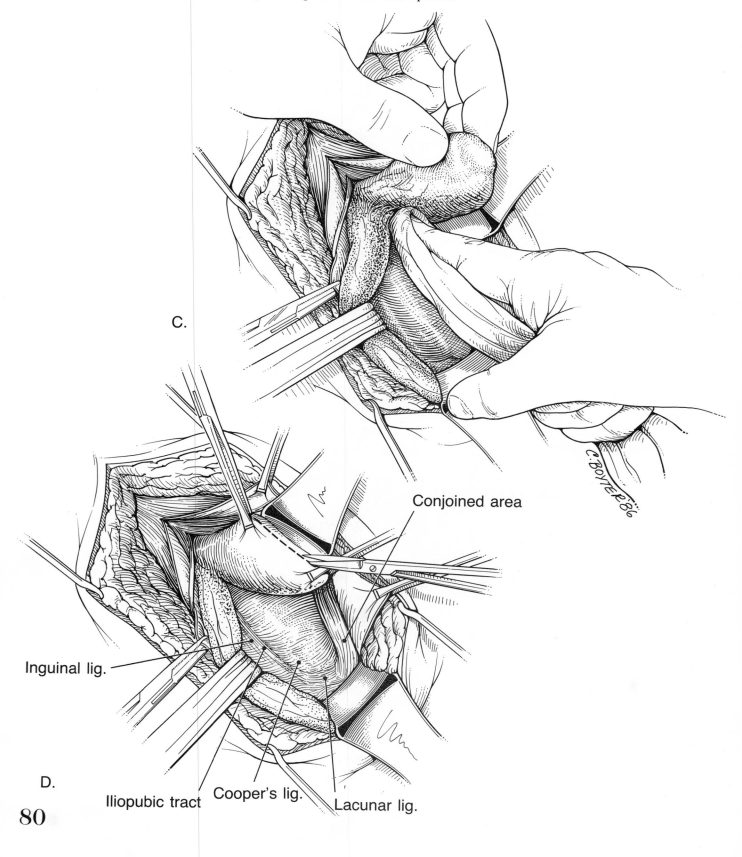

C.

Conjoined area

Inguinal lig.

D.

Iliopubic tract   Cooper's lig.   Lacunar lig.

E. *Step 5.* Perform a digital examination within the sac. Check for
- Omental or viscus adhesions into the sac
- Possible femoral hernia
- Posterior wall weakness and possible direct or external supravesical hernia

F. *Step 6.* Ligate and amputate the sac. Occasionally if there is too much relaxation at the internal ring, the ligated sac is fixed under the transversus abdominis muscle, which is the upper boundary of the internal ring *(Inset)*.

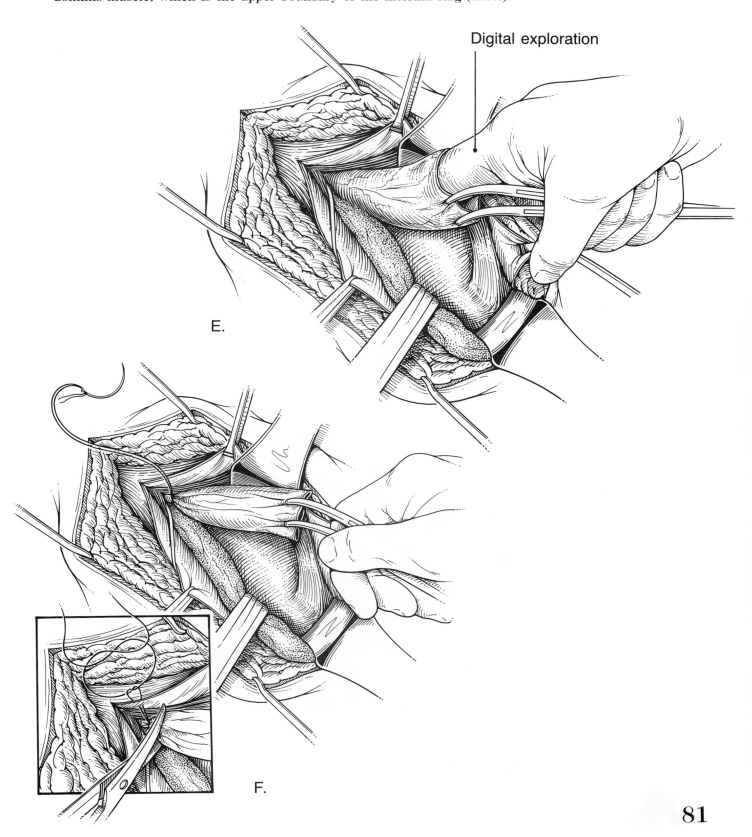

Digital exploration

E.

F.

PLATE 23 (*Continued*)

Repair of Indirect Inguinal Hernia

We agree with Nyhus that a single suturing technique is not appropriate for all patients. The following illustrates our technique:

G. *Step 7*

1. Suture the conjoined area to the ligament of Gimbernat with 0 Surgilon or 0 silk.
2. Suture the conjoined area to the ligament of Cooper, including the iliopubic arch and occasionally the ligament of Poupart (shelving edge) if the ligament of Cooper is deep.
3. After good palpation of the femoral arteries to avoid injury to the femoral vein, place this transitional suture as in no. 2 above, incorporating the femoral sheath.
4. Suture as above or suture the arch to the shelving edge of the inguinal ligament, including the iliopubic tract.

The remainder of the sutures incorporate the arch, iliopubic tract, and inguinal ligament.

Be careful with the deep inguinal ring. The suture in this area starts with the arch and incorporates the crura of the transversalis fascia (if present), the iliopubic tract, and shelving edge of the inguinal ligament. The distal phalanx of the fifth finger should be inserted with ease into the deep ring, thereby ensuring that the closure is not too snug.

This drawing shows the ligature of the sac. Usually it will not be visible.

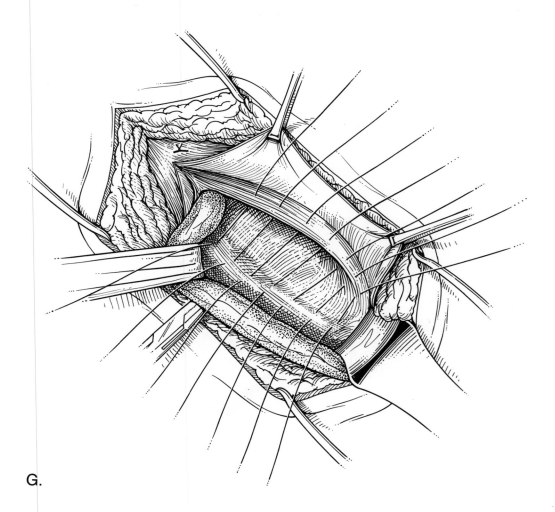

G.

H. *Step 8.* Tie all sutures.

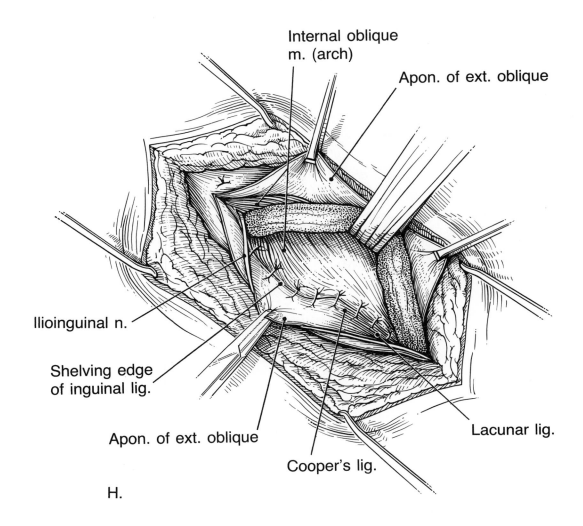

Internal oblique
m. (arch)

Apon. of ext. oblique

Ilioinguinal n.

Shelving edge
of inguinal lig.

Apon. of ext. oblique

Cooper's lig.

Lacunar lig.

H.

PLATE 23 (*Continued*)
Repair of Indirect Inguinal Hernia

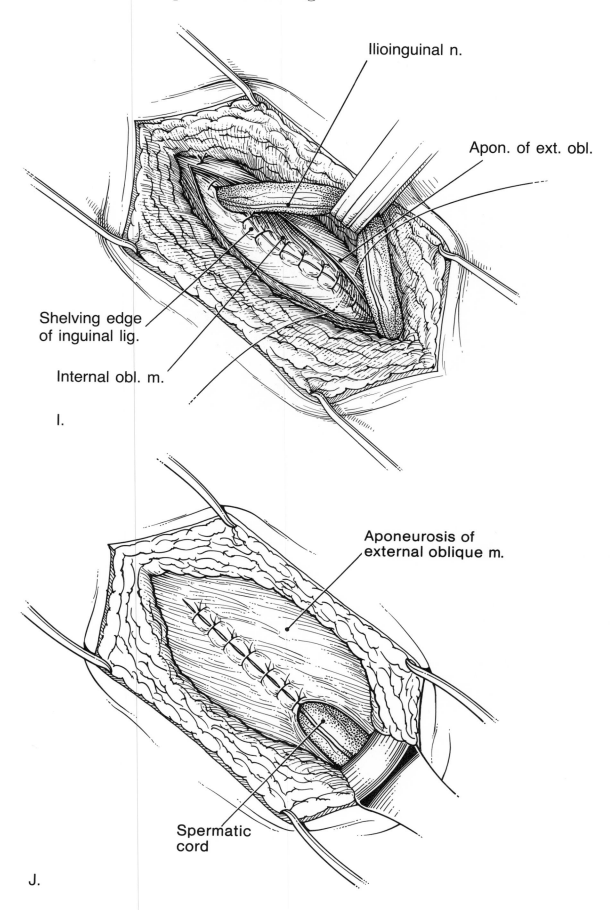

Ilioinguinal n.

Apon. of ext. obl.

Shelving edge
of inguinal lig.

Internal obl. m.

I.

Aponeurosis of
external oblique m.

Spermatic
cord

J.

84

I. *Step 9.* Close the aponeurosis of the external oblique muscle with interrupted 00 Surgilon. Occasionally we incorporate with deep bites the arch which was previously sutured to the inguinal ligament. This drawing shows the sutures below the spermatic cord.

J. In most cases, the spermatic cord is placed under the aponeurosis of the external oblique muscle. Occasionally one more suture is placed just above the spermatic cord at the lateral apex.

K. *Step 10.* Close Scarpa's fascia with continuous or interrupted 000 plain catgut. In this drawing sutures begin at the medial apex. Be careful not to traumatize the ilioinguinal nerve, which should be placed under Scarpa's fascia.

L. *Step 11.* Close the skin with clips.

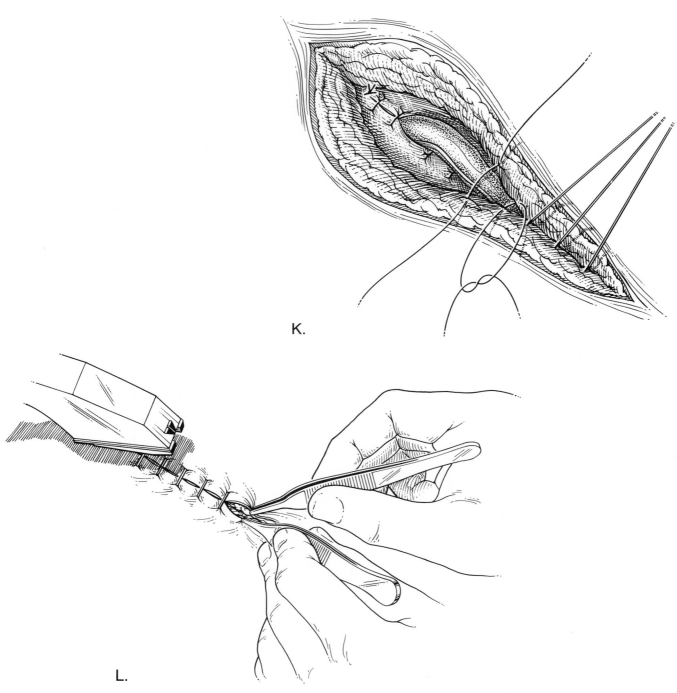

K.

L.

85

Sliding Indirect Inguinal Hernia

Definition

A sliding indirect inguinal hernia contains the herniated viscus which makes up all or some of the posterior wall of the sac. Most typically, sliding hernias involve the colon, but they can involve the bladder and, in the female, the ovaries and uterine tube.

PLATE 24

Repair of Sliding Indirect Inguinal Hernia

A,B. Communicating and noncommunicating sliding hernias. The internal ring is wider than usual due to the thick spermatic cord. Coincidental direct hernia or weakness of the posterior wall is a strong possibility.

C. The hernia sac is located anterior and medial to the cord as in an indirect hernia. It contains the cecum or sigmoid colon. Rarely the urinary bladder may be a part of the sac wall. An ovary, a uterine tube, and a portion of the uterus have been encountered in an infant with a sliding hernia. The descending viscus forms the posterior wall of the empty processus.

   Step 1. Mobilize the sac and open it high and anteriorly. Do not dissect the viscus from the posterior wall of the sac.

D. *Step 2.* If there is excess anterior wall of the sac, trim it carefully.

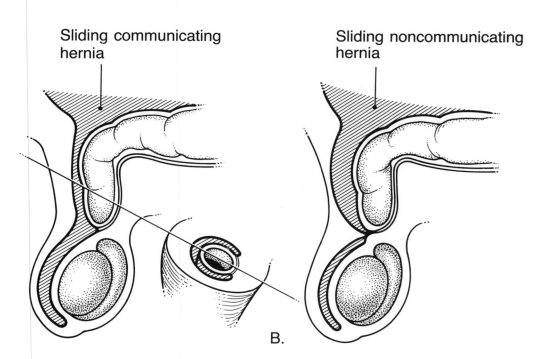

Sliding communicating hernia

Sliding noncommunicating hernia

A.

B.

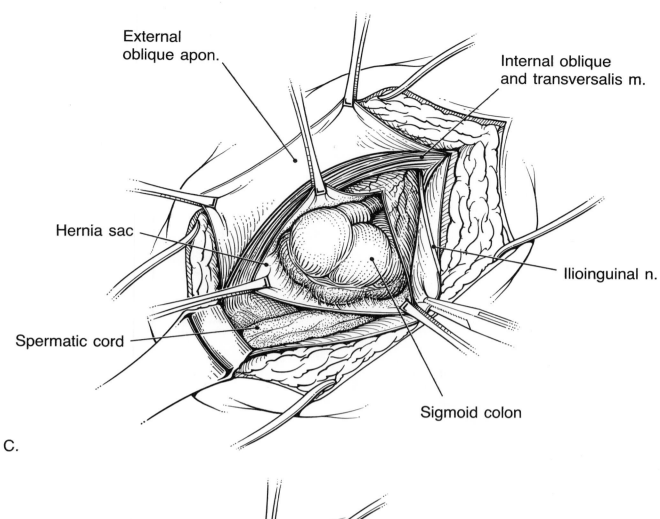

External
oblique apon.

Internal oblique
and transversalis m.

Hernia sac

Ilioinguinal n.

Spermatic cord

Sigmoid colon

C.

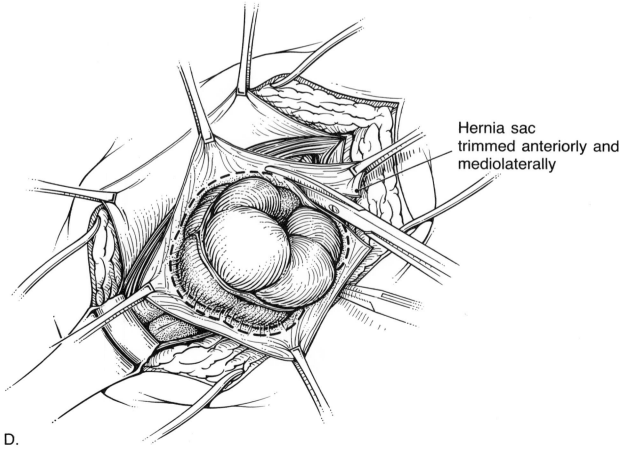

Hernia sac
trimmed anteriorly and
mediolaterally

D.

PLATE 24 (*Continued*)

Repair of Sliding Indirect Inguinal Hernia

E. *Step 3.* Close the remnants of the sac. Finish the repair as in indirect inguinal hernia.

Closure of the remnants
of the hernia sac
with purse-string
or continuous suture

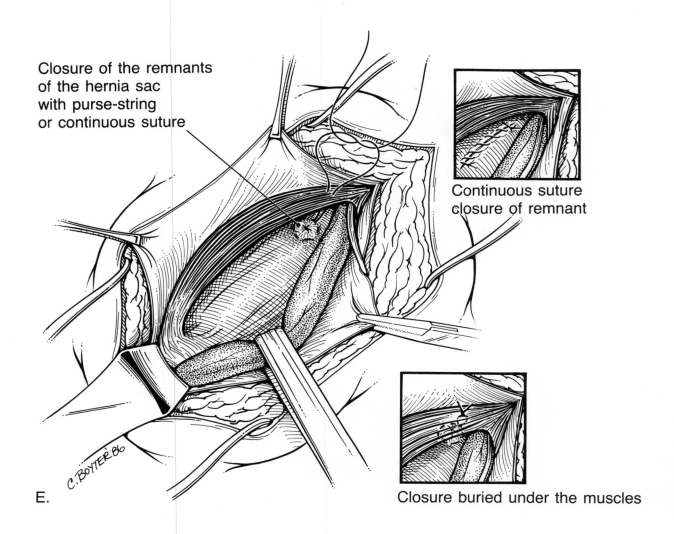

Continuous suture
closure of remnant

Closure buried under the muscles

E.

Direct Inguinal Hernia

Definition

A direct inguinal hernia passes through the floor of the inguinal canal in Hesselbach's triangle, which is covered by the transversalis fascia and aponeurosis of the transversus abdominis muscle. The hernia path lies behind the spermatic cord and does not enter the internal ring but may exit through the external ring. A direct hernia rarely enters the scrotum.

PLATE 25
Repair of Direct Inguinal Hernia

The Hoguet maneuver to convert a direct hernia sac to an indirect hernia is not described among the following procedures since the direct hernia sac is not opened but only closed by a purse string. Cooper's ligament, the iliopubic tract, and also the conjoined area were used for the repair of practically all inguinofemoral hernias.

A. *Step 1.* Incise the skin, subcutaneous layers, and external oblique aponeurosis. Elevate the spermatic cord or round ligament as in indirect inguinal hernia.

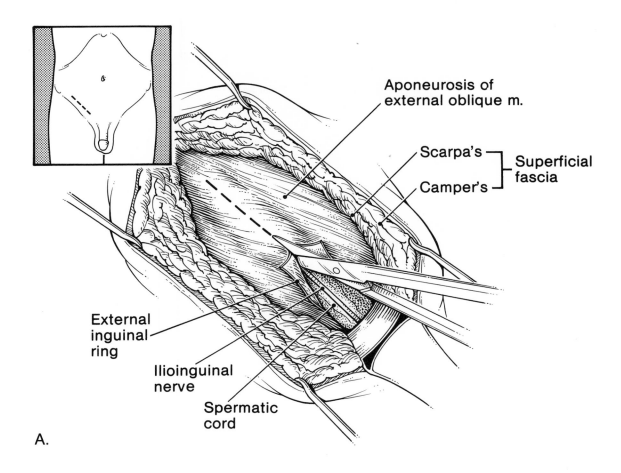

Aponeurosis of external oblique m.

Scarpa's ⎤
          ⎬ Superficial fascia
Camper's ⎦

External inguinal ring

Ilioinguinal nerve

Spermatic cord

A.

89

PLATE 25 (*Continued*)

Repair of Direct Inguinal Hernia

B. Bulging of the direct hernia with the cord pulled medially.

C. Bulging of the direct hernia with the cord pulled laterally.

D. *Step 2.* Using 000 silk, make a purse-string suture at the base of the un-opened sac.

    Inset: Tie the suture.

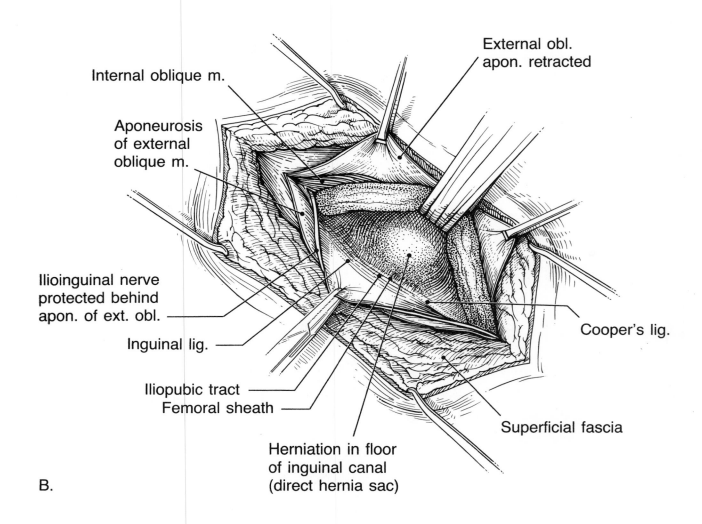

Internal oblique m.

External obl.
apon. retracted

Aponeurosis
of external
oblique m.

Ilioinguinal nerve
protected behind
apon. of ext. obl.

Inguinal lig.

Cooper's lig.

Iliopubic tract
Femoral sheath

Superficial fascia

Herniation in floor
of inguinal canal
(direct hernia sac)

B.

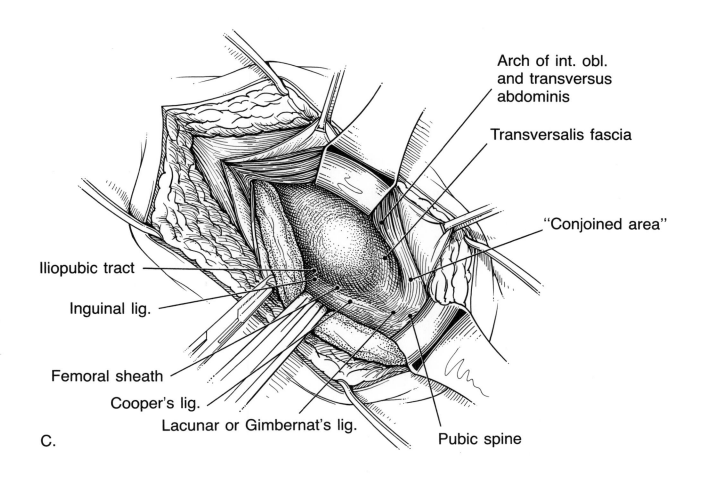

Arch of int. obl. and transversus abdominis

Transversalis fascia

"Conjoined area"

Iliopubic tract

Inguinal lig.

Femoral sheath

Cooper's lig.

Lacunar or Gimbernat's lig.

Pubic spine

C.

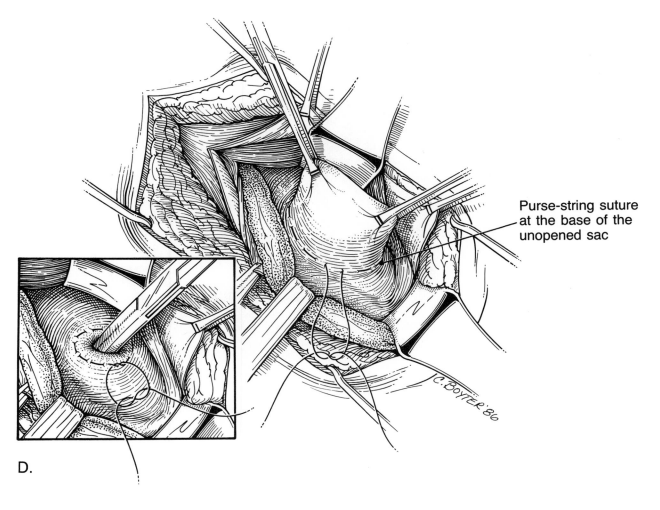

Purse-string suture at the base of the unopened sac

C. BOYTER '86

D.

91

PLATE 25 (*Continued*)
Repair of Direct Inguinal Hernia

The suturing technique for direct inguinal hernia is the same as for indirect hernia. Follow the precautions outlined in the indirect inguinal hernia section.

E. *Step 3*

1. Suture the conjoined area or the transversus abdominis arch to Gimbernat's ligament with 0 Surgilon or 0 silk.
2. Suture the conjoined area or the transversus abdominis arch to Cooper's ligament, including the iliopubic tract and occasionally Poupart's ligament (shelving edge).
3. Palpate the femoral artery and suture as in No. 2 above, placing a transition suture in the femoral sheath.
4. Suture as above or suture the arch to the shelving edge of the inguinal ligament or to the iliopubic tract.

F. *Step 4.* Tie all sutures.

G. *Step 5.* Close the aponeurosis of the external oblique muscle with interrupted 00 Surgilon.

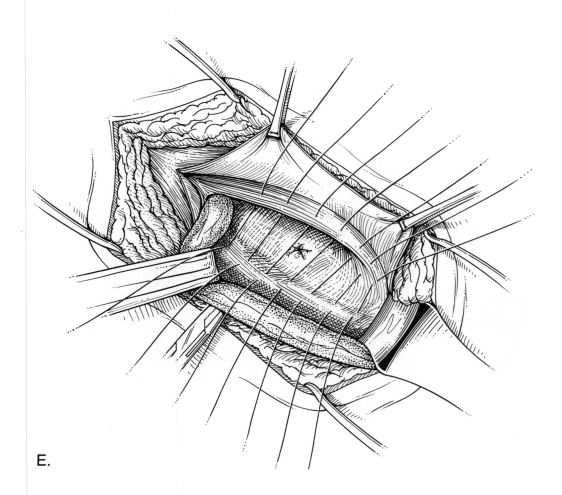

E.

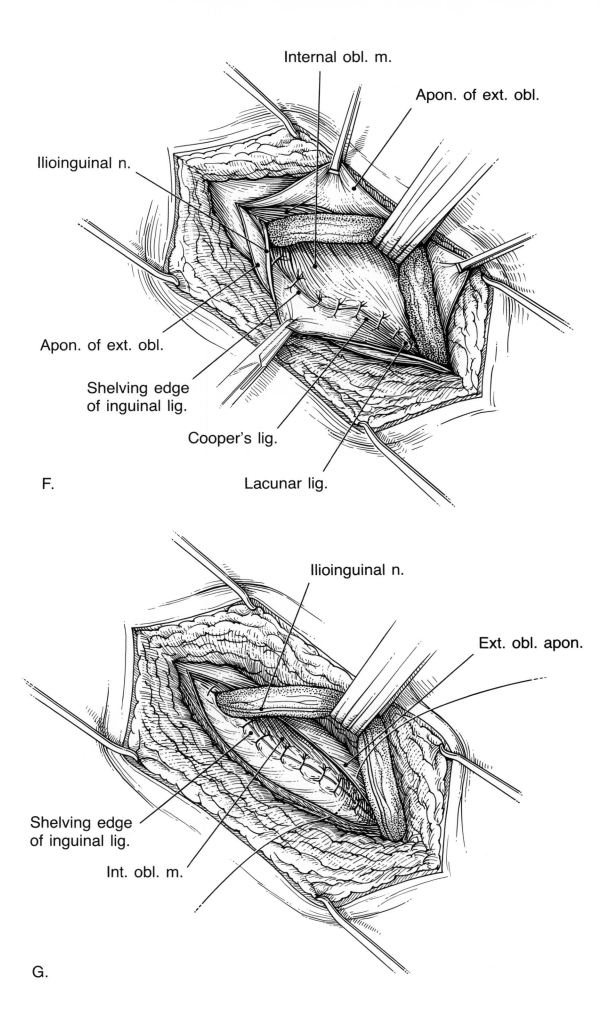

Internal obl. m.

Apon. of ext. obl.

Ilioinguinal n.

Apon. of ext. obl.

Shelving edge
of inguinal lig.

Cooper's lig.

Lacunar lig.

F.

Ilioinguinal n.

Ext. obl. apon.

Shelving edge
of inguinal lig.

Int. obl. m.

G.

93

PLATE 25 (*Continued*)

Repair of Direct Inguinal Hernia

H. *Step 6.* Close Scarpa's fascia with continuous or interrupted 000 plain catgut.

I. *Step 7.* Close the skin with clips.

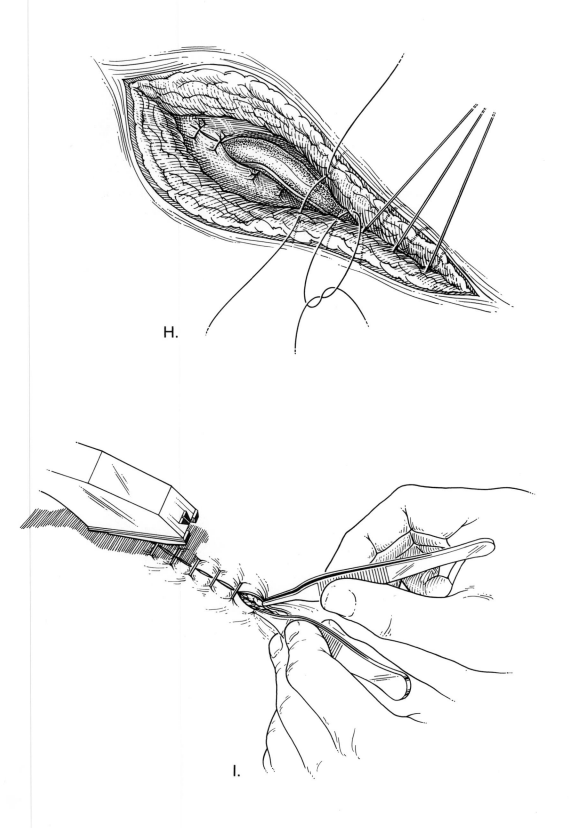

H.

I.

The Relaxing Incision

The surgeon should be familiar with the formation of the anterior lamina of the rectus sheath:

- Below the semicircular line (Douglas or arcuate) there is no posterior aponeurotic layer of the rectus sheath.
- The anterior layer is formed by the aponeuroses of the internal oblique and transversus abdominis muscles and reinforced by the aponeurosis of the external oblique muscle.
- The aponeurosis of the external oblique muscle may "touch down" at the lateral half or at the medial half of the anterior lamina. It almost never does so at the linea semilunaris (lateral border of the rectus abdominis) or at the linea alba.

INCISION

The relaxing incision is made just lateral to the line of attachment ("touch down") of the external oblique aponeurosis to the anterior lamina of the sheath. This is at the point where the fused internal oblique and transversus abdominis aponeuroses form the rectus sheath.

The incision starts at the pubic crest and extends upward 5 to 8 cm. The length of the incision depends on the local anatomy and pathology (Ponka).

A good anatomical relaxing incision will protect the external oblique aponeurosis and will not permit the rectus muscle to form a myocele. It will not allow the formation of a true hernia.

Avoid:

- A linea alba incision or an incision at the linea semilunaris. This is done by careful elevation of the medial flap of the aponeurosis of the external oblique muscle.
- The iliohypogastric nerve.

PLATE 26
The Relaxing Incision

A. Diagrammatic drawing of the relaxing incision.
X = Point of relaxing incision at the anterior lamina of the rectus sheath
▲ = "Touch down" of the external oblique aponeurosis, always between the linea alba and semilunar line

B. The completed direct hernia repair demonstrates that the relaxing incision allows the transversus abdominis to slide inferiorly. As the relaxing incision opens, the rectus muscle is exposed, but the overlying intact superficial lamina (external oblique aponeurosis) of the rectus sheath prevents the development of a hernia.

Source: Plate 26B from Condon RE: Anterior iliopubic tract repair, in *Hernia*, 2d ed. Nyhus LM, Condon E (eds). Lippincott, Philadelphia, 1978, p. 210, Fig. 8-11.

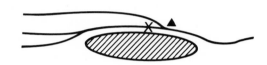

A.

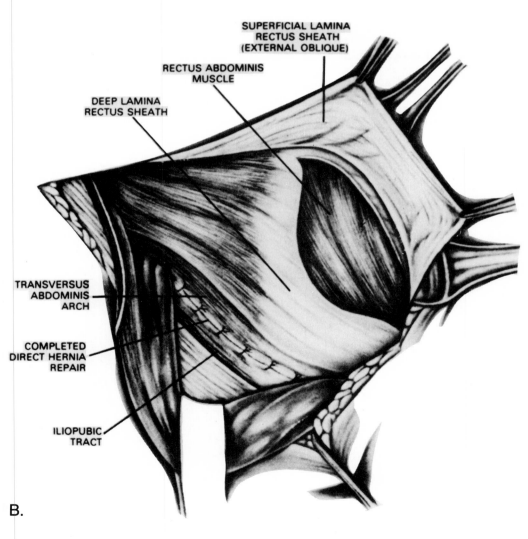

B.

External Supravesical Hernia

Definition

An external supravesical hernia leaves the peritoneal cavity through the supravesical fossa, which lies medial to the site of direct inguinal fossae. Its subsequent course is that of a direct inguinal hernia.

The repair procedure is the same as for direct inguinal hernia. The surgeon should be careful to protect the iliohypogastric nerve, which is located medial to the superior edge of the surgical ellipse.

PLATE 27

Diagram of the Fossae of the Anterior Abdominal Wall and Their Relation to the Sites of Groin Hernia

A, umbilicus; B, median umbilical ligament (obliterated urachus); C, medial umbilical ligament (obliterated umbilical arteries); D, lateral umbilical ligament containing inferior (deep) epigastric arteries; and E, falciform ligament. Sites of possible hernias: (1) lateral fossa (indirect inguinal hernia); (2) medial fossa (direct inguinal hernia); (3) supravesical fossa (supravesical hernia); and (4) femoral ring (femoral hernia).

Source: Rowe JS Jr., Skandalakis JE, Gray SW: Multiple bilateral inguinal hernias. *Am Surg* 39(5):269–270, 1973, Fig. 2.

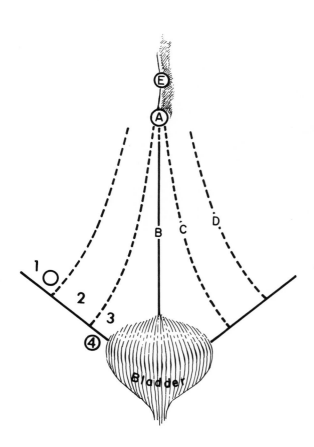

Femoral Hernia

Definition

A femoral hernia is a protrusion of preperitoneal fat or intraperitoneal viscus through a weak transversalis fascia into the femoral ring and the femoral canal.

PLATE 28

Pathways of Femoral Hernia

A. Femoral hernia. Typical and atypical pathways taken by the femoral hernial sac. Note the possible relations to the femoral artery (A) and femoral vein (V).

B. Femoral hernia. The left half of the drawing shows an aberrant obturator artery passing medial to the hernial sac, making it dangerous to incise the lacunar ligament. The right half of the drawing shows an aberrant obturator artery passing lateral to the hernial sac, making it safe to incise the lacunar ligament.

Source: Plate 28B from Skandalakis JE, Gray SW, Akin JT Jr.: The surgical anatomy of hernial rings. *Surg Clin North Am* 54(6):1227–1246, 1974, Fig. 3.

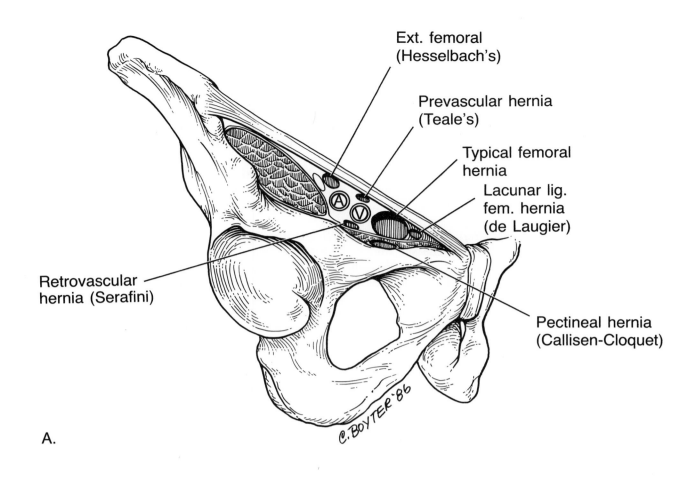

Ext. femoral
(Hesselbach's)

Prevascular hernia
(Teale's)

Typical femoral
hernia

Lacunar lig.
fem. hernia
(de Laugier)

Retrovascular
hernia (Serafini)

Pectineal hernia
(Callisen-Cloquet)

A.

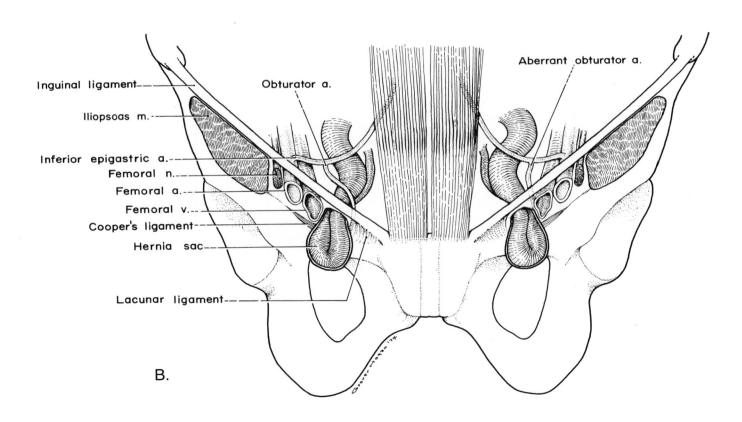

Inguinal ligament

Iliopsoas m.

Inferior epigastric a.

Femoral n.

Femoral a.

Femoral v.

Cooper's ligament

Hernia sac

Lacunar ligament

Obturator a.

Aberrant obturator a.

B.

99

PLATE 29
Repair of Femoral Hernia

A. *Step 1.* Incise the skin and divide the external oblique aponeurosis as in other inguinal hernias. Elevate the spermatic cord or round ligament of the uterus and separate it from the posterior wall. Incise the internal oblique and transversus abdominis muscles. Incise the transversalis fascia without entering the peritoneum. This maneuver exposes the preperitoneal space.

Blunt dissection in the preperitoneal space will direct the surgeon to the neck of the hernia sac. Cut any adhesions and remnants of the attenuated transversalis fascia very carefully. Do not open the sac at this time.

B. *Step 2.* Insert one index finger under the subcutaneous fat to palpate and isolate the sac under the inguinal ligament and the fossa ovalis. With the index and middle finger of the other hand, gently push the unopened sac upward through the femoral canal into the inguinal canal.

If the hernia is not strangulated, this pressure is very useful. If the hernia is incarcerated or strangulated, the contents of the sac should be examined and not permitted to return to the abdominal cavity.

C. The femoral hernia now becomes a direct hernia.

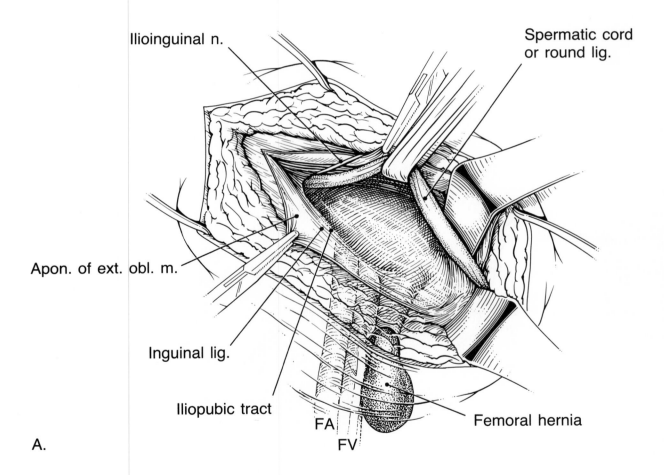

Ilioinguinal n.

Spermatic cord or round lig.

Apon. of ext. obl. m.

Inguinal lig.

Iliopubic tract

FA

FV

Femoral hernia

A.

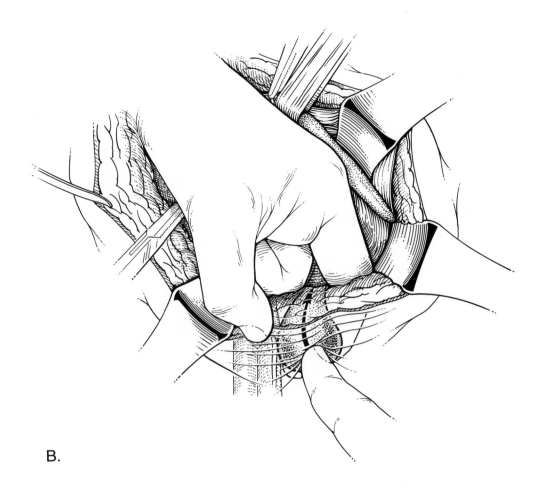

B.

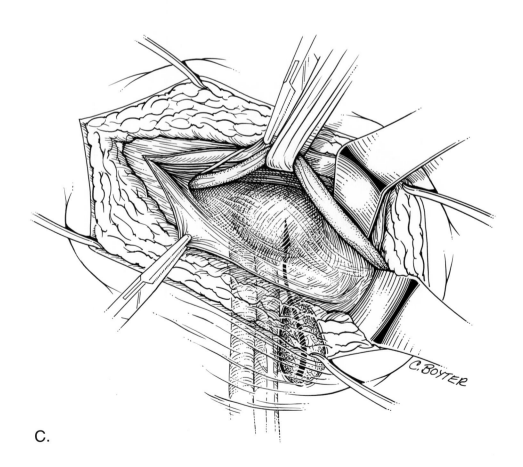

C. BOYTER

C.

101

PLATE 29 (*Continued*)

Repair of Femoral Hernia

D. *Step 3.* Make a purse-string suture at the base of the unopened sac.

    Inset: Tie the suture and continue the repair as for direct hernia.

    An alternative method of repair accomplishes tightening of the femoral canal by suturing the iliopubic tract (above) to Cooper's ligament (below). Care must be taken to avoid constriction of the femoral vein.

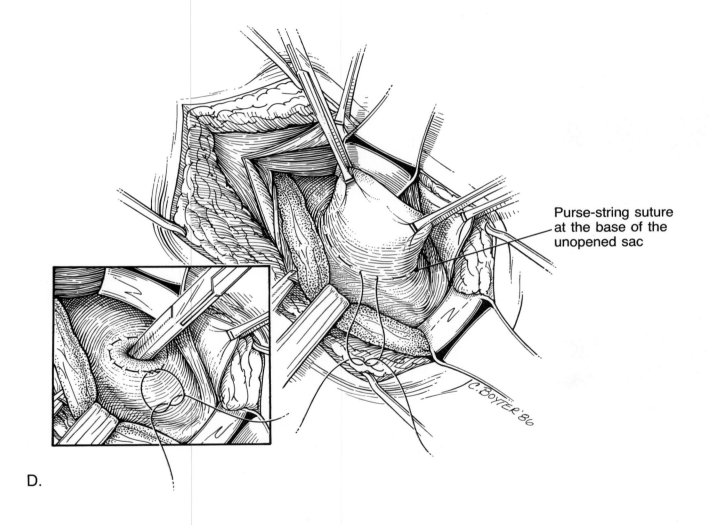

Purse-string suture
at the base of the
unopened sac

D.

E. If there is heavy fixation of the neck to the transversalis fascia, make a small incision at the transversalis fascia around the neck.

F. Free the sac.

G. Place a purse-string suture at the base of the sac as for direct inguinal hernia.

H. With two or three sutures, close the previous incision of the transversalis fascia and repair as for direct hernia.

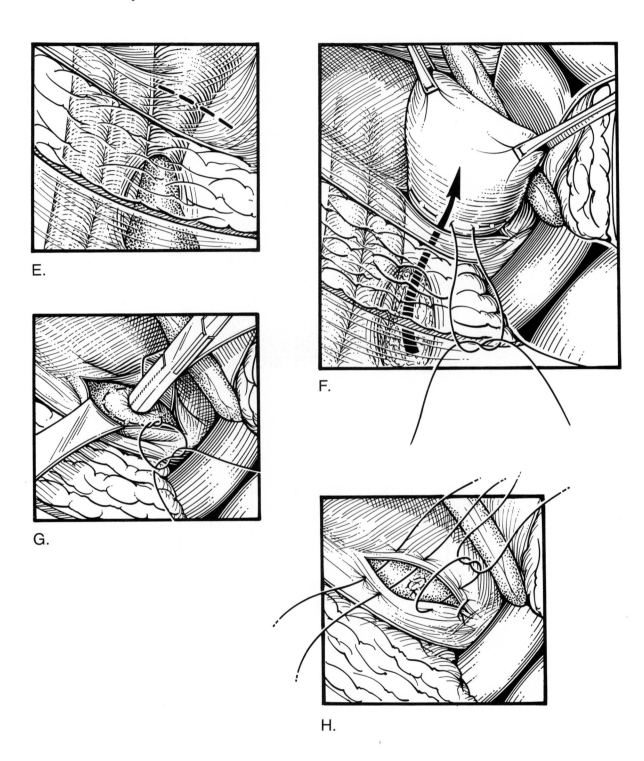

E.

F.

G.

H.

PLATE 29 (*Continued*)
Repair of Femoral Hernia

I. The sac has remained in the upper part of Scarpa's triangle. A Kelly clamp may be used to bring the sac into the inguinal canal.

Inset: If the hernia is strangulated, elevate the inguinal ligament by inserting a hemostat underneath it. Then cut the ligament to liberate the viscus.

An alternative method of reduction requires sectioning of the lacunar ligament. The surgeon must be certain that an aberrant obturator artery is not present before severing the ligament.

J. Gently manipulate the sac into the posterior wall without losing the contents. An assistant should hold the mass firmly with the thumb and index finger.

K. Open the sac and inspect the contents.

L. If the viscus is vital, trim and ligate the sac. Proceed with the repair as in direct inguinal hernia. If the viscus is not vital, resection and anastomosis with the usual repair should follow.

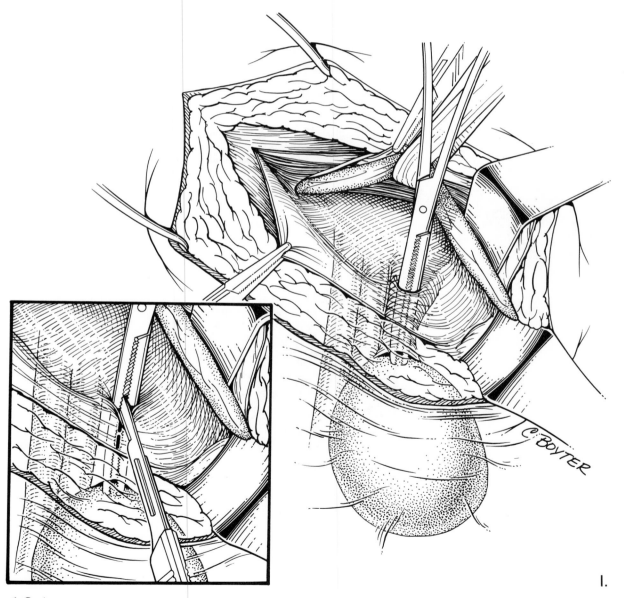

I.

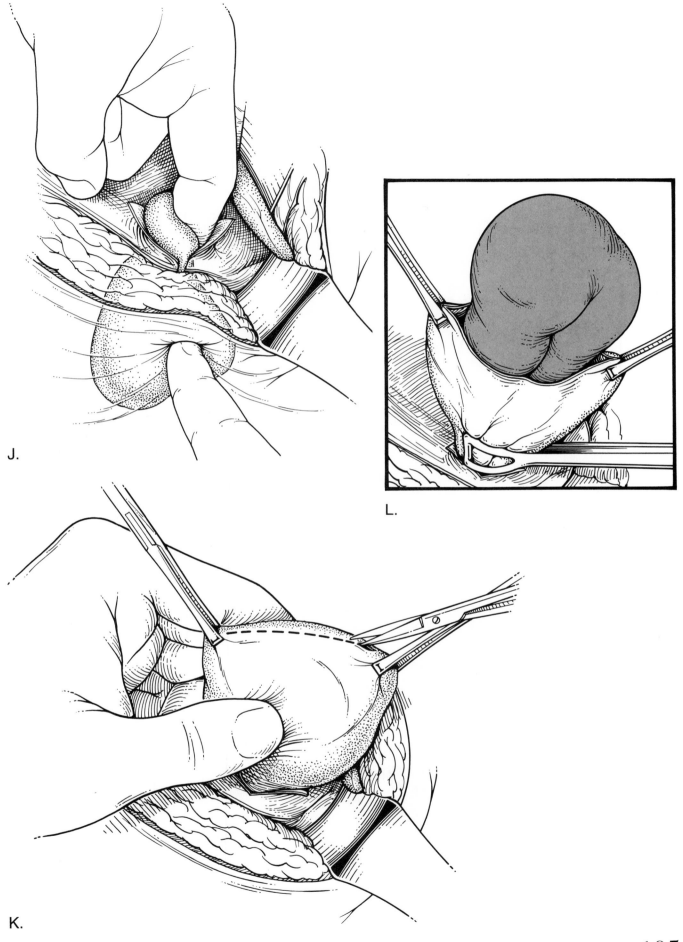

J.

K.

L.

105

PLATE 30

Femoral Hernia Repair Below the Inguinal Ligament

A. *Step 1.* Make a vertical or transverse incision just above the femoral swelling with extension to the subcutaneous tissues.

B. *Step 2.* Isolate the swelling by careful sharp dissection and digital maneuver until the sac is exposed.

C. *Step 3.* Carefully open the sac. Fluid (which is always present) is sent to the lab for culture and sensitivity testing.

Step 4. Inspect the contents of the sac. If they are viable, push them gently into the abdominal cavity. If constriction of the neck does not permit the return of the viscus into the peritoneal cavity, the hernia ring should be cut. It is our opinion that the best anatomical entity to sacrifice in this situation is the inguinal ligament, not the lacunar ligament.

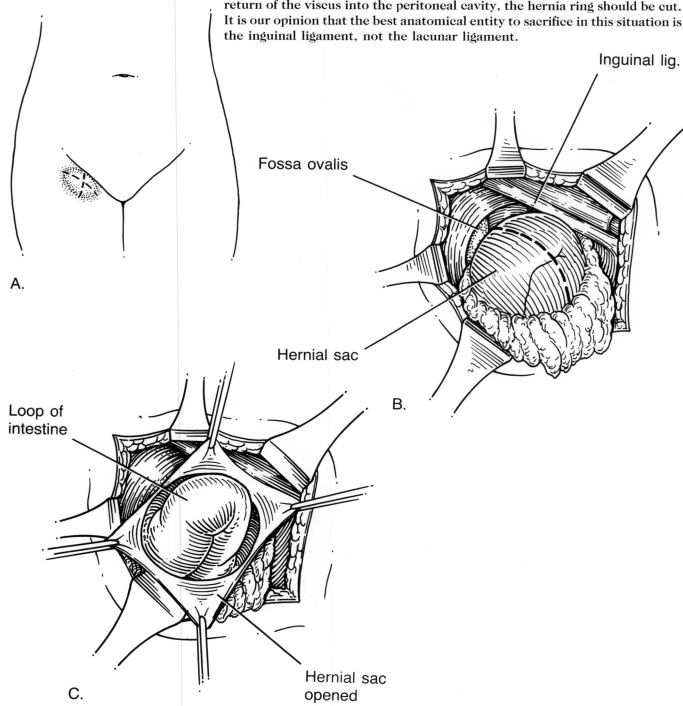

A.

Inguinal lig.

Fossa ovalis

Hernial sac

B.

Loop of intestine

Hernial sac opened

C.

D. *Step 5.* Ligate the sac with 00 Surgilon and excise it. Gently push the sac into the peritoneal cavity so that the canal is as clean as possible.

E,F. *Step 6.* Using 00 or 000 Surgilon, suture the inguinal ligament to the pectineal fascia or to Cooper's ligament. We prefer to use Cooper's ligament.

Step 7. Close the subcutaneous fat and skin.

If the contents of the sac (bowel) are not viable, the assistant should keep the loop in situ, holding it firmly. Make a lower midline incision immediately; resection and anastomosis of the bowel must be done from above.

Use of drains or wound closure depends upon the contamination of the fossa ovalis or of the peritoneal cavity.

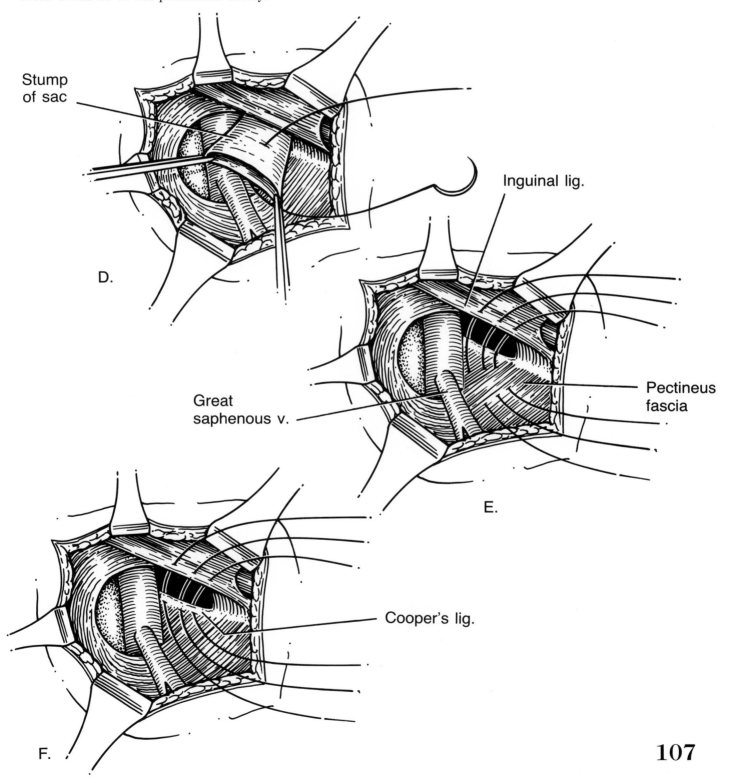

Stump of sac

D.

Inguinal lig.

Great saphenous v.

Pectineus fascia

E.

Cooper's lig.

F.

107

PLATE 31
Repair of Male Pediatric Inguinal Hernia

A. *Step 1.* Make a transverse inguinal crease incision.

B. *Step 2.* Divide Scarpa's fascia.

C. *Step 3.* Identify the external inguinal ring and divide the external oblique aponeurosis. Identification of the ring is enhanced by palpating the pubic tubercle, which corresponds to the base of the triangular aperture of the superficial (external) ring, which is covered by the external oblique and rectus fascia (Gallaudet). Open the external ring in the direction of the fibers.

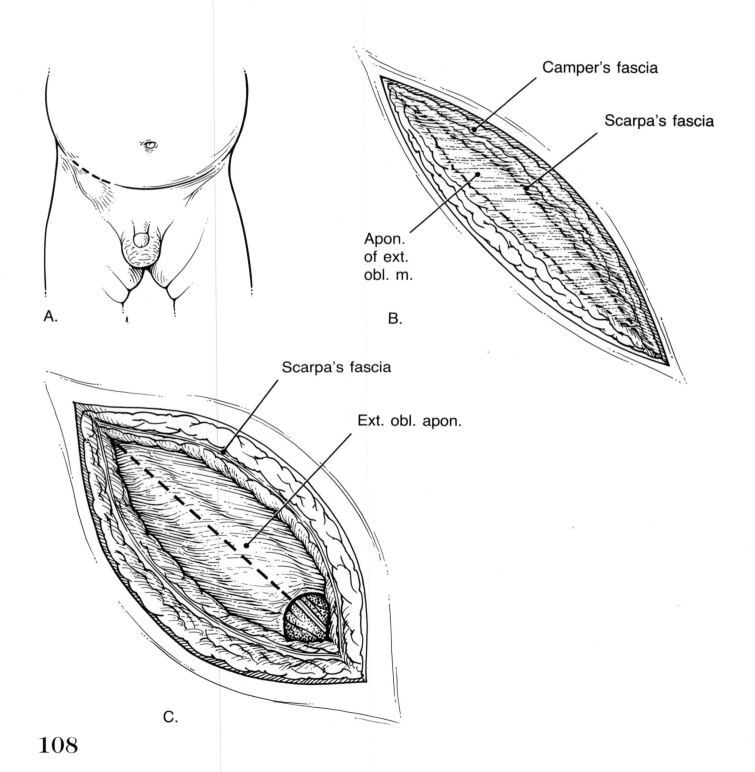

Camper's fascia

Scarpa's fascia

Apon. of ext. obl. m.

A.

B.

Scarpa's fascia

Ext. obl. apon.

C.

D. The ilioinguinal nerve and the cremaster muscle fibers can be identified.

E. *Step 4.* Dissect the sac from the cremaster muscle fibers. Then dissect it carefully from the vas deferens and the spermatic artery and veins.

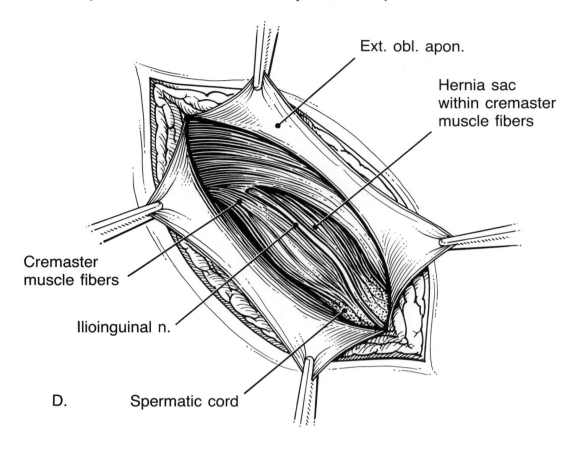

Ext. obl. apon.

Hernia sac within cremaster muscle fibers

Cremaster muscle fibers

Ilioinguinal n.

D.

Spermatic cord

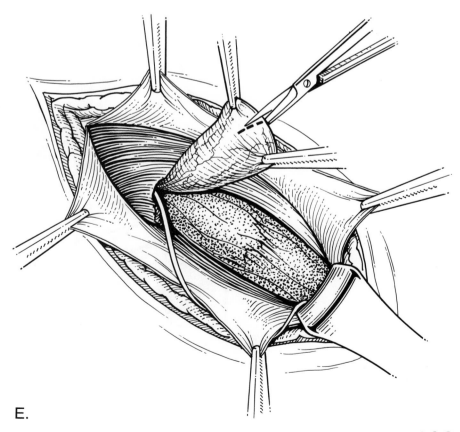

E.

PLATE 31 (*Continued*)

Repair of Male Pediatric Inguinal Hernia

F. *Step 5.* Dissect the sac down to the internal ring and ligate it at that point with 000 silk.

    Step 6. Inset: Transect the excess sac.

G. Alternatively, suture the internal oblique muscle (arch) to the shelving edge of Poupart's ligament.

H. *Step 7.* Close the external oblique fascia with interrupted 000 silk sutures.

I. *Step 8.* Close the skin with either continuous or interrupted absorbable sutures such as 0000 vicryl on a cutting needle.

    Inset: Place SteriStrips perpendicular to the wound edges.

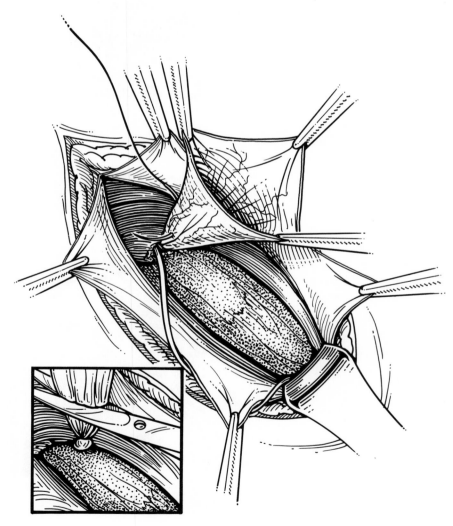

F.

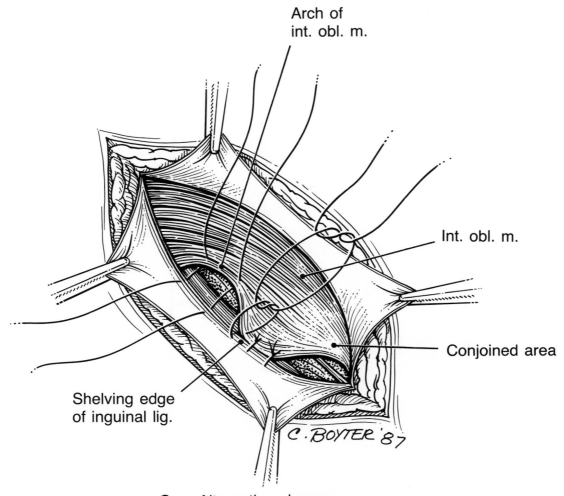

Arch of
int. obl. m.

Int. obl. m.

Conjoined area

Shelving edge
of inguinal lig.

C. BOYTER '87

G.   Alternative closure

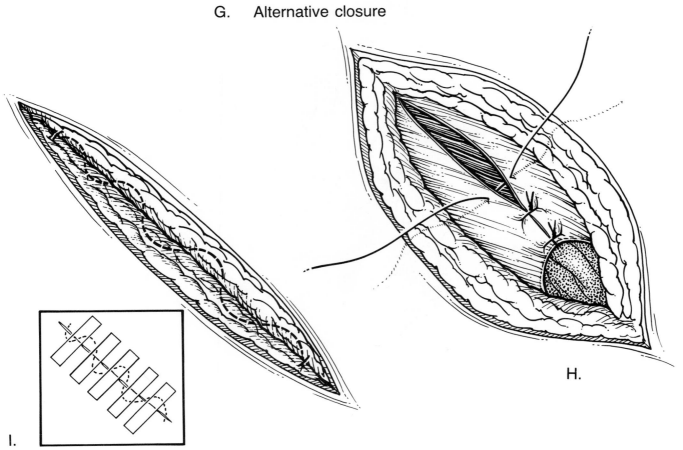

I.

H.

111

PLATE 32
Repair of Female Pediatric Inguinal Hernia

The approach to the repair of female pediatric inguinal hernia is identical to that of male pediatric hernia.

A. *Step 1.* Separate the cremasteric fibers from the hernia sac. The round ligament is within the sac.

B. *Step 2.* Open the sac. The uterine tube adheres to the posterior wall of the sac.

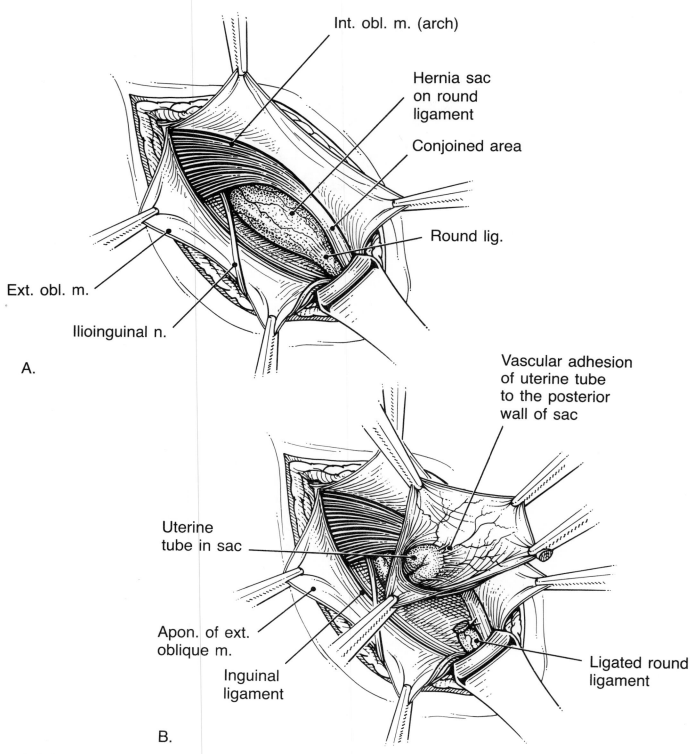

Int. obl. m. (arch)

Hernia sac
on round
ligament

Conjoined area

Round lig.

Ext. obl. m.

Ilioinguinal n.

A.

Vascular adhesion
of uterine tube
to the posterior
wall of sac

Uterine
tube in sac

Apon. of ext.
oblique m.

Inguinal
ligament

Ligated round
ligament

B.

112

C. *Step 3.* Divide the sac around the tube. Ligate the round ligament and grasp it with a clamp.

D. *Step 4.* Invert the posterior portion of the sac with the fixed uterine tube so that the sac is imbricated below the level of the internal ring.

E. *Step 5.* Close the hernia sac by suturing its anterior wall to the outer margin of the inverted sac with 000 or 0000 silk.

Step 6. Close the external oblique aponeurosis with interrupted 000 sutures. Close the subcutaneous tissues and skin as in male pediatric inguinal hernia.

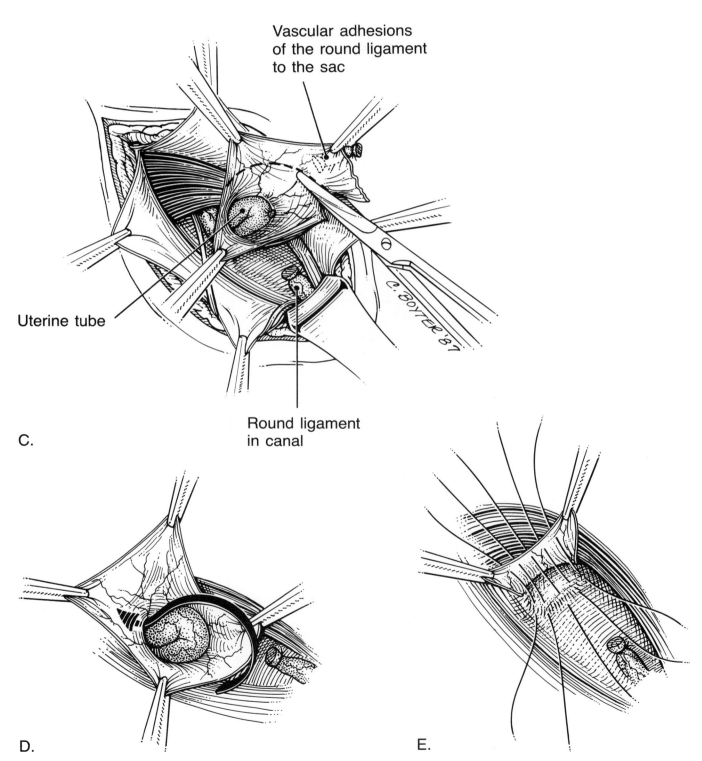

Vascular adhesions
of the round ligament
to the sac

Uterine tube

Round ligament
in canal

C.

D.

E.

113

PLATE 33
Repair of Undescended Testis

The incision for the repair of undescended testis is the same as that for male pediatric inguinal hernia (in the distal abdominal crease) except that it is slightly longer.

Open Scarpa's fascia and the external oblique aponeurosis as in male pediatric inguinal hernia; divide the cremaster muscle.

A. *Step 1.* Dissect the hernia sac and the testis off the posterior wall of the inguinal canal. Clamp the gubernaculum for traction.

B. *Step 2.* Divide the transversalis fascia (and the transversus abdominis aponeurosis). Divide the internal oblique muscle.

C. *Step 3.* Dissect the hernia sac off the cord structures and upward toward the internal ring. The inferior epigastric vessels can be seen beneath the level of the transversalis fascia and floor of the inguinal canal.

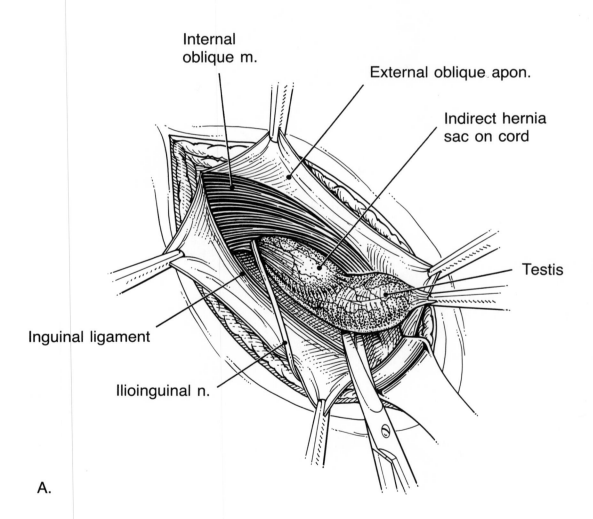

Internal oblique m.

External oblique apon.

Indirect hernia sac on cord

Testis

Inguinal ligament

Ilioinguinal n.

A.

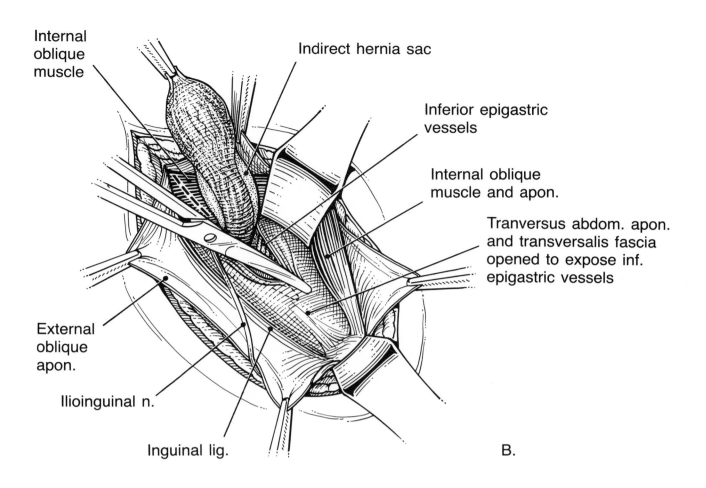

Internal oblique muscle

Indirect hernia sac

Inferior epigastric vessels

Internal oblique muscle and apon.

Tranversus abdom. apon. and transversalis fascia opened to expose inf. epigastric vessels

External oblique apon.

Ilioinguinal n.

Inguinal lig.

B.

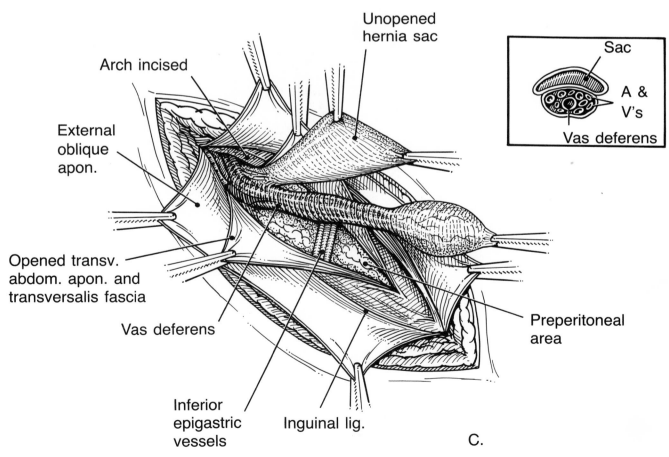

Arch incised

Unopened hernia sac

Sac

A & V's

Vas deferens

External oblique apon.

Opened transv. abdom. apon. and transversalis fascia

Vas deferens

Inferior epigastric vessels

Inguinal lig.

Preperitoneal area

C.

115

PLATE 33 (*Continued*)

Repair of Undescended Testis

D. *Step 4.* Divide and ligate the inferior epigastric artery and vein.

E. *Step 5.* Carefully separate the testis and hernia sac from the cremaster muscle and fasciae

F. *Step 6.* Enlarge the internal ring by a small incision to permit better mobilization of the spermatic cord. Open the sac distal to the enlarged deep ring to avoid residual tunica vaginalis, which could be sealed and produce a hydrocele.

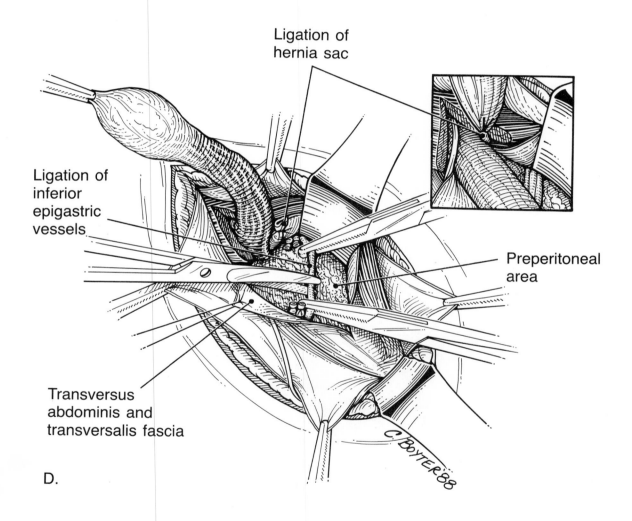

Ligation of hernia sac

Ligation of inferior epigastric vessels

Preperitoneal area

Transversus abdominis and transversalis fascia

D.

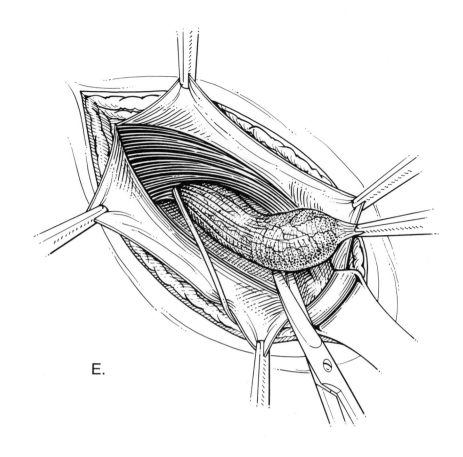

E.

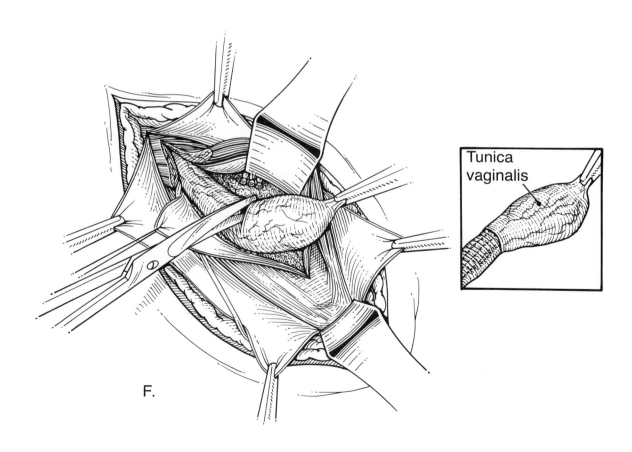

F.

Tunica vaginalis

117

PLATE 33 (*Continued*)

Repair of Undescended Testis

G. *Step 7.* Carefully dissect the sac from the spermatic cord.

H. *Step 8.* Divide the inferior epigastric vessels. Dissect the vas deferens both proximally and distally toward the seminal vesicles and the vessels toward the renal level. In this way, more length is achieved so that the testis can be brought down to its proper place in the scrotum without tension.

I. *Step 9.* Insert a finger into the scrotal pouch, trying not to form a false pathway.

J. Layers of the scrotal pouch. The tunica vaginalis is separated from the surrounding spermatic fascia for subsequent insertion of the testis.

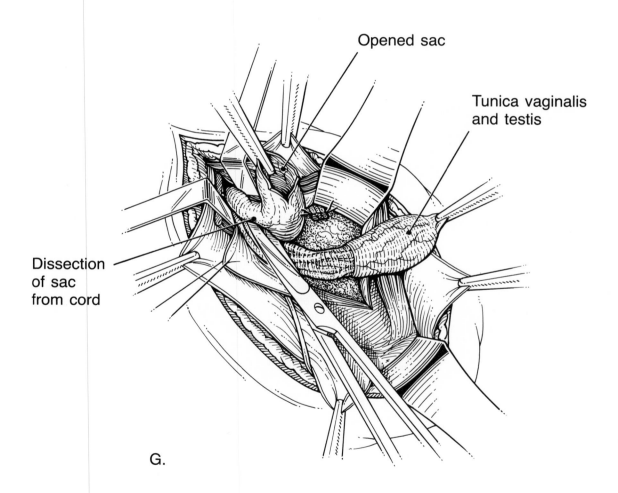

Opened sac

Tunica vaginalis and testis

Dissection of sac from cord

G.

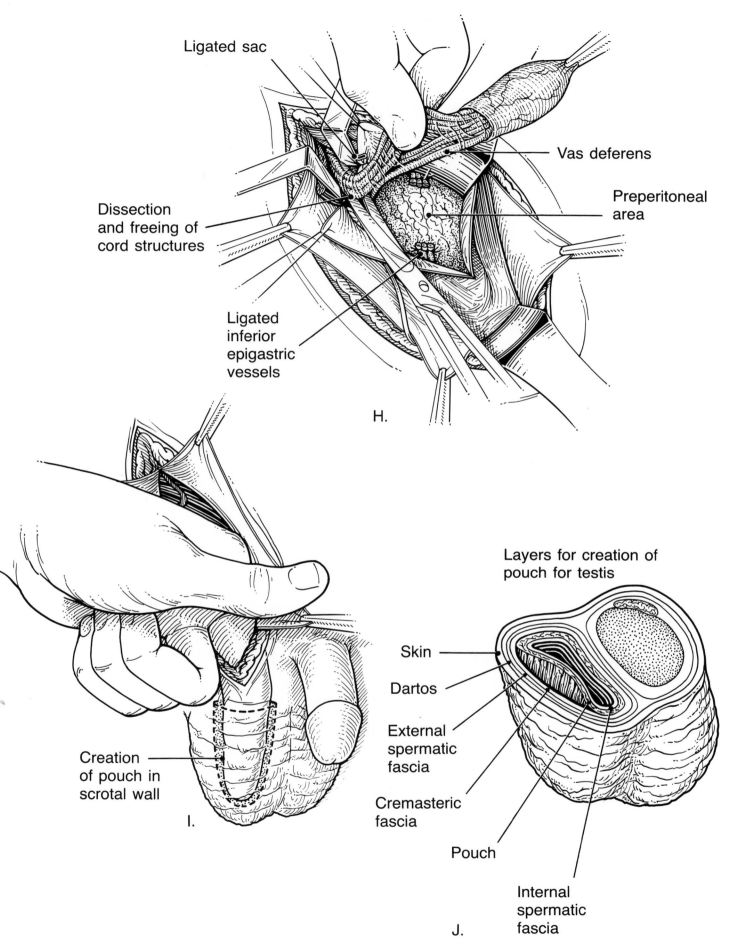

Ligated sac

Vas deferens

Dissection
and freeing of
cord structures

Preperitoneal
area

Ligated
inferior
epigastric
vessels

H.

Creation
of pouch in
scrotal wall

I.

Layers for creation of
pouch for testis

Skin

Dartos

External
spermatic
fascia

Cremasteric
fascia

Pouch

Internal
spermatic
fascia

J.

119

PLATE 33 (*Continued*)

Repair of Undescended Testis

K. *Step 10.* Close the transversalis fascia and the internal oblique and external oblique aponeuroses. Pierce the testis through the tunica albuginea with a Keith needle and 00 silk. Bring the silk out with the Keith needle through the tip of the scrotal skin; tie over a button.

L. An additional procedure to apply increased tension to the testis is done by attaching the 00 silk suture which was tied around the button to a rubber band, and then attaching the rubber band to some cloth tape on the thigh.

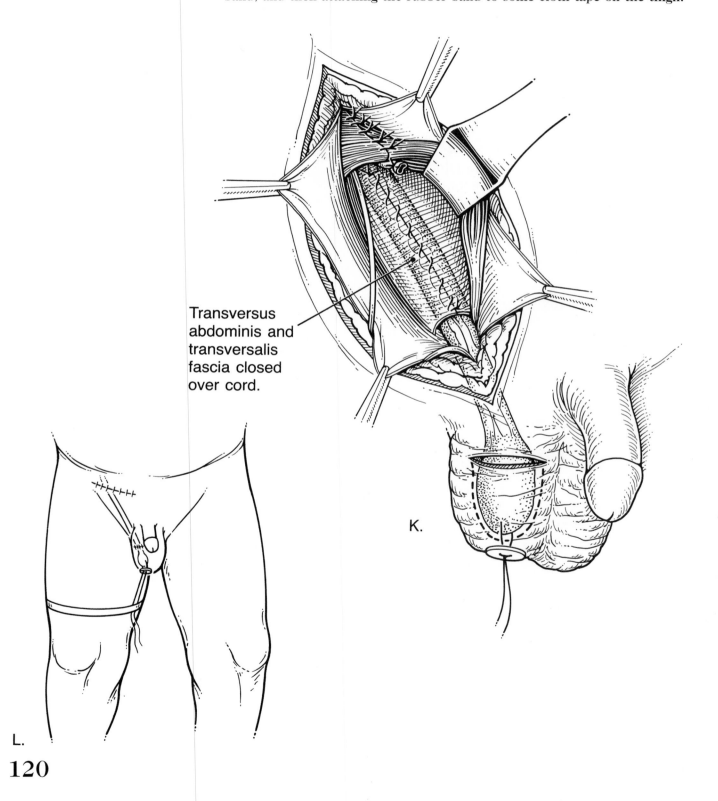

Transversus abdominis and transversalis fascia closed over cord.

K.

L.

Alternative Procedures for Inguinal Hernia Repair

*We have to strive to keep our mind receptive, and to
examine suggestions made by others fairly and on their
own merits, seeking arguments for as well as against
them. We must be critical, certainly, but beware lest ideas
be rejected because an automatic reaction causes us to
see only the arguments against them. We tend especially to
resist ideas competing with our own.*

SEYMOUR I. SCHWARTZ, M.D.

The Nyhus Procedure (Preperitoneal Approach and Iliopubic Tract Repair)

PLATE 34

The Nyhus Procedure—Anatomy of the Preperitoneal Approach

A. Parasagittal section through the right midinguinal region, illustrating the separation of the musculoaponeurotic lamina into the anterior and posterior inguinal walls.

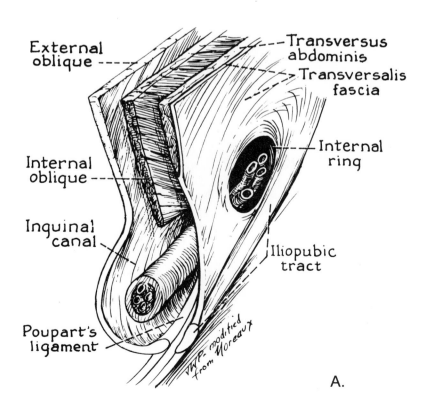

A.

PLATE 34 (*Continued*)

The Nyhus Procedure—Anatomy of the Preperitoneal Approach

B. Diagrammatic representation of important anatomical structures of the posterior inguinal wall as seen from the preperitoneal approach.

C. The same view demonstrating sites of groin hernias.

D. The operative approach to the preperitoneal space. It is rarely necessary to ligate and sever the inferior epigastric artery and vein.

Source: Plate 34A, B, C, D from Nyhus LM: The preperitoneal approach and iliopubic tract repair of inguinal, hernia, in Nyhus LM, Condon RE (eds): *Hernia,* 2d ed. Lippincott, Philadelphia, 1978, Chap. 9, p. 216, 218, 222, Figs. 9-1, 9-2A, B, 9-6.

E. Cross section of the distorted groin anatomy in a direct inguinal hernia. Compare with Plate 20R, S, and T.

Source: Plate 34E from Lampe EW: Experiences with preperitoneal hernioplasty, in Nyhus LM, Condon RE (eds): *Hernia,* 2d ed. Lippincott, Philadelphia, 1978, p. 244, Fig. 9-11.

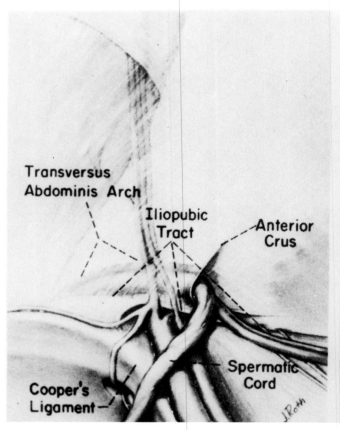

B.

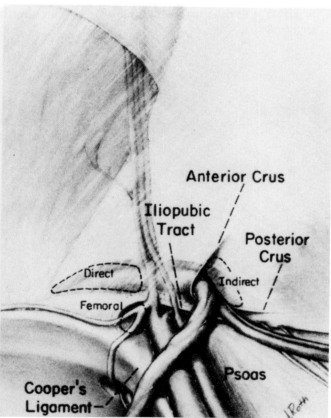

C.

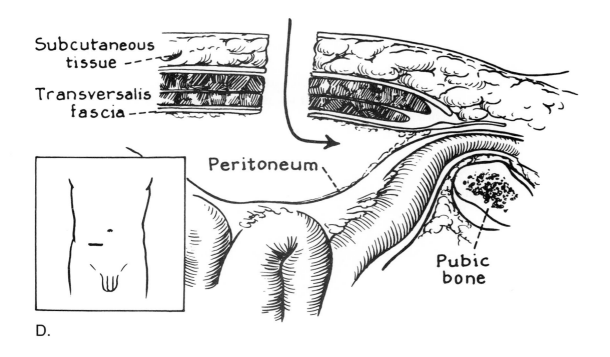

Subcutaneous tissue

Transversalis fascia

Peritoneum

Pubic bone

D.

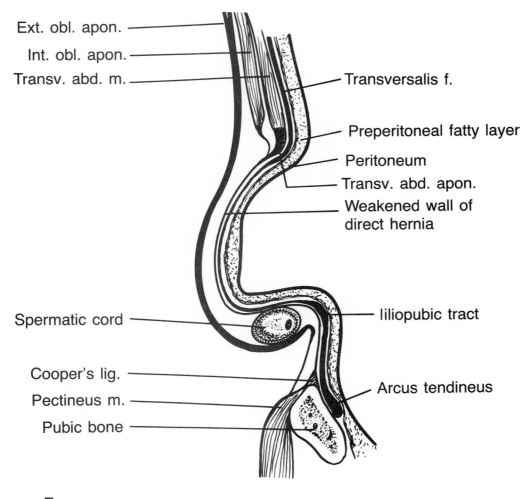

Ext. obl. apon.

Int. obl. apon.

Transv. abd. m.

Transversalis f.

Preperitoneal fatty layer

Peritoneum

Transv. abd. apon.

Weakened wall of direct hernia

Spermatic cord

Iliopubic tract

Cooper's lig.

Pectineus m.

Arcus tendineus

Pubic bone

E.

PLATE 35

Nyhus Procedure—Iliopubic Tract Repair, Direct Inguinal Hernia

A. *Step 1.* Make a transverse skin incision two finger breadths above the symphysis pubis.
(Some of the following description includes direct quotation from Dr. Nyhus.)

B. *Step 2.* After the skin and subcutaneous tissues have been incised and the rectus sheath exposed, the level of the internal ring may be estimated by insertion of the left index finger into the external ring. This simple maneuver allows the surgeon to visualize the location of the internal ring in his or her mind's eye. The incision in the anterior rectus fascia should be placed so that it will pass just superior (cephalad) to the internal ring.

C. *Step 3.* Make a transverse fascial incision beginning over the midrectus of the affected side.

D. *Step 4.* Enlarge the incision by separating and cutting the fascia and muscle fibers of the external oblique, internal oblique, and transversus abdominis muscles. The transversalis fascia is seen in the depth of the wound. When the transversalis fascia is cut, the preperitoneal space is entered and the proper plane of dissection is achieved.

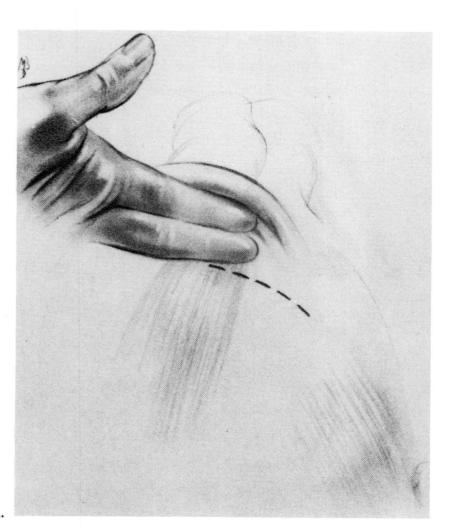

A.

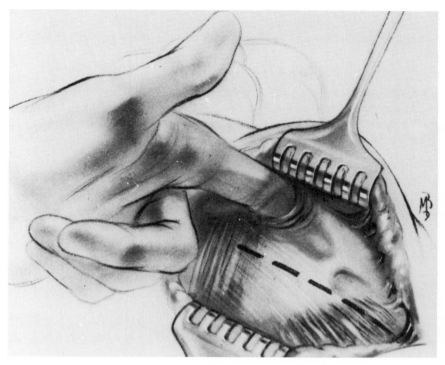

B.

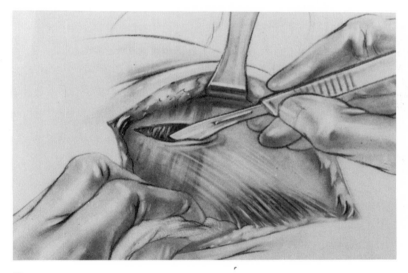

C.

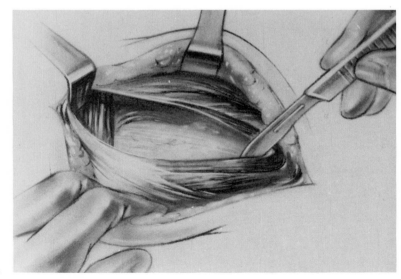

D.

125

PLATE 35 (*Continued*)

Nyhus Procedure—Iliopubic Tract Repair, Direct Inguinal Hernia

E. *Step 5.* Isolate, but do not open, the sac and redundant peritoneum. Invert the sac, using a purse-string suture, if necessary. Suture the superior edge of the direct defect (transversalis fascia–transversus abdominis aponeurosis) above to the iliopubic tract below.

Source: Plate 35 A through E from Nyhus LM: The preperitoneal approach and iliopubic tract repair of inguinal hernia, in *Hernia,* 2d ed. Nyhus LM, Condon RE (eds). Lippincott, Philadelphia, 1978, pp. 219, 220, 221, 223, Figs. 9-3, 9-4, 9-5, 9-7 B.

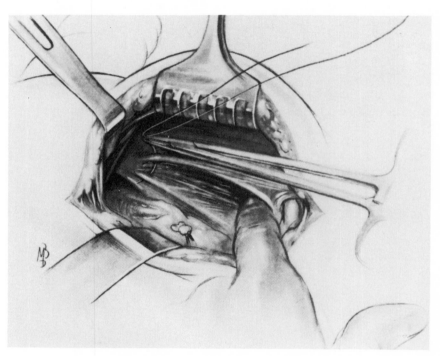

E.

PLATE 36

Nyhus Repair—Indirect Hernia

A,B. *Step 1.* The approach is the same as in direct hernia. Isolate, prepare, open,, close, and excise the indirect sac.

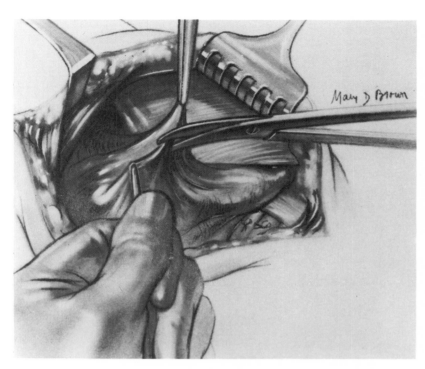

A.

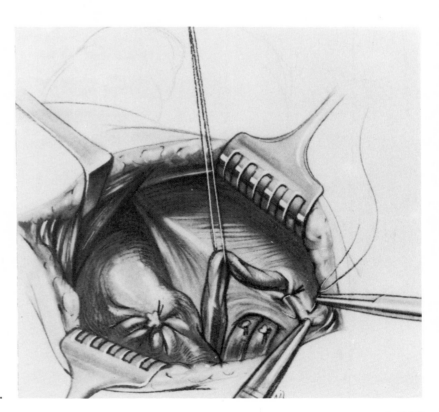

B.

PLATE 36 (*Continued*)

Nyhus Repair—Indirect Hernia

C. *Step 2.* Close the defect medially by suturing the fused edge of the transversalis fascia and transversus abdominis aponeurosis to the iliopubic tract. Also suture laterally, creating a new abdominal ring by suturing the anterior crus of the sling to the posterior crus (iliopubic tract). Use 00 silk.

The spermatic cord is resting at the area of the femoral vessels. Close the wound in layers with interrupted 0000 silk.

Source: Plate 36 A, B, C from Nyhus, LM: The preperitoneal approach and iliopubic tract repair of the inguinal hernia, in *Hernia*, 2d ed. Nyhus LM, Condon RE (eds). Lippincott, Philadelphia, 1978, pp. 224, 225, 226, Figs. 9-8A, 9-8D, 9-8E.

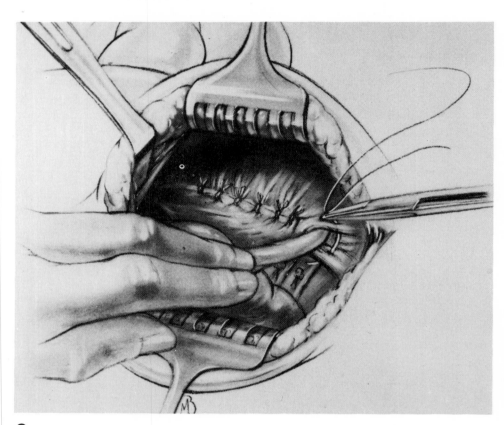

C.

PLATE 37
Nyhus Approach—Femoral Hernia

The approach is the same as that described previously for direct and indirect inguinal hernia repair.

A. *Step 1.* Reduce the femoral hernia sac by traction and blunt dissection. If the exposure is not adequate, ligate the inferior epigastric vessels.

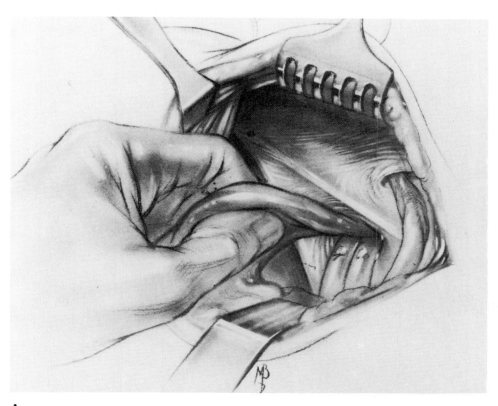

A.

PLATE 37 (*Continued*)
Nyhus Approach—Femoral Hernia

B. *Step 2.* Ligate and excise the femoral sac. Start the repair of the femoral canal by suturing the iliopubic tract above to Cooper's ligament below. Close the wound in layers as usual.

Source: Plate 37 A, B from Nyhus, LM: The preperitoneal approach and iliopubic tract repair for femoral hernia, in *Hernia,* 2d ed. Nyhus LM, Condon RE (eds). Lippincott, Philadelphia, 1978, pp. 253, 254, Figs. 10-2, 10-5.

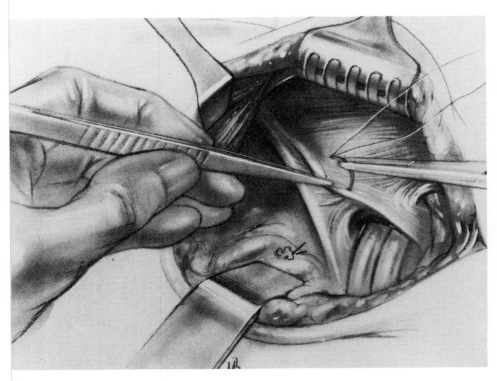

B

PLATE 38
Condon Procedure—Repair of Indirect Inguinal Hernia

A,B. Reconstruct the posterior wall of the inguinal canal by suturing the transversus abdominis arch to the iliopubic tract from the pubic tubercle to the deep inguinal ring. Also suture lateral to the cord for reconstruction of the deep inguinal ring. Use 00 Dacron or nylon sutures.

Source: Plate 38, B from Condon RE: Anterior iliopubic tract repair, in *Hernia*, 2d ed. Nyhus LM, Condon RE (eds). Lippincott, Philadelphia, 1978, Chap. 8, pp. 204, Fig. 8-7.

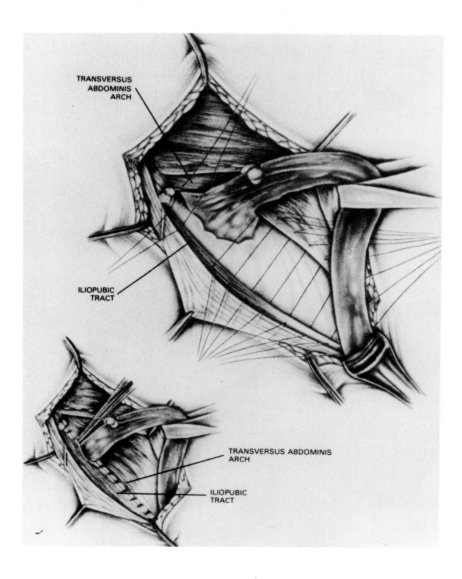

PLATE 39
Condon Procedure—Repair of Direct Inguinal Hernia

A. *Step 1.* Make an incision at the bulging posterior wall of the inguinal canal. Excise all redundant and weakened tissue.

B. *Step 2.* Place sutures between the transversus abdominis arch above and Cooper's ligament and the iliopubic tract below.

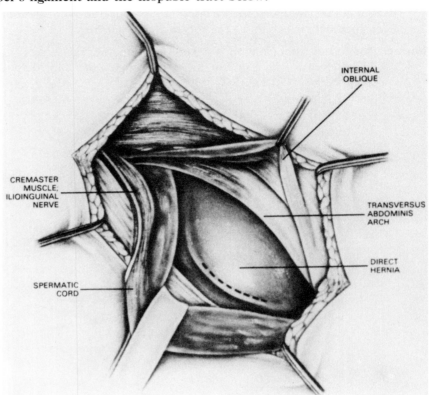

A.

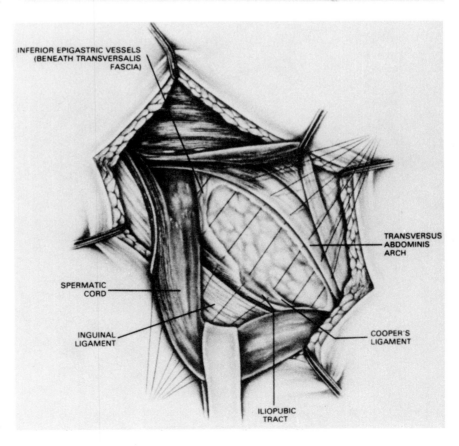

B.

C. *Step 3.* Make a relaxing incision; use additional sutures if necessary.

D. *Step 4.* Complete the relaxing incision. Tie the sutures that were placed previously.

Source: Plate 39A through D from Condon RE: Anterior iliopubic tract repair, in *Hernia,* 2d ed. Nyhus LM, Condon RE (eds). Lippincott, Philadelphia, Chap. 8, pp. 206, 207, 209, 210, Figs. 8-8, 8-9, 8-10, 8-11.

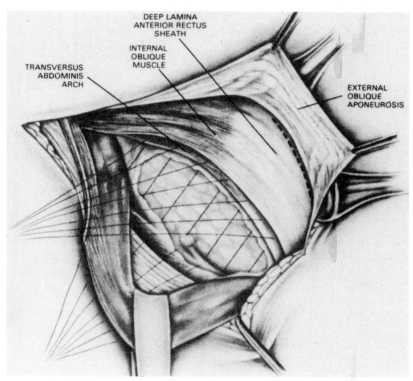

C.

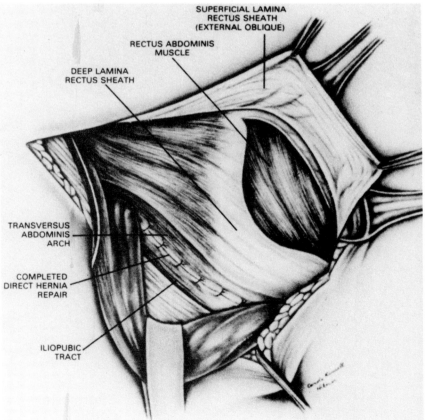

D.

The Shouldice Repair

According to Glassow,[1] the Shouldice repair is comprehensive in that it is applicable to the cure of indirect, direct, or recurrent inguinal hernias because it treats the posterior wall of the inguinal canal as well as the internal ring.

Glassow also emphasized the skeletonization of the spermatic cord by excision of the cremaster muscle. In addition, he pointed out that, for sliding hernias, the sac is usually not opened or ligated.

[1]Glassow, F. The Shouldice repair for inguinal hernia, in *Hernia,* 2nd ed. Nyhus LM, Condon RE (eds). Lippincott, Philadelphia, 1978, Chap. 6, p. 163.

PLATE 40
Shouldice Technique

Follow steps 1 through 6 as for indirect inguinal hernia repair (Plate 23).

A. *Step 1.* Incise the posterior wall of the inguinal canal. Carefully divide the attenuated but fused transversus abdominis aponeurosis and transversalis fascia of the posterior wall (floor). The line for incision starts laterally at the internal ring, avoiding the deep epigastric vessels, and travels downward medially, ending at the pubic tubercle.

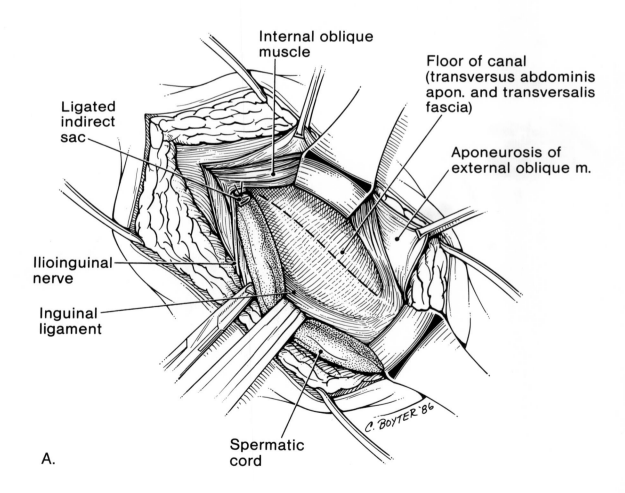

A.

B. *Step 2.* The posterior wall is divided. Elevate the narrower medial flap as much as possible, but do not elevate the lower lateral flap.

C. *Step 3.* Start the first suture line at the pubic bone. Use 000 continuous Prolene and approximate the deep part (white line) of the elevated medial flap to the free edge of the lateral flap. Tie the continuous suture at the internal ring, but *do not cut.*

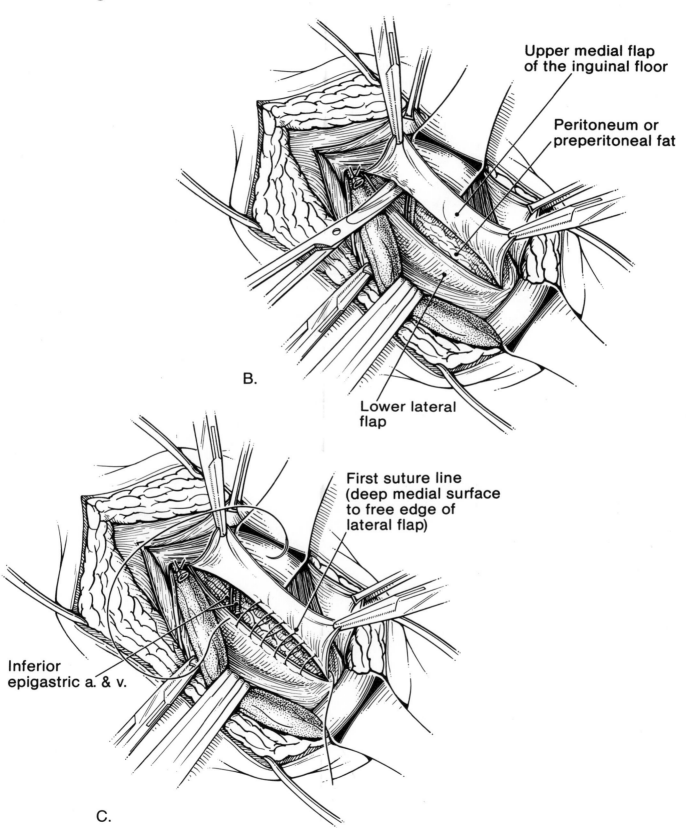

Upper medial flap of the inguinal floor

Peritoneum or preperitoneal fat

Lower lateral flap

B.

First suture line (deep medial surface to free edge of lateral flap)

Inferior epigastric a. & v.

C.

135

PLATE 40 (*Continued*)

Shouldice Technique

D. *Step 4.* Using the same uncut suture, approximate the free edge of the medial flap in a continuous way to the shelving edge of the inguinal ligament, traveling downward from the internal ring to the pubic bone. Tie and cut the suture at the pubic bone. In some cases an additional row of stitches is used.

E. *Step 5.* Using 000 Prolene, start the third suture line at the internal ring, approximating the internal oblique and transversus arch and the conjoined area to the inguinal ligament. Tie the suture at the area of the pubic tubercle, but do not cut.

F. *Step 6.* Using the same suture, reapproximate the same anatomical entities as in step 5 from the pubic tubercle to the internal ring.

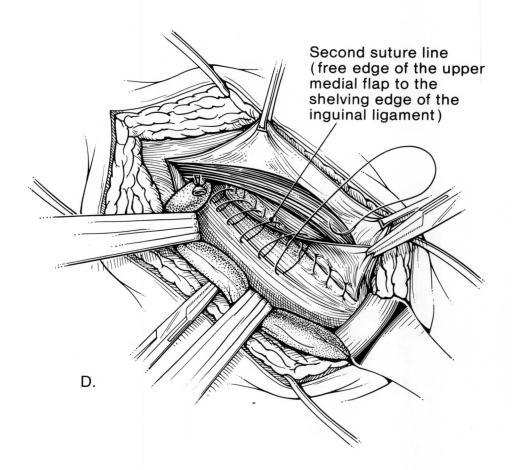

Second suture line
(free edge of the upper
medial flap to the
shelving edge of the
inguinal ligament)

D.

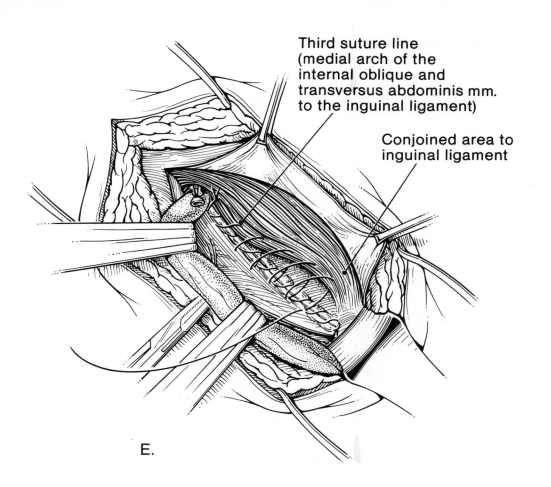

Third suture line
(medial arch of the
internal oblique and
transversus abdominis mm.
to the inguinal ligament)

Conjoined area to
inguinal ligament

E.

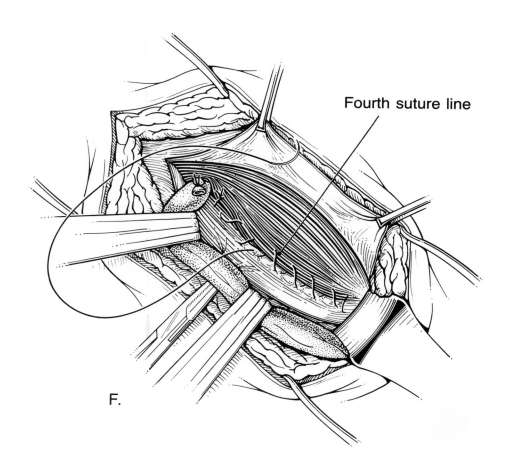

Fourth suture line

F.

137

PLATE 40 (*Continued*)

Shouldice Technique

G. *Step 7.* Close the external oblique aponeurosis above the spermatic cord. Occasionally if there is too much tension, the aponeurosis is closed under the spermatic cord.

Step 8. Close the superficial fascia and skin as described previously.

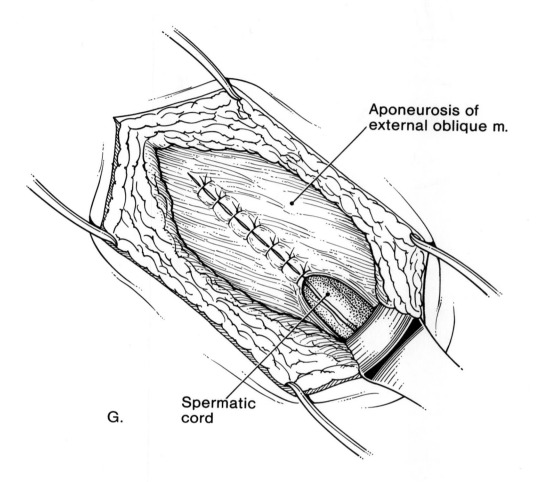

Aponeurosis of external oblique m.

G.

Spermatic cord

Other Repair Procedures for Inguinal Hernia

The Inguinal Darn
Darning the floor (posterior wall) of the inguinal canal can be accomplished by using continuous no. 1 nylon and suturing between the conjoined area and the arch above and the iliopubic tract and/or the shelving edge of the inguinal ligament below. One or two rows of stitches may be used.

Prosthesis
A sheet of Mersilene, Marlex mesh, or other synthetic prosthetic material is placed at the posterior wall of the inguinal canal and secured with interrupted 0000 silk sutures to the arch and conjoined area above and to the iliopubic tract and/or shelving edge of the inguinal ligament below.

Ponka[1] reported that synthetic mesh may also be placed in intraperitoneal, preperitoneal, subaponeurotic, or subcutaneous locations as well.

Uses of the Anterior Rectus Lamina
The anterior lamina of the rectus sheath may be rotated, producing a flap which is sutured to the inguinal ligament or the iliopubic tract or both.

Recurrent Inguinal and Femoral Hernia

Definition
A recurrent hernia is one that appears at the site of the initial operation with pathology identical to that for which repair was previously undertaken.

Pathology of Recurrence
Every recurrent hernia has its problems, peculiarities, and distorted topographical anatomy. The defect may be large or small and may be a direct, indirect, external supravesical, or femoral hernia. It may be located close to the pubic tubercle, at the posterior wall of the inguinal canal, at the internal inguinal ring, or at the femoral ring and canal.

Frequency of Recurrence
Figures from several series have been listed by Ponka[1] and by Nyhus and Condon.[2] They show recurrence rates ranging from 5 to 11 percent for indirect hernia, 5 to 16 percent for direct hernia, and 1 to 9 percent for femoral hernia. Unless the recurrence of the hernia occurs immediately postoperatively, it may never be recorded. The figures are probably too low because, as Ponka has observed, "Too often, when a patient has a recurrence, he is likely to report to another physician or hospital in the hope that a successful repair will be achieved."[3]

[1]Ponka JL: *Hernias of the Abdominal Wall.* Saunders, Philadelphia, 1980, p. 553.

[2]Nyhus LM, Condon RE (eds): *Hernia, 2d ed. Lippincott, Philadelphia, 1978.*

[3]Ponka JL: *Hernias of the Abdominal Wall.* Saunders, Philadelphia, 1980, p. 176.

Procedure for Repair of Recurrent Inguinal or Femoral Hernia

1. Examine the inguinal area well.
2. Try to understand the previous repair. Ask for the report of the repair or reread your own.
3. Remove the skin scar.
4. Carefully dissect to locate the spermatic cord in males. It is essential to locate, protect, and preserve the spermatic cord, thereby avoiding complications such as bleeding and possible atrophy or necrosis of the testis.
5. The spermatic cord may be found
   a. Under the skin and subcutaneous tissue
   b. Under the aponeurosis of the external oblique muscle
   c. Deep to the muscle layers in extremely rare cases
6. Identify the inguinal ligament.
7. Identify, if possible, the genital branch of the genitofemoral nerve, the ilioinguinal nerve, and the iliohypogastric nerve. Sacrifice the nerves if it is absolutely necessary to avoid neuroma.
8. Palpate and locate the defect.
9. Find the sac. In an indirect hernia, open it and perform a digital exploration. Ligate and transfix the sac. In a direct or external supravesical hernia, the sac should not be opened but should be purse-stringed.
10. Meticulously dissect the anatomic entities and strata involved by removing old sutures and scar tissue and by reaching good aponeurotic, not fascial, edges around the defect, if possible.
11. Locate Cooper's ligament.
12. Satisfy yourself that this is a recurrent hernia, not a new one.
13. After you find the "good stuff," use whichever technique or modification will best restore the local distorted anatomy and make you personally satisfied with the repair.
14. The repair should be effected with no tension. If tension is anticipated, consider the use of a prosthesis, such as one or two layers of Marlex mesh.

    Here the surgeon should be familiar with the surgical ellipse. (See Plate 21.) Unfortunately, in cases of recurrent hernia, some anatomic elements—such as the inguinal ligament, Cooper's ligament, or the iliopubic tract—are occasionally unidentifiable. Usually the superior medial (above) part of the ellpise is in better condition than the inferior lateral (lower) part. If the inguinal ligament, iliopubic tract, or Cooper's ligament are unidentifiable, the prosthetic material may be anchored to the remnants of the conjoined area and the arch. The mesh should correspond to a line from the anterior superior iliac spine to the pubic tubercle including, of course, the pectineal line.

    From an anatomic standpoint, we think that the best procedure for curing this problem is the preperitoneal approach of Nyhus.
15. If the patient is old or has had several procedures for recurrent hernia, do not hesitate to perform an orchiectomy. Removal, not severance, of the spermatic cord and testis will facilitate permanent closing of the internal ring.

Multiple Hernias

Bilateral inguinal hernias are common, and as many as three different hernias on one side have been reported. In 1804, Sir Astley Cooper illustrated a specimen with six hernia openings in the abdominal wall; two were in the supravesical fossae. We have seen a patient with eight coexisting hernias, four on each side. They were indirect, direct, femoral, and external supravesical. We have also seen a patient with indirect, direct, interstitial, and external supravesical hernias, all on the same side. Remarkably, there was no hernia on the other side.

The surgeon must keep in mind that the presence of an inguinal hernia does not preclude the presence of another such hernia in the same or contralateral groin. Occasionally, a coexisting hernia is overlooked at operation and the second hernia is mistaken for a recurrence.

PLATE 41

Diagram of the Landmarks in Four Types of Groin Hernia

A, indirect inguinal hernia; B, direct inguinal hernia; C, femoral hernia; D, external supravesical hernia emerging from beneath the rectus abdominis muscle.

Some landmarks are (1) inguinal ligament, (2) external iliac artery, (3) inferior epigastric artery, (4) medial umbilical ligament, and (5) testis.

Source: Skandalakis JE, Gray SW, Rowe JS Jr: *Anatomical Complications in General Surgery.* McGraw-Hill, New York, 1983, p. 266, Fig. 13-14.

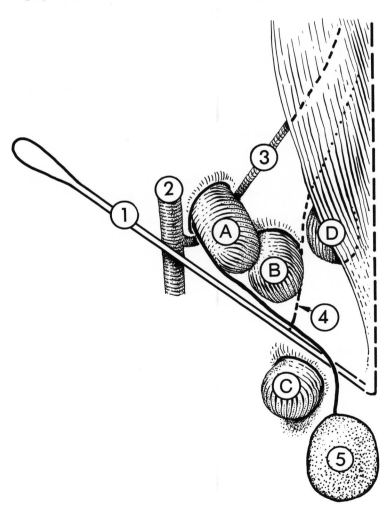

Hydrocele

Definition

A hydrocele is a collection of abnormal fluid within the sac of the tunica vaginalis. It may be associated with a hernia. There are several varieties.

If the hydrocele changes in size (as determined by patient observation), it is a communicating hydrocele and requires a high ligation of the sac in addition to partial excision of the hydrocele.

PLATE 42

Defects of the Closure of the Processus Vaginalis

Inset shows appearance in cross section. X = processus vaginalis.

A. Completely unclosed processus. An intestinal loop or omentum may follow the testis into the scrotum (congenital indirect hernia).

B. The cranial (funicular) portion of the processus remains unclosed. Herniation may occur later in life (acquired indirect hernia).

C. All but the cranial portion is unclosed. Serous fluid accumulates to form an infantile hydrocele.

D. The midportion of the processus is unclosed, forming a cyst (cystic hydrocele).

E. Normally closed processus. Fluid may accumulate in the tunica vaginalis (adult hydrocele).

F. Sliding indirect inguinal hernia. The descending viscus, usually colon, remains retroperitoneal. The sac (processus vaginalis) remains unclosed.

Source: Plate 42A through F from Skandalakis JE, Gray SW, Rowe JS Jr: *Anatomical Complications in General Surgery.* McGraw-Hill, New York, 1983, p. 284, Fig. 14-2.

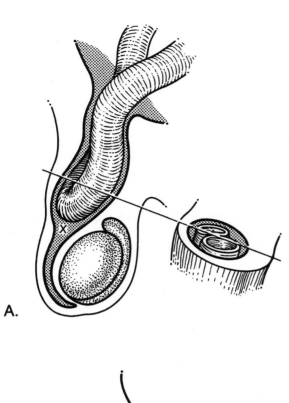

A.

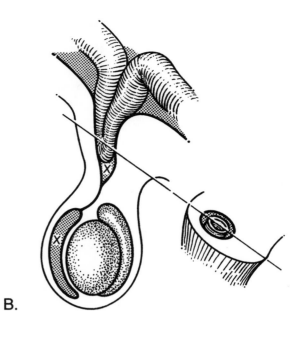

B.

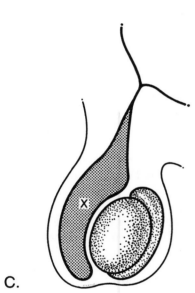

C.

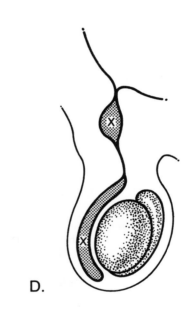

D.

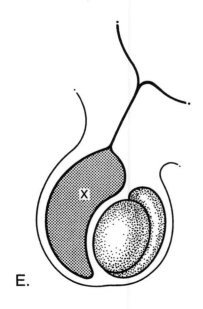

E.

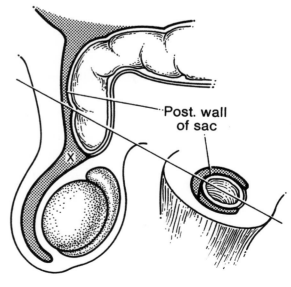

Post. wall
of sac

F.

143

PLATE 43

Repair of Pediatric Hydrocele—Inguinal Approach

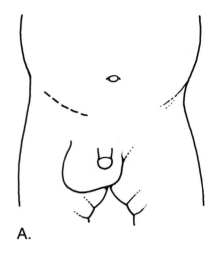

A.

A. *Step 1.* Incise above and parallel to the inguinal ligament. Divide the superficial fascia.

B. *Step 2.* Deliver the testis into the inguinal wound by external pressure of the scrotum. If this is difficult, make a small opening in the aponeurosis of the external oblique muscle at the external ring or aspirate the hydrocele.

Remember:
- The epididymis is fixed to the posterior border and upper pole of the testis.
- There are four layers in this area:
  1. External spermatic fascia
  2. Cremaster muscle
  3. Internal spermatic fascia
  4. Tunica vaginalis

Step 3. Make a vertical incision dividing the first three layers and finally the tunica vaginalis. For all practical purposes, layers 1, 2, and 3 are fused and are difficult and unnecessary to separate. However, separating these layers from the tunica vaginalis is a must.

Choose one of the following procedures:

C. *Step 4.* Evert the cut edges of the opened sac and suture behind the testis and spermatic cord using interrupted 000 or 0000 chromic catgut (bottleneck of Andrew). This procedure is seldom used at present.

D. Perform a subtotal removal of the sac leaving a small amount of tunica vaginalis, which is sutured in situ for good hemostasis (Winklemann's procedure). This is the preferred method of repair.

Perform a subtotal removal of the sac leaving enough tunica vaginalis to be sutured behind the testis (Jaboulay method). This method (not illustrated) is of historical interest but is no longer used.

E. *Step 5.* Gently push the testis down into the scrotum with its normal covering. Be sure that there is no torsion of the spermatic cord. A 24-h drain is advisable.

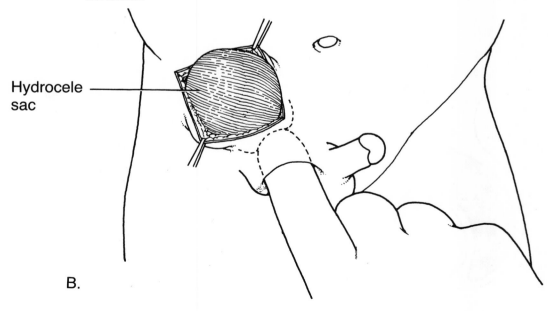

Hydrocele sac

B.

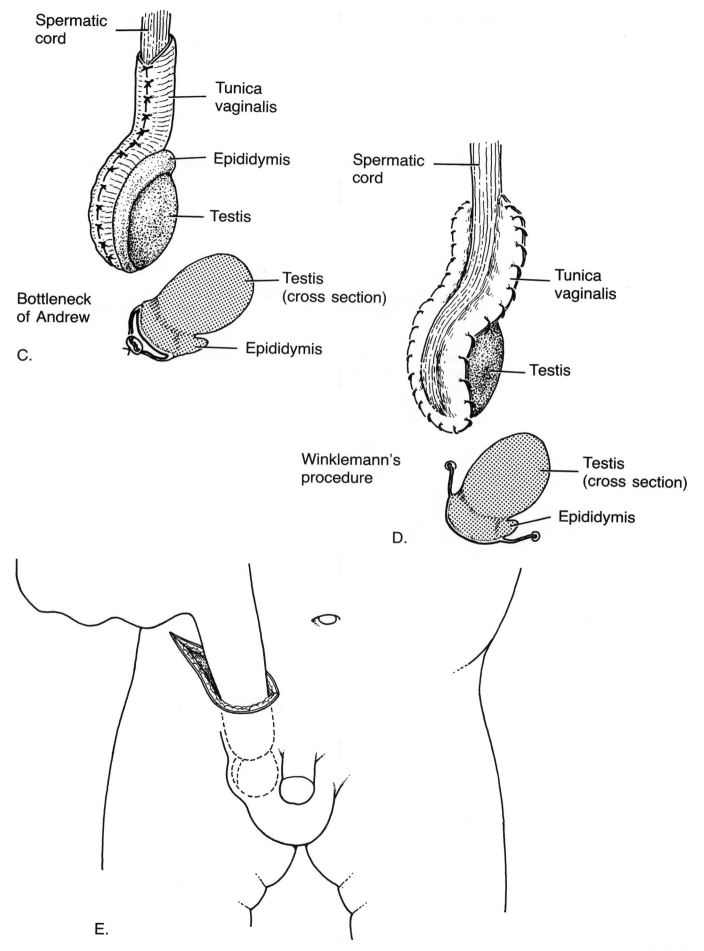

Spermatic cord

Tunica vaginalis

Epididymis

Testis

Bottleneck of Andrew

C.

Testis (cross section)

Epididymis

Spermatic cord

Tunica vaginalis

Testis

Winklemann's procedure

Testis (cross section)

Epididymis

D.

E.

145

PLATE 44

Repair of Adult Noncommunicating Hydrocele

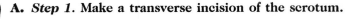

A. *Step 1.* Make a transverse incision of the scrotum.

Remember: The terminal vascular branches in the scrotum lie transversely; therefore, to minimize bleeding, explore the scrotum through a transverse incision.

B. *Step 2.* Carefully divide the three uppermost layers of the testis. Deliver the testis with its covering outside the scrotum.

C. *Step 3.* Withdraw the fluid from the sac.

D. The covering of the spermatic cord.

E. Testis with opened tunica vaginalis.

Step 4. Choose one of the procedures (bottleneck of Andrew, Winklemann's procedure) described previously and continue the repair as with the inguinal approach.

F. *Step 5.* Approximate the dartos and close the skin. Use few catgut sutures to approximate the dartos, thereby avoiding skin inversion due to dartos retraction.

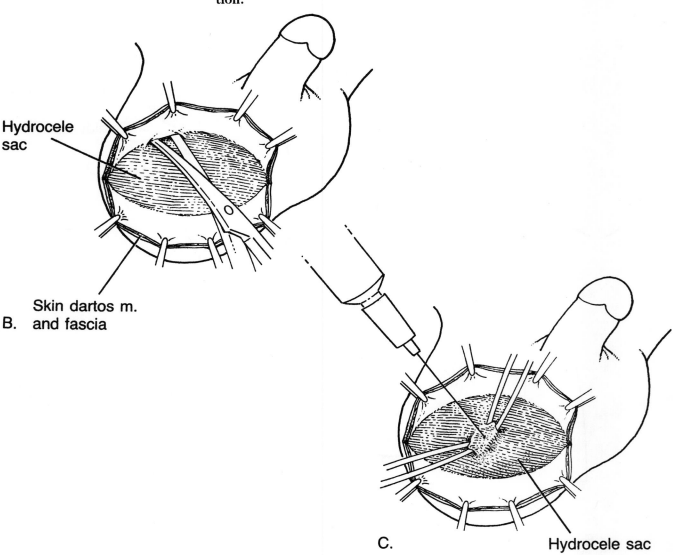

Hydrocele sac

Skin dartos m. and fascia

B.

C.

Hydrocele sac

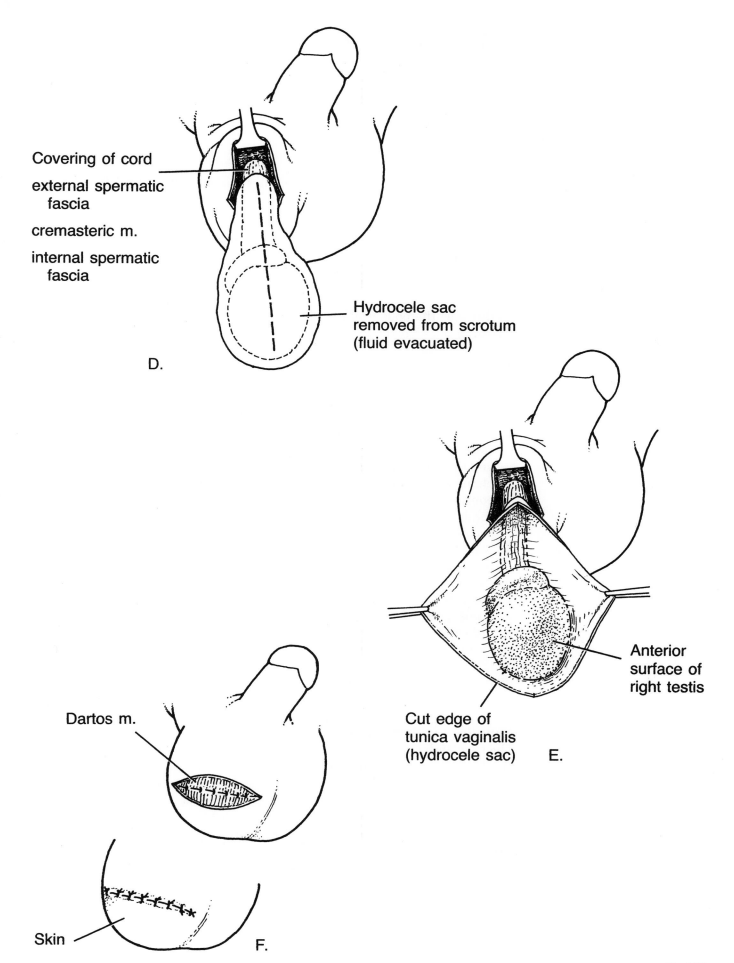

Covering of cord
external spermatic fascia
cremasteric m.
internal spermatic fascia

Hydrocele sac removed from scrotum (fluid evacuated)

D.

Dartos m.

Anterior surface of right testis

Cut edge of tunica vaginalis (hydrocele sac)

E.

Skin

F.

147

POSTERIOR (LUMBAR) BODY WALL

Surgical Anatomy of the Posterior (Lumbar) Body Wall

The lumbar area of the posterior body wall is bounded:
Superiorly, by the twelfth rib.
Inferiorly, by the crest of the ilium.
Posteriorly, by the erector spinae (sacrospinalis) muscles.
Anteriorly, by the posterior border of the external oblique muscle.

In this area the body wall is composed of the following layers of muscle and fascia:

1. Thick, tough skin.
2. Superficial fascia: two layers of fibrous tissue with fat between them.
3. A superficial muscle layer composed of the latissimus dorsi muscle postero-laterally and the external oblique muscle anterolaterally.
4. Thoracolumbar fascia containing three layers: posterior, middle, and anterior. The posterior and middle layers envelop the sacrospinalis muscle, and the middle anterior layer envelops the quadratus lumborum. Another characteristic of the middle layer of the thoracolumbar fascia is its lateral continuation to the transversus abdominis aponeurosis by fusion of all three layers. Therefore, the transversus abdominis aponeurosis should be accepted on faith as part of the thoracolumbar fascia.
5. A middle muscular layer of sacrospinalis, internal oblique, and serratus posterior inferior muscles.
6. The deep muscular layer, composed of the quadratus lumborum and psoas muscles.
7. Transversalis fascia.
8. Preperitoneal fat.
9. Peritoneum.

Within this area, two triangles may be described.

Superior Lumbar Triangle (of Grynfelt)
The base of the triangle is the twelfth rib and serratus posterior inferior muscle. The anterior (abdominal) boundary is the posterior border of the internal oblique muscle; the posterior (lumbar) boundary is the anterior border of the sacrospinalis muscle. The floor of the triangle is formed by the aponeurosis of the transversus abdominis muscle arising by fusion of the layers of the thoracolumbar fascia. The roof of the triangle is formed by the external oblique and latissimus dorsi muscles.

148

Inferior Lumbar Triangle (of Petit)

The base of the triangle is the iliac crest. The anterior (abdominal) boundary is the posterior border of the external oblique muscle. The posterior (lumbar) boundary is the anterior border of latissimus dorsi muscle. The floor of the triangle is formed by the internal oblique muscle with contributions from the transversus abdominis muscle and posterior lamina of the thoracolumbar fascia and the internal oblique muscle. The triangle is covered by superficial fascia and skin.

The two triangles may be compared as follows:

Superior Triangle	Inferior Triangle
Inverted triangle (apex down)	Upright triangle (apex up)
Larger	Smaller
More constant	Less constant
Most common site of lumbar hernia	Less common site of lumbar hernia
Twelfth thoracic nerve	No nerves
First lumbar nerve	No nerves
Avascular	More vascular
Covered by latissimus dorsi muscle	Covered by superficial fascia and skin
Floor: union of the layers of the thoracolumbar fascia to form the aponeurosis of transversus abdominis	Floor: thoracolumbar fascia and internal oblique and partially transversus abdominis

Lumbar Hernia

Hernia through the Superior Lumbar Triangle

Definition
A superior lumbar hernia is a protrusion of preperitoneal fat, peritoneum with sac formation, or a viscus through the lumbar area just below the twelfth rib (Plate 45A).

Boundaries
If the hernia is small, the hernia ring is formed by the aponeurosis of the transversus abdominis only; if it is large, it may occupy the entire superior triangle. It may be necessary to enlarge the ring by a medial or lateral incision, or both, midway between the twelfth rib and the crest of the ilium.

Hernia through the Inferior Lumbar Triangle

Definition
An inferior lumbar hernia is a protrusion of preperitoneal fat, or a peritoneal sac with or without a herniated viscus through the lumbar area just above the iliac crest (Plate 45A).

Boundaries
If the hernia is small, the ring is formed by the thoracolumbar fascia and fibers of the internal oblique muscle. If it is larger, the ring may include the boundaries of the whole inferior triangle. Enlargement of the ring is by section of the fascia.

Anatomical Complications of Lumbar Hernia

Vascular Seroma or hematoma.

Neurological Injury of the T_{12} or L_1 nerves during repair of hernia through the superior lumbar triangle.

Organ Injury of viscus (most likely the colon) if hernia is incarcerated or sliding, during the opening of the sac, or by taking deep bites of the protruding fat.

Recurrence Possible but rare.

PLATE 45
Sites of Lumbar Hernias

A. *Left:* An inferior hernia through Petit's triangle. The base of the triangle is formed by the iliac crest. *Right:* A superior hernia through Grynfelt's triangle. The base of the inverted triangle is formed by the twelfth rib.

B. A diagrammatic cross section through the posterior body wall in the lumbar region. The pathway of a superior lumbar hernia is indicated by the arrow.

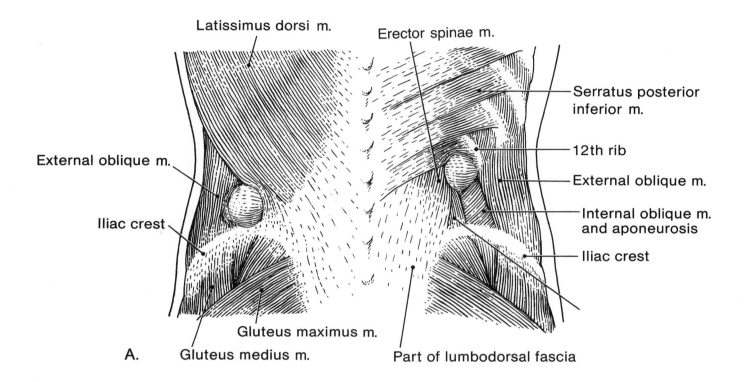

Latissimus dorsi m.
Erector spinae m.
Serratus posterior inferior m.
External oblique m.
12th rib
External oblique m.
Iliac crest
Internal oblique m. and aponeurosis
Iliac crest
Gluteus maximus m.
Gluteus medius m.
Part of lumbodorsal fascia

A.

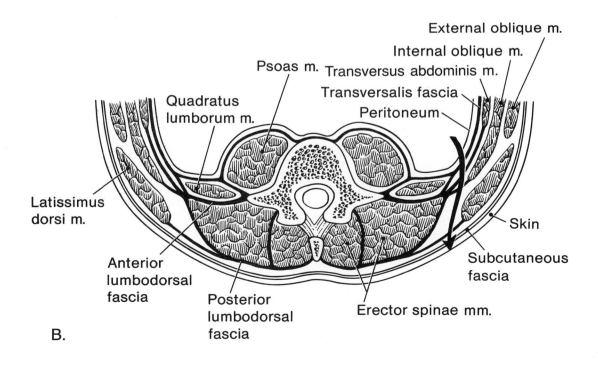

External oblique m.
Internal oblique m.
Psoas m. Transversus abdominis m.
Quadratus lumborum m.
Transversalis fascia
Peritoneum
Latissimus dorsi m.
Skin
Anterior lumbodorsal fascia
Subcutaneous fascia
Posterior lumbodorsal fascia
Erector spinae mm.

B.

151

PLATE 45 (*Continued*)
Sites of Lumbar Hernias

C. Hernia through the inferior lumbar triangle. A, Normal relations of the descending colon and the left posterior abdominal wall in cross section; B, Herniation of the descending colon through the inferior lumbar triangle. (1) External oblique muscle, (2) internal oblique muscle, (3) transversus abdominis muscle, (4) psoas muscle, (5) quadratus lumborum muscle, (6) latissimus dorsi muscle, (7) sacrospinalis muscle, (8) posterior layer of lumbodorsal fascia, (9) anterior layer of lumbodorsal fascia, (10) transversus abdominis aponeurosis.

Source: Plate 45C from Skandalakis JE, Gray SW, Akin JT Jr: The surgical anatomy of hernial rings. *Surg Clin North Am* 54(6):1227–1246, Fig. 8.

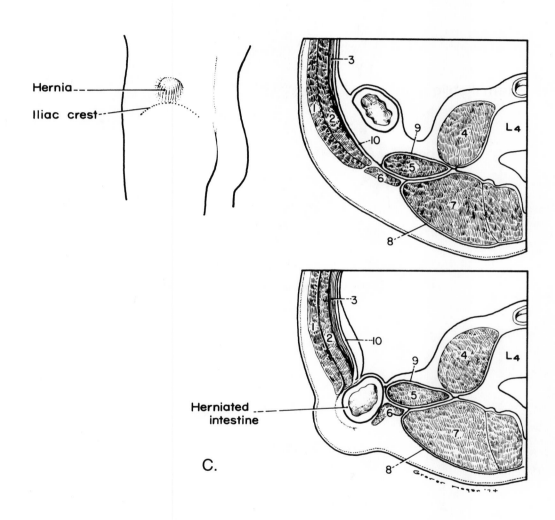

C.

Repair of Lumbar Hernia

Treatment prior to surgery calls for

1. Intravenous pyelogram, barium enema and gastrointestinal series, and small bowel series
2. Bowel preparation
3. Dorsal and lumbosacral x-rays to rule out vertebral pathology
4. Operation as soon as the diagnosis is made except in poor-risk patients

Place the patient in the lateral position with the hernia side up. The lower extremity of the hernia side is extended, and the opposite extremity is flexed at the knee. It is advisable to place a pillow between the lower extremities. If the patient is short and fat, use a kidney elevator.

The choice of the repair material depends upon the size of the defect:

- For small defects, close the thoracolumbar fascia and muscles with 00 Surgilon.
- For large hernias, use mesh, single or double, flap graft, or both, if necessary.

PLATE 46
Repair of Lumbar Hernia (Dowd-Ponka Repair)

A. *Step 1.* Make an incision, oblique or vertical, over the hernia site. Remember that in the upper hernia, the sac lies beneath skin, superficial fascia, and latissimus dorsi muscle; in the lower hernia, there is no layer of muscle.

B. *Step 2.* Using 000 silk, ligate the hernial sac, if present, and replace it in the abdomen. If a large lipoma is present, a purse-string suture or several interrupted sutures will keep the fat "down."

Step 3. Place a Marlex or Prolene patch over the defect, and suture to the external oblique and latissimus dorsi muscles and lumbar periosteum using 000 interrupted Surgilon.

Incisions:

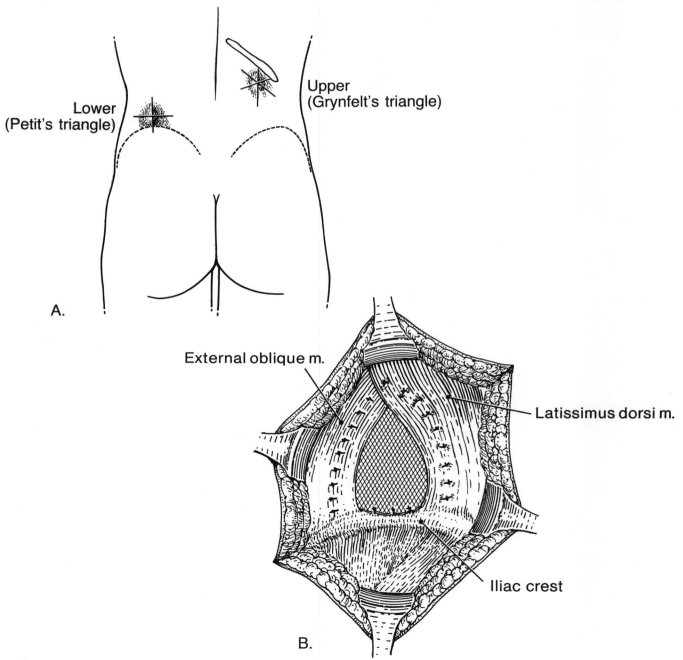

154

C. *Step 4.* Approximate the external oblique and latissimus dorsi muscles over the Marlex patch as far as possible without tension. Cut a flap of gluteal fascia (along dashed line).

D. *Step 5*
    a. Use the flap of gluteal fascia turned up to cover the defect remaining, and secure it with 000 Surgilon interrupted sutures to the present muscles.

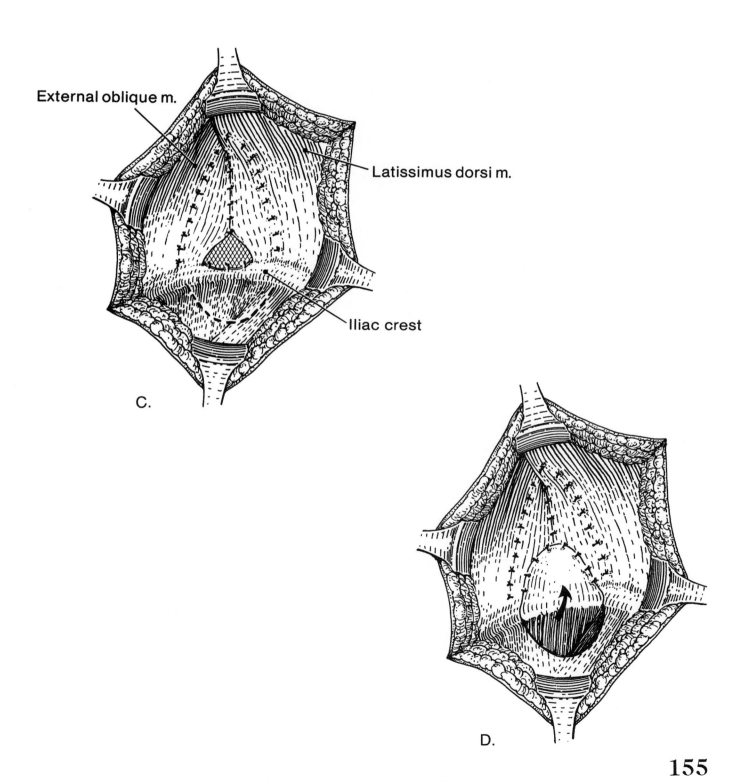

External oblique m.

Latissimus dorsi m.

Iliac crest

C.

D.

PLATE 46 (*Continued*)

Repair of Lumbar Hernia (Dowd-Ponka Repair)

E. b. A large hernial ring may require a second layer of Marlex mesh sutured to the muscles.

F. Diagram of the interrupted stitches used for two layers of Marlex. One or two J-P drains may be necessary.

Step 6. Close the subcutaneous fat and skin.

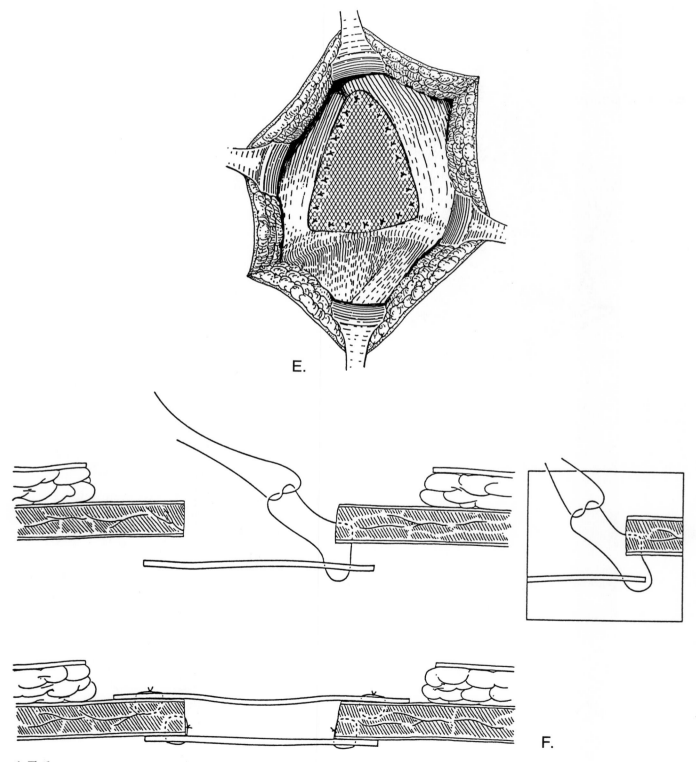

E.

F.

SECTION TWO

HERNIAS OF THE PELVIC WALL, PERINEUM, AND PELVIC FLOOR

Were I to place a man of proper talents, in the most direct road for becoming truly great in his profession, I would choose a good practical Anatomist and put him into a large hospital to attend the sick and dissect the dead.

WILLIAM HUNTER (1718–1783)
Two Introductory Lectures . . . to His Last Course of Anatomical Lectures, Lecture 2

Hernias of the Pelvic Wall

Surgical Anatomy of the Pelvic Wall

Peritoneum

The peritoneum of the pelvic wall is complicated by folds and fossae as it is reflected over organs of the urinary, genital, and digestive tracts.

URINARY TRACT REFLECTIONS

A number of folds of peritoneum are associated with the urinary bladder. Where these folds or ligaments seem to have some support function, they have been called *true ligaments;* where they seem less supportive, they have been called *false ligaments*. The distinction is arbitrary and unconvincing. The most important of these peritoneal ligaments are listed in Table 10 in the section on internal supravesical hernias.

GENITAL TRACT REFLECTIONS

The paragenital fossa lies between the broad ligament and the uterosacral ligament. The uterosacral ligaments extend backward from the cervix, embracing the rectum in their course and, with overlying peritoneum, forming the rectouterine fold, which bounds the rectouterine pouch (of Douglas) on each side.

DIGESTIVE TRACT REFLECTIONS

Between the uterosacral folds and the lateral rectal wall is the pararectal fossa, which communicates with the rectouterine pouch.

The Pelvic Blood Vessels (Internal Iliac Vessels)

These are the unpaired median sacral and the superior rectal arteries and the paired internal iliac arteries. All enter the pelvis retroperitoneally and all can be safely ligated.

The pelvis is drained by the rectal venous plexus, which is formed by the superior and middle rectal veins. From this plexus, drainage is to the inferior mesenteric vein (portal) and internal iliac vein (systemic). The uterine venous plexus drains to the internal iliac vein (systemic).

Pelvic Fascia

PARIETAL LAYER

According to Last,[1] this is a strong, membranous layer of fascia that provides a wallpaperlike covering for both the pelvic wall and the pelvic floor. It covers the muscles that form the pelvic wall—the obturator internus and the piri-

---

[1] Last RJ: *Anatomy: Regional and Applied,* 7th ed. Churchill Livingstone, Edinburgh, 1984.

formis—and is firmly attached to the peritoneum at their margins. (An exception is the fascia of Waldeyer, which extends from the sacrum to the ampulla of the rectum.) It also covers the "cracks" in the wall that are formed by the foramina. The superior and inferior blood vessels pierce this fascia to go to the buttocks.

VISCERAL LAYER

This layer is somewhat weaker and may be labeled according to the organ it covers, such as vesical, rectal, or prostatic. The visceral fascia is loose or dense in conformity with the distensibility of the organ.

Nerves of the Pelvis

These are the obturator nerve; the pelvic splanchnic nerves; the pelvic, sacral, and coccygeal plexuses; and the sacral part of the sympathetic nervous system.

Muscles

The pelvic muscles may be divided into lateral pelvic muscles (piriformis, obturator internus) and the muscles of the pelvic diaphragm. The piriformis muscle lies partly within and partly outside the bony pelvis, passing through the greater sciatic foramen. Outside the pelvis, the muscle forms part of the gluteal musculature (Plate 47C, D, E). It is related to the posterior surface of the ischium; the capsule of the hip joint; and the gluteus maximus, gluteus medius, and coccygeus muscles. Within the pelvis, the piriformis is related to the rectum, sacral plexus, and branches of the internal iliac vessels.

Remember that the pelvic surface of the obturator internus muscle forms the lateral boundary of the ischiorectal fossa. Outside the pelvis, the muscle is covered by the gluteus maximus and is crossed by the sciatic nerve.

PLATE 47

Anatomy of the Pelvic Wall and Pelvic Diaphragm

A. Diagram of the elements of the pelvic wall: Skin to peritoneum.

B. Frontal section of the pelvis showing the fasciae of the pelvic diaphragm, the obturator fascia, and the pudendal (Alcock's) canal. Parietal fascia is strong on the pelvic wall and floor, but not strong enough to hold sutures well. Therefore, Prolene mesh should be considered a possible means of correcting the local defect.

Source: Plate 47C inset from Skandalakis JE, Gray SW, Rowe JS Jr: *Anatomical Complications in General Surgery.* 1983, p. 270, Fig. 13-18.

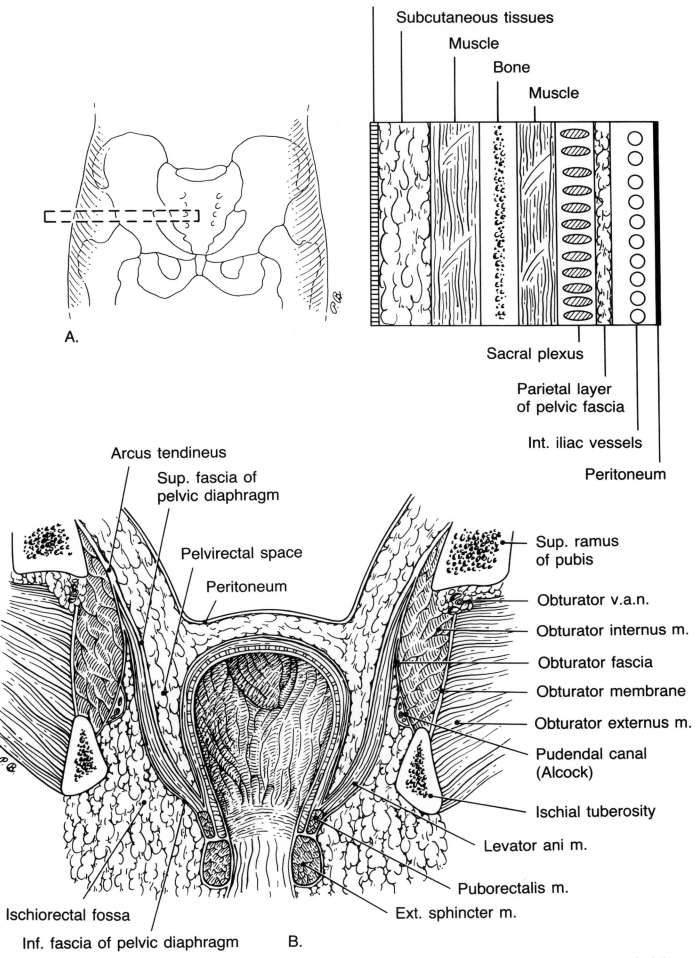

Skin

Subcutaneous tissues

Muscle

Bone

Muscle

Sacral plexus

Parietal layer
of pelvic fascia

Int. iliac vessels

Peritoneum

A.

Arcus tendineus

Sup. fascia of
pelvic diaphragm

Pelvirectal space

Peritoneum

Sup. ramus
of pubis

Obturator v.a.n.

Obturator internus m.

Obturator fascia

Obturator membrane

Obturator externus m.

Pudendal canal
(Alcock)

Ischial tuberosity

Levator ani m.

Puborectalis m.

Ext. sphincter m.

Ischiorectal fossa

Inf. fascia of pelvic diaphragm

B.

161

PLATE 47 (*Continued*)

Anatomy of the Pelvic Wall and Pelvic Diaphragm

C. Right lateral external view of pelvis. The greater sciatic foramen transmits the piriformis muscle and sciatic nerve. *Inset:* Sites of potential hernias through the sciatic foramina. A, Suprapiriformic sciatic hernia; B, infrapiriformic sciatic hernia; C, subspinous sciatic hernia through the lesser sciatic foramen.

D. Right pelvic wall with deep muscles and sciatic foramina.

E. Right gluteal region with sites of sciatic hernias. Gluteus maximus has been transected and reflected.

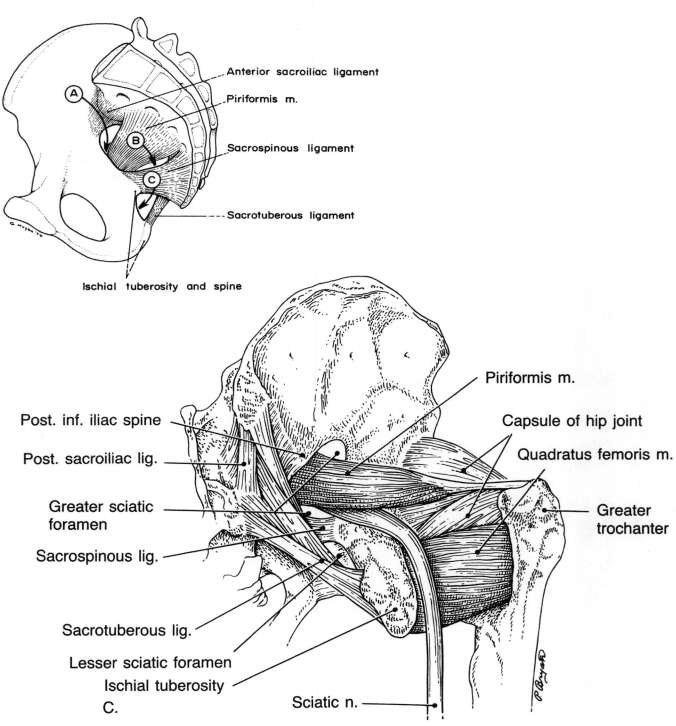

Anterior sacroiliac ligament

Piriformis m.

Sacrospinous ligament

Sacrotuberous ligament

Ischial tuberosity and spine

Post. inf. iliac spine

Post. sacroiliac lig.

Greater sciatic foramen

Sacrospinous lig.

Sacrotuberous lig.

Lesser sciatic foramen

Ischial tuberosity

C.

Piriformis m.

Capsule of hip joint

Quadratus femoris m.

Greater trochanter

Sciatic n.

162

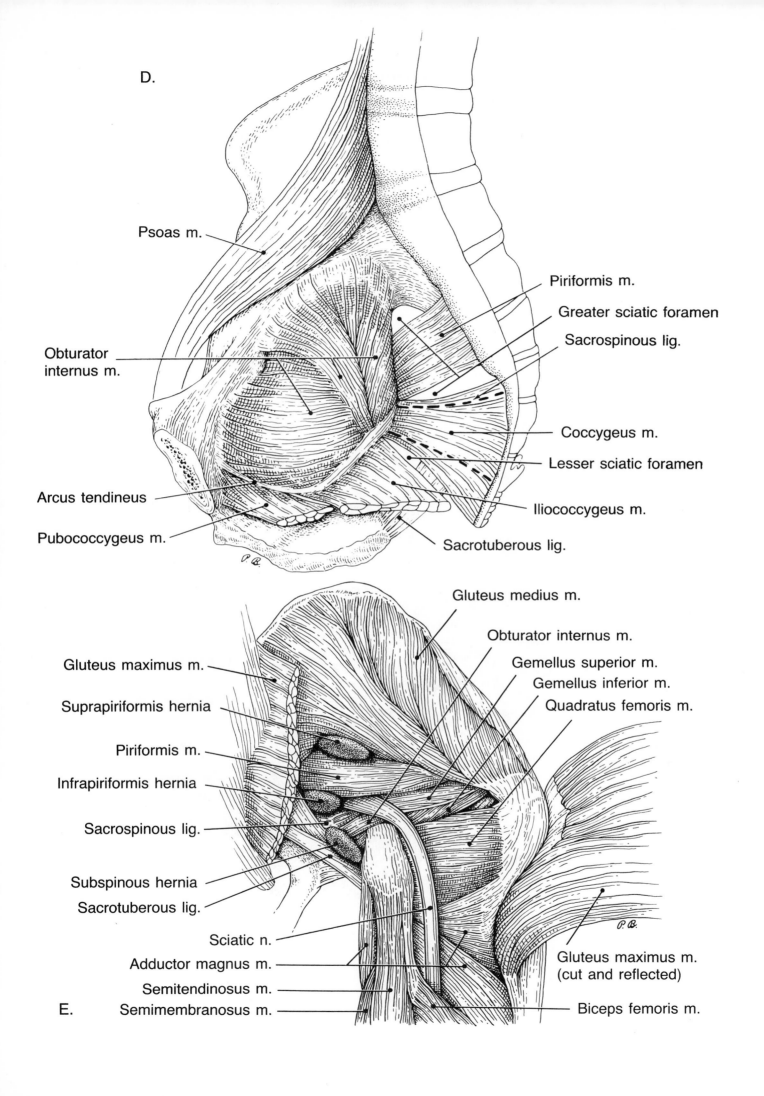

D.

Psoas m.

Piriformis m.

Greater sciatic foramen

Sacrospinous lig.

Obturator
internus m.

Coccygeus m.

Lesser sciatic foramen

Arcus tendineus

Iliococcygeus m.

Pubococcygeus m.

Sacrotuberous lig.

Gluteus medius m.

Obturator internus m.

Gluteus maximus m.

Gemellus superior m.

Suprapiriformis hernia

Gemellus inferior m.

Quadratus femoris m.

Piriformis m.

Infrapiriformis hernia

Sacrospinous lig.

Subspinous hernia

Sacrotuberous lig.

Gluteus maximus m.
(cut and reflected)

Sciatic n.

Adductor magnus m.

Semitendinosus m.

E.

Semimembranosus m.

Biceps femoris m.

PLATE 47 (*Continued*)
Anatomy of the Pelvic Wall and Pelvic Diaphragm

F. The superior gluteal nerve passes through the superior (suprapiriformic) portion of the greater sciatic foramen. The inferior gluteal nerve and the posterior cutaneous nerve of the thigh pass, with the sciatic nerve, through the inferior (infrapiriformic) portion of the greater foramen. The lesser sciatic foramen is traversed by the pudendal nerve, the nerve to the internal obturator muscle and the internal pudendal artery and vein.

G. Right pelvic wall and nerve supply. The sacral and coccygeal plexus. *Inset:* Course of pudendal nerve.

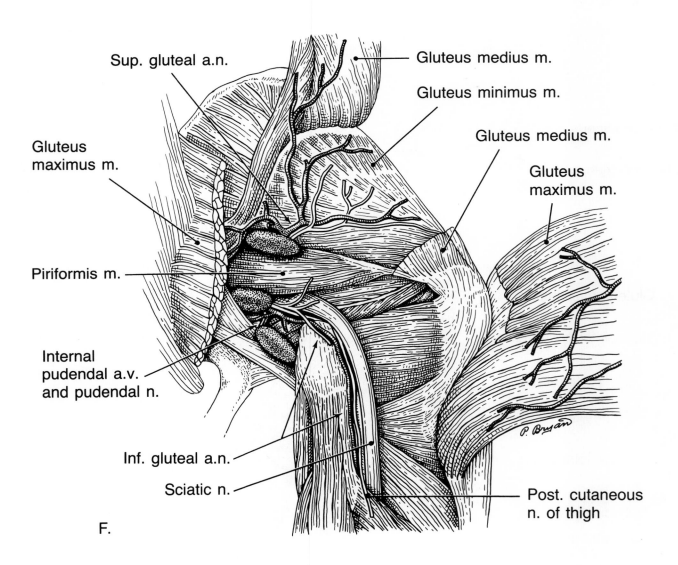

Sup. gluteal a.n.

Gluteus medius m.

Gluteus minimus m.

Gluteus medius m.

Gluteus maximus m.

Gluteus maximus m.

Piriformis m.

Internal pudendal a.v. and pudendal n.

Inf. gluteal a.n.

Sciatic n.

Post. cutaneous n. of thigh

F.

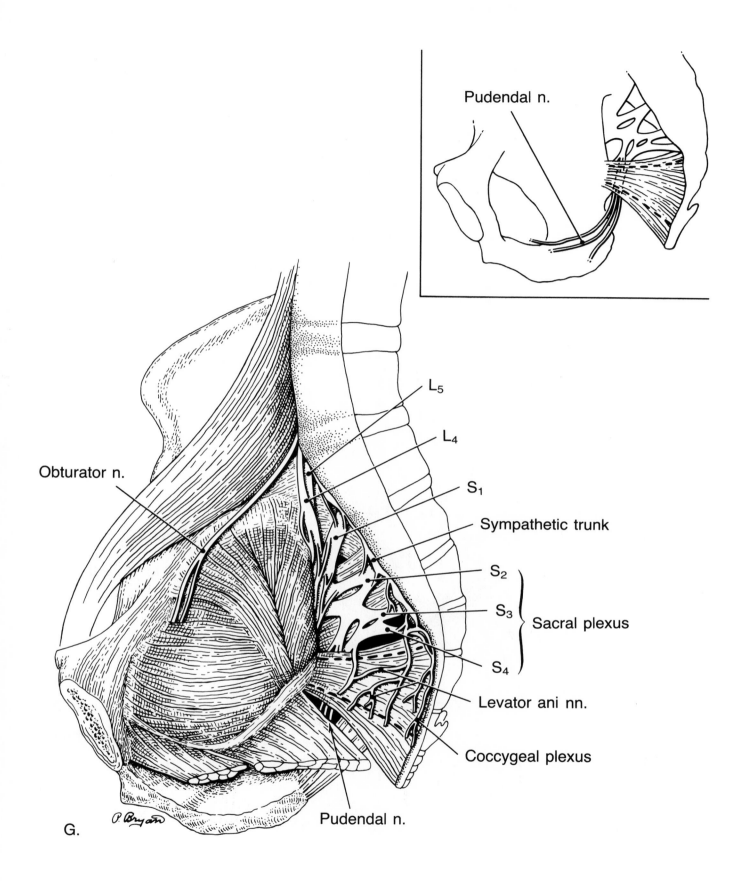

Pudendal n.

Obturator n.

L₅

L₄

S₁

Sympathetic trunk

S₂

S₃ } Sacral plexus

S₄

Levator ani nn.

Coccygeal plexus

Pudendal n.

G.

P. Bryan

165

PLATE 47 (*Continued*)
Anatomy of the Pelvic Wall and Pelvic Diaphragm

H. The internal iliac (hypogastric) artery branches into an anterior and a posterior division. In the chapter on sciatic hernia, we are concerned with those branches that are related to the sac and to the repair: the superior gluteal artery, which passes through the superior portion of the greater sciatic foramen; and the inferior gluteal artery, which enters the foramen below the piriformis muscle. The inferior gluteal artery gives off the superior and inferior vesical arteries and the obturator artery before entering the foramen. Two unpaired arteries in the pelvis, the median sacral and superior rectal arteries, are not shown. All of these arteries enter the pelvis extraperitoneally and may be ligated with impunity.

I. The superior and inferior gluteal veins emerge through the suprapiriformic and infrapiriformic apertures of the greater sciatic foramen to form the internal iliac (hypogastric) vein. The internal pudendal vein emerges through the lesser sciatic foramen to join the external iliac vein. There are many variations of the venous drainage.

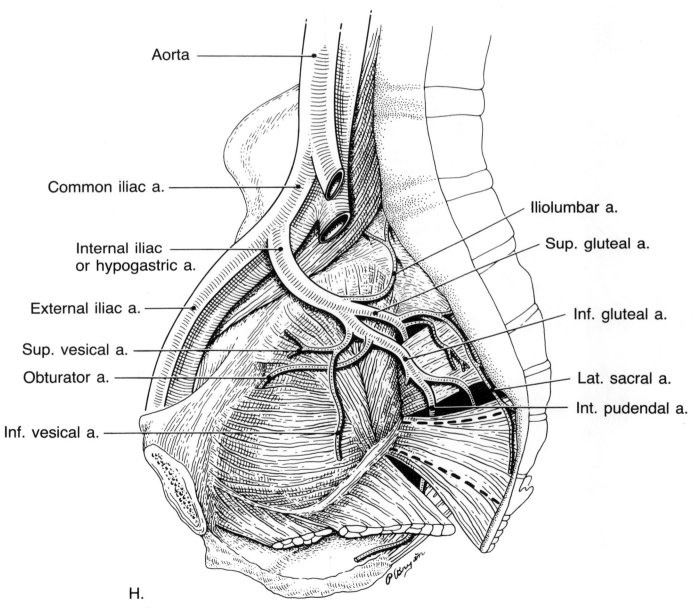

Aorta

Common iliac a.

Internal iliac or hypogastric a.

External iliac a.

Sup. vesical a.

Obturator a.

Inf. vesical a.

Iliolumbar a.

Sup. gluteal a.

Inf. gluteal a.

Lat. sacral a.

Int. pudendal a.

H.

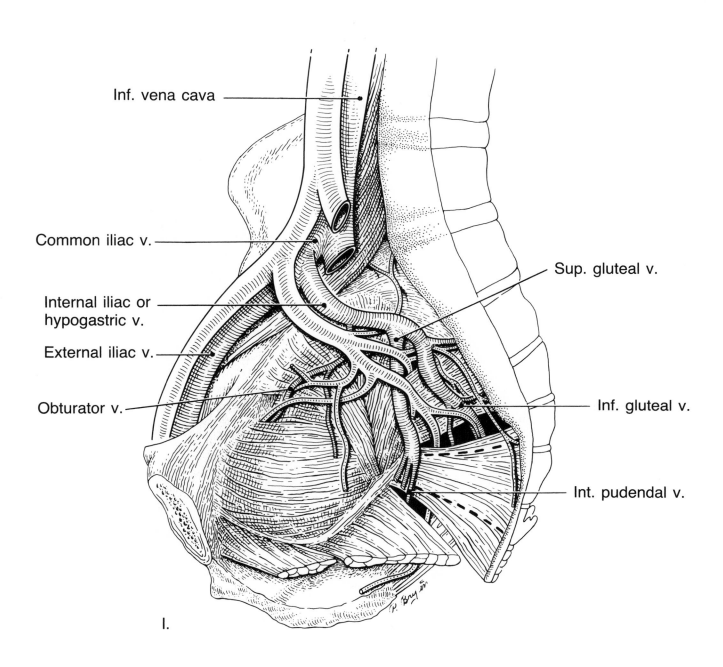

Inf. vena cava

Common iliac v.

Internal iliac or
hypogastric v.

External iliac v.

Obturator v.

Sup. gluteal v.

Inf. gluteal v.

Int. pudendal v.

I.

167

Sciatic Hernia

Definition

A sciatic hernia is a protrusion of a peritoneal sac and its contents through the greater or lesser sciatic foramen. It has also been called "sacrosciatic," "gluteal," or "ischiatic" hernia.

Surgical Anatomy of the Sciatic Region

There are three potential apertures through which a sciatic hernia may occur (Plate 47C and inset). Two are through the greater sciatic foramen above (suprapiriformic) or below (infrapiriformic) the piriformis muscle, which also passes through the foramen. A third potential hernia (subspinous) may pass through the lesser sciatic foramen below the sacrospinous ligament. All three hernial sites are covered by the gluteus maximus muscle.

The suprapiriformic hernial ring is composed of the anterior sacroiliac ligament anteriorly, the upper border of the piriformis muscle inferiorly, the ilium laterally, and the sacrotuberous ligament and the upper part of the sacrum medially.

Infrapiriformic hernia is bounded above by the lower border of the piriformis muscle, below by the sacrospinous ligament, posteriorly by the sacrotuberous ligament, and anteriorly by the ilium.

Subspinous hernia, through the lesser foramen, has a ring composed of the ischial tuberosity anteriorly, the sacrospinous ligament and ischial spine superiorly, and the sacrotuberous ligament posteriorly. Through the lesser foramen pass the tendon of the internal obturator muscle, the nerve supplying this muscle, the pudendal nerve, and the internal pudendal vessels.

The relations of the sac to nerves and vessels at its exit from the pelvis are:

Suprapiriformic   The superior gluteal nerve and vessels are anterior to the sac.

Infrapiriformic   The sciatic nerve
The inferior gluteal nerve and vessels and the pudendal nerve and vessels are lateral to the sac.

Subspinous   The sciatic nerve and the internal pudendal nerve and vessels are lateral to the sac.

168

PLATE 48
Repair of Sciatic Hernia—Transabdominal Approach

This is recommended when the diagnosis is uncertain, reduction of the hernia may be difficult, or other abdominal or pelvic procedures are contemplated.

The abdomen is entered by a low midline or a paramedian incision; the patient is placed in a Trendelenburg position and the abdomen explored.

A. *Step 1.* Liberate the intestinal loop by cutting the ring, if necessary, and reduce the contents. The vitality of the bowel will govern the surgeon's subsequent procedure.

Step 2. Transect the piriformis muscle by a posterior and inferior incision. Remember the proximity of the vessels and nerves passing through the greater sciatic foramen. If reduction cannot be accomplished otherwise, incise the internal obturator muscle. (See plate 47D.)

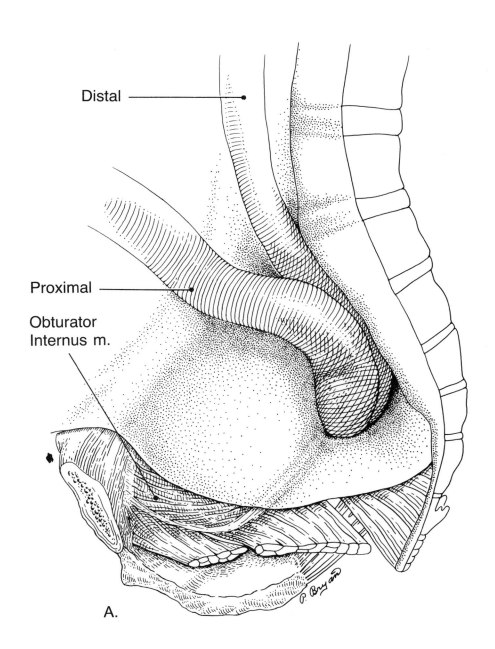

Distal

Proximal

Obturator
Internus m.

A.

PLATE 48 (*Continued*)

Repair of Sciatic Hernia—Transabdominal Approach

B. *Step 3.* Reduce the hernia and evert the empty sac.

C. *Step 4.* Ligate and excise the sac.

D. *Step 5.* Cover the area of the peritoneal defect and the ring with Prolene mesh, which may be secured by continuous or interrupted Prolene 000 sutures.

Step 6. Close the abdominal wall in layers.

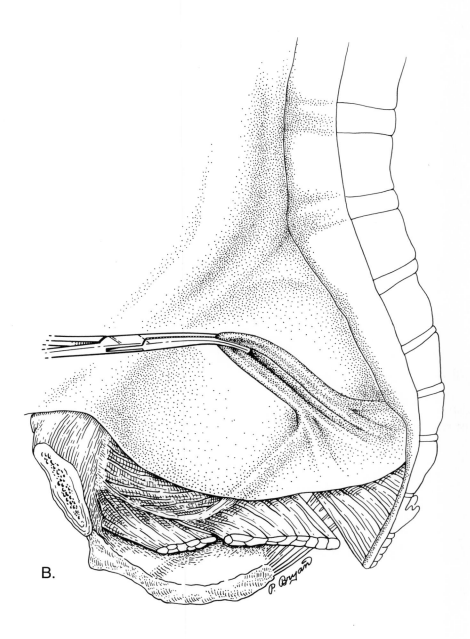

B.

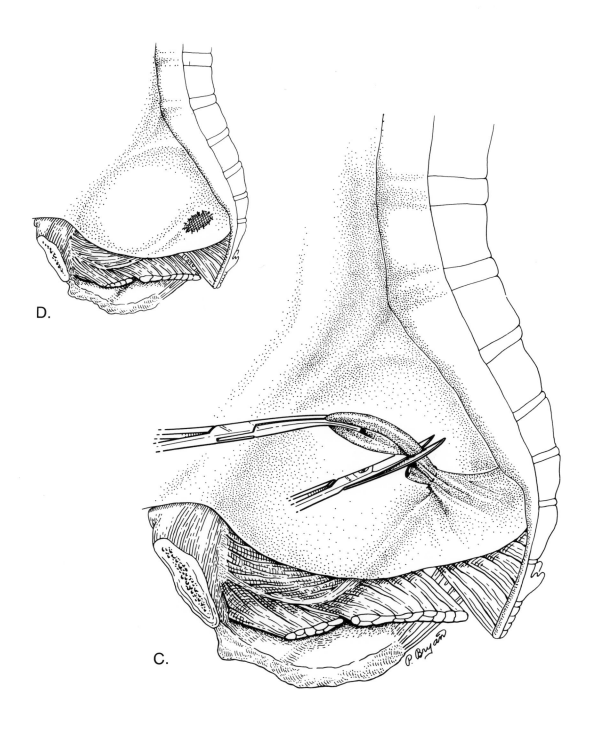

D.

C.

P. Bryan

171

PLATE 49
Repair of Sciatic Hernia—Transgluteal Approach

This is recommended when the diagnosis is certain, reduction of the hernia is easy, and there is no intestinal obstruction.

A. *Step 1.* The patient is in a prone position with pillows under the knees to produce complete relaxation of the gluteus maximus. Make an oblique incision over the palpable mass. Alternatively, make the incision from the top of the greater trochanter to the midpoint of a line between the posterior superior iliac spine and the tip of the coccyx. (The lesion shown is a right suprapiriformic hernia.)

B. *Step 2.* Split the gluteus maximus and expose and open the hernial sac. Avoid nerve and vascular injury by careful dissection of the sac.

C. *Step 3.* Return the contents of the sac to the abdomen if necessary; ligate and excise the sac.

D. *Step 4.* Close the muscular defect with interrupted sutures of 000 silk, approximating the gluteus maximus and medius muscles to the piriformis muscle.

E. *Step 5.* If the muscular defect is large, use a patch of Prolene mesh and 000 Prolene sutures, continuous or interrupted.

Remember to Avoid:

In the suprapiriformic hernia:
    The superior gluteal nerve and vessels
    The posterior femoral cutaneous nerve
    The nerve to the internal obturator muscle
    The nerve to the quadratus femoris muscle
    The sciatic nerve

In the infrapiriformic hernia:
    Inferior gluteal nerve and vessels
    Pudendal nerve and vessels

In the subspinous hernia:
    Internal pudendal nerve and vessels
    Sciatic nerve

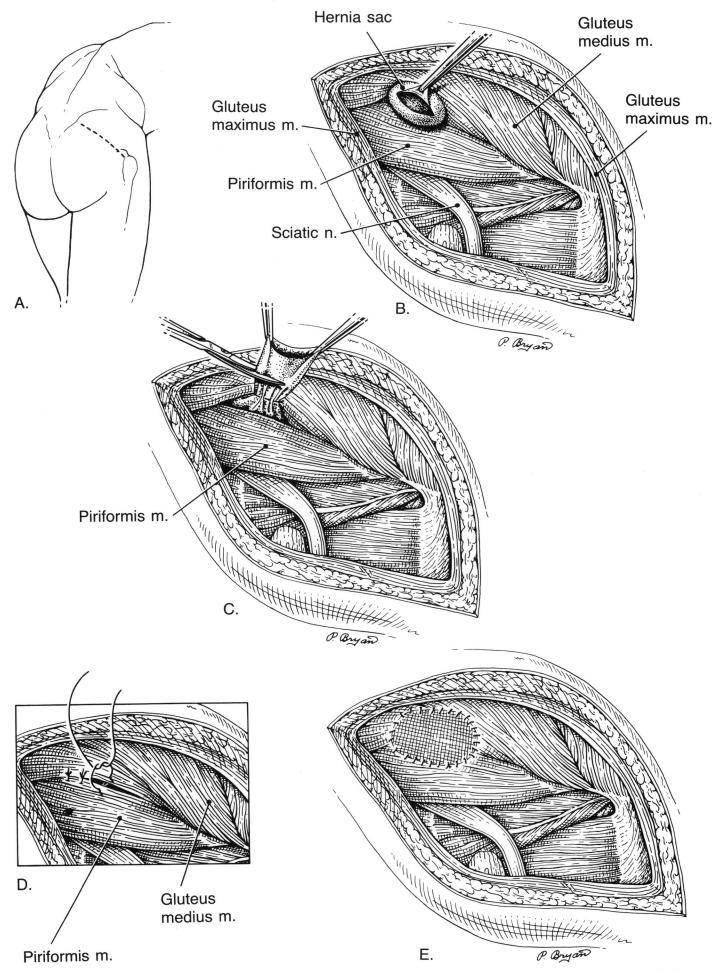

A.

Hernia sac

Gluteus
medius m.

Gluteus
maximus m.

Gluteus
maximus m.

Piriformis m.

Sciatic n.

B.

Piriformis m.

C.

D.

Gluteus
medius m.

Piriformis m.

E.

173

Obturator Hernia

Definition

An obturator hernia is an abnormal protrusion of preperitoneal fat or an intestinal loop through the obturator foramen. It characteristically affects the right side of middle-aged women. Its relation to groin hernias is seen in Plate 50A.

Surgical Anatomy of the Obturator Region

The obturator *region* is bounded superiorly by the horizontal ramus of the pubic bone, laterally by the hip joint and the shaft of the femur, medially by the pubic arch, the perineum, and the gracilis muscle,[1] and inferiorly by the insertion of the adductor magnus on the adductor tubercle of the femur.

The obturator *foramen* is the largest bony foramen in the body and is formed by the rami of the ischium and pubis. It lies inferior to the acetabulum on the anterolateral wall of the pelvis. Except for a small area, the obturator canal, the foramen is closed by the obturator membrane. Fibers of the membrane are continuous with the periosteum of the surrounding bones and with the tendons of the internal and external obturator muscles. Embryologically, the foramen and its membrane represent an area of potential bone formation that never proceeds to completion. In this sense the obturator foramen is a lacuna and the obturator canal is the true foramen.

The obturator *canal* is a tunnel 2 to 3 cm long beginning in the pelvis at the defect in the obturator membrane. It passes obliquely downward to end outside the pelvis in the obturator region of the thigh. The canal is bounded above and laterally by the obturator groove of the pubis and inferiorly by the free edge of the obturator membrane and the internal and external obturator muscles. Through this canal pass the obturator artery, vein, and nerve (Plate 50B).

The obturator nerve is usually superior to the artery and vein (Plate 50C). The nerve separates into anterior and posterior divisions as it leaves the canal (Plate 50D). The hernial sac may follow either division of the nerve (Plate 50E). The obturator artery divides to form an arterial ring around the foramen (Plate 50F).

The herniated fat or ileal loop or, rarely, the urinary bladder, compresses the obturator nerve, affecting either or both divisions to produce the characteristic hip-knee pain (Howship-Romberg sign) present in about one-half of the patients with obturator hernia (Plate 50G).[1]

The formation of an obturator hernia begins with a "pilot tag" of retroperitoneal fat in the first stage, followed by the appearance of a peritoneal dimple in the second stage into which a knuckle of viscus may be partially incarcerated (Richter's hernia) in the third stage (Plate 50H). Eventually, the incarceration of an ileal loop produces complete obstruction. The frequency of pilot tags in cadavers and the rarity of actual obturator hernias in patients suggest that most obturator hernias do not progress beyond the first and second stages of development.[1]

[1]Gray SW, Skandalakis JE, Soria RE, Rowe JS Jr: Strangulated obturator hernia. *Surgery* 75:20–27, 1974.

PLATE 50
Surgical Anatomy of the Obturator Region

A. Lateral view of the right side of the pelvis showing the sites of inguinal, femoral, and obturator hernias.

B. View of the medial wall of the male pelvis showing the obturator canal and structures passing through it.

C. Diagrammatic coronal section of the lateral wall of the male pelvis showing the relation of obturator nerve, artery, and vein to other pelvic structures.

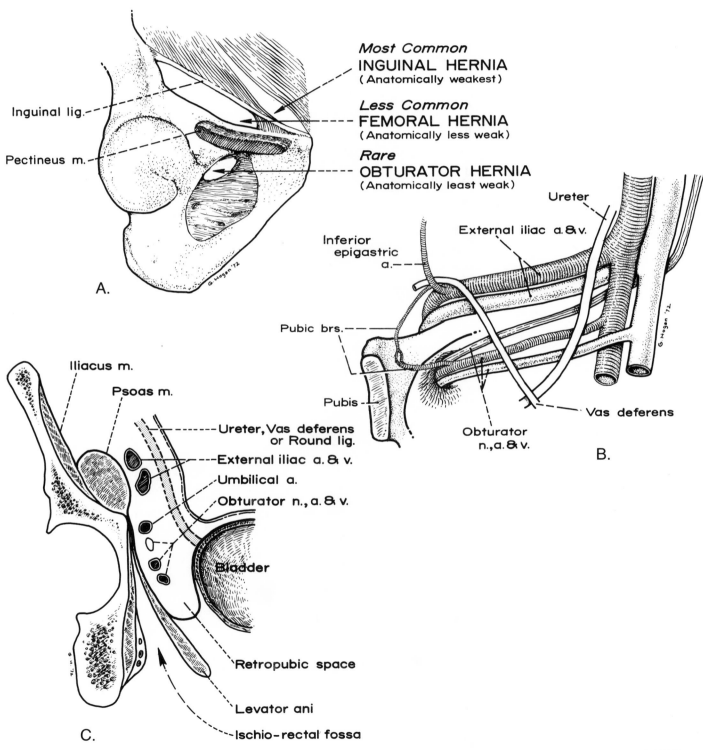

175

PLATE 50 (*Continued*)
Surgical Anatomy of the Obturator Region

D. The course and distribution of the right obturator nerve.

E. Diagram of long section of the upper thigh through the obturator foramen showing the potential paths of obturator hernia. The hernia may follow the anterior or posterior division of the nerve.

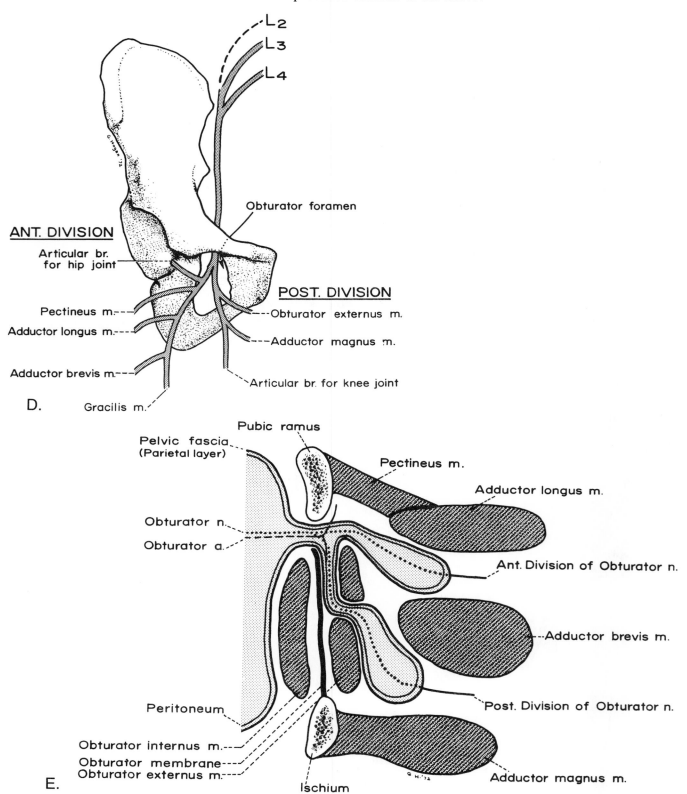

L₂
L₃
L₄

Obturator foramen

ANT. DIVISION

Articular br. for hip joint

POST. DIVISION

Pectineus m.
Adductor longus m.
Adductor brevis m.

Obturator externus m.
Adductor magnus m.
Articular br. for knee joint

D.

Gracilis m.

Pubic ramus

Pelvic fascia (Parietal layer)

Pectineus m.

Adductor longus m.

Obturator n.
Obturator a.

Ant. Division of Obturator n.

Adductor brevis m.

Peritoneum

Post. Division of Obturator n.

Obturator internus m.
Obturator membrane
Obturator externus m.

E.

Ischium

Adductor magnus m.

F. As it emerges through the obturator canal, the obturator artery divides to form an arterial ring around the obturator foramen.

G. Compression of either or both divisions of the obturator nerve by the hernia may produce pain (Howship-Romberg sign). Palpation by vagina or rectum may confirm the presence of a hernia.

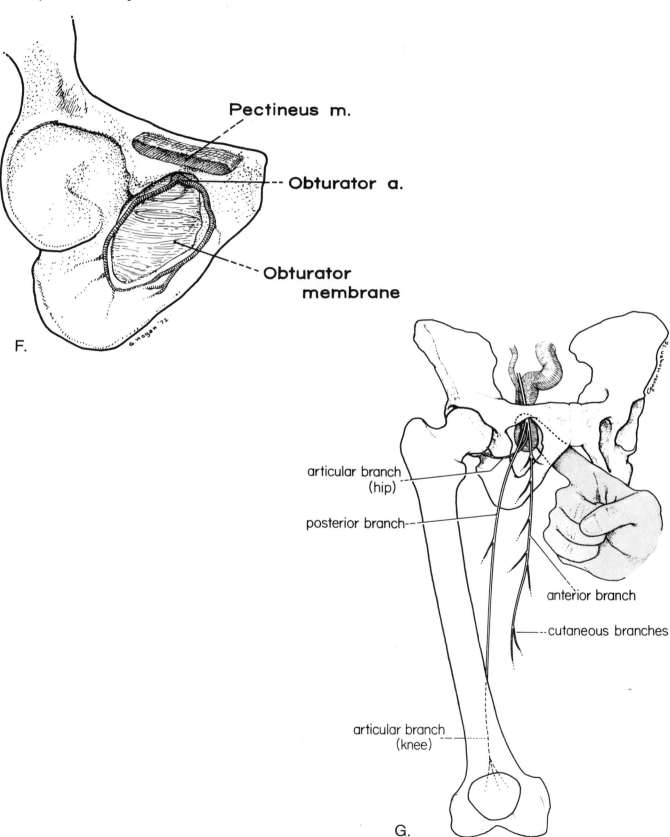

Pectineus m.

Obturator a.

Obturator membrane

F.

articular branch (hip)

posterior branch

anterior branch

cutaneous branches

articular branch (knee)

G.

PLATE 50 (*Continued*)

Surgical Anatomy of the Obturator Region

H. Diagrammatic section through the obturator canal showing the genesis of an obturator hernia. *Left:* Normal (no hernia). First stage: Pilot tag of retroperitoneal connective tissue in canal. Second stage: A peritoneal dimple has been found. Third stage: Partial intermittent incarceration (Richter's hernia) of an ileal loop followed by complete herniation of the loop.

Source: Plate 50A, D, H, F, and G from Gray SW, Skandalakis JE: Strangulated obturator hernia, in *Hernia,* 2d ed. Nyhus LM, Condon RE (eds). Lippincott, Philadelphia, 1978, p. 428, Fig. 25-1; p. 432, Fig 25-7; p. 433, Fig. 25-8; p. 436, Fig. 25-11. Plate 50B, C, and E from Gray SW, Skandalakis JE, Soria RE, Rowe JS: Strangulated obturator hernia. *Surgery* 75:20–27, 1974, Figs. 1, 2, 4.

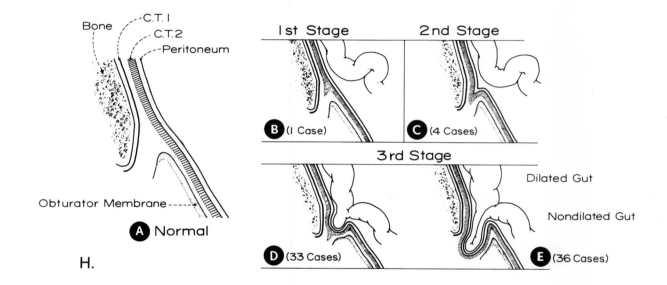

H.

PLATE 51
Repair of Obturator Hernia

A. *Step 1.* Make a transverse suprapubic incision one finger breadth above the pubic symphysis. Divide both Camper's and Scarpa's fasciae.

B. *Step 2.* Incise the anterior lamina of the rectus sheath transversely on both sides.

C. *Step 3.* Minimally mobilize the anterior lamina of the rectus sheath.

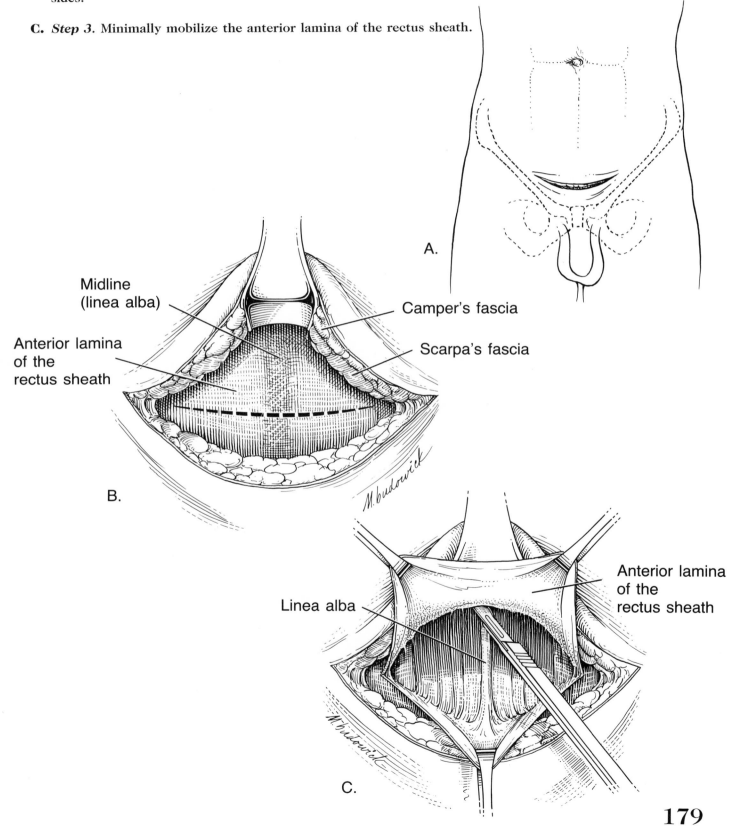

179

PLATE 51 (*Continued*)

Repair of Obturator Hernia

D. *Step 4.* Divide the tendinous insertion of the right or left rectus muscle on the pubic rami.

E. *Step 5.* Further mobilize the anterior lamina of the rectus sheath. Incise the linea alba and retract the recti laterally. If the surgeon needs more room, the transverse incision may be extended laterally to the aponeuroses of the external and internal oblique and the transversus abdominis muscles.

F. *Step 6.* Divide the transversalis and prevesical fasciae without opening the peritoneum.

G. The urinary bladder is visualized.

H. *Step 7.* Push the preperitoneal fat upward with a sponge or sponge stick.

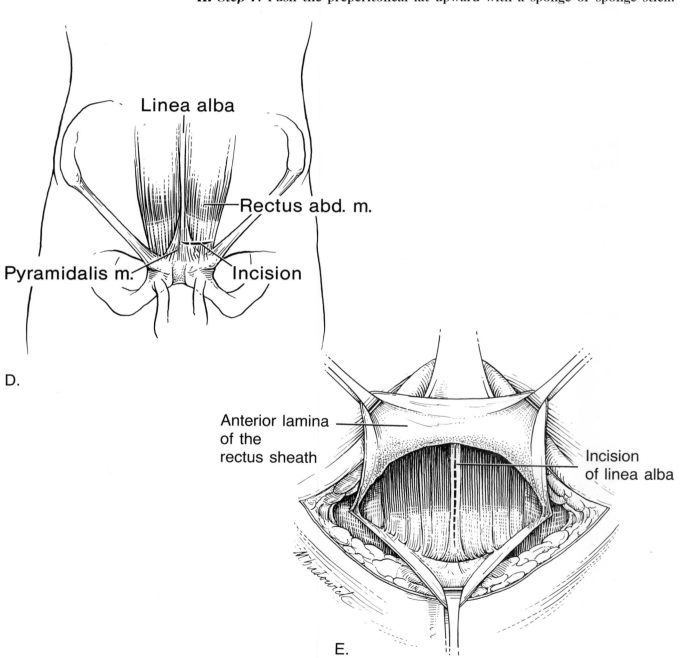

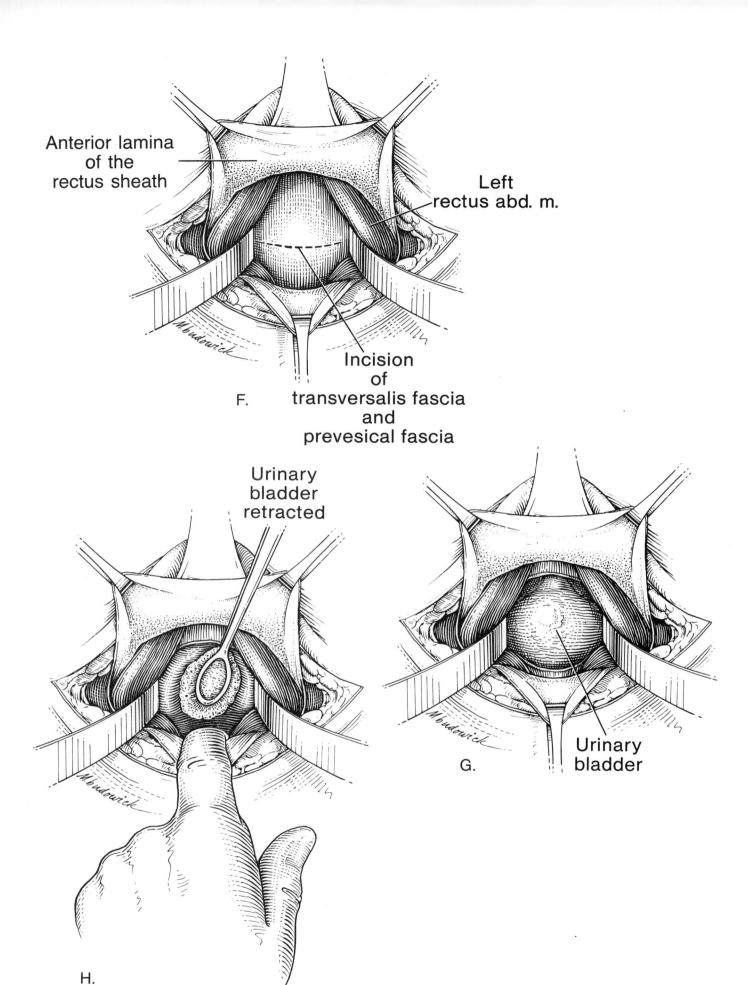

Anterior lamina of the rectus sheath

Left rectus abd. m.

F.

Incision of transversalis fascia and prevesical fascia

Urinary bladder retracted

G.

Urinary bladder

H.

181

PLATE 51 (*Continued*)

Repair of Obturator Hernia

I. Sagittal section showing the perivesical space and the prevesical (retropubic) space (of Retzius).

J. *Step 8*. Introduce a finger into the retropubic space to identify the structures entering the obturator foramen.

K. *Step 9*. Medial view of right pelvis. Insert the finger into the retropubic space under the pubic ramus just lateral to the pubic symphysis. A cordlike formation containing the obturator nerve, artery, and vein can be felt. The nerve appears as a shiny silver cord.

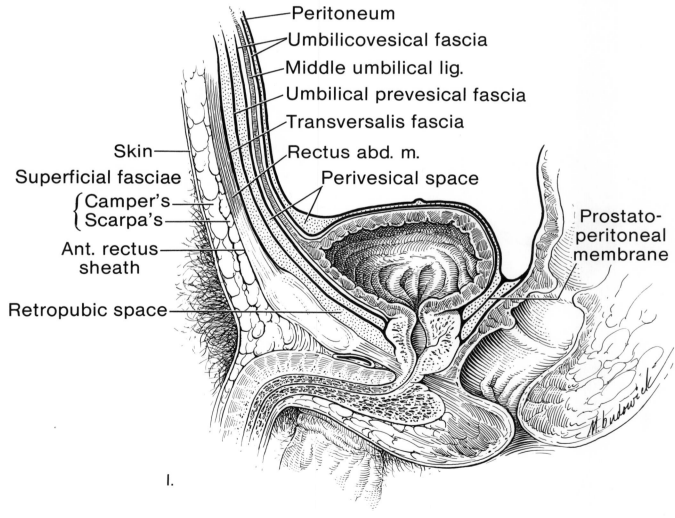

Peritoneum
Umbilicovesical fascia
Middle umbilical lig.
Umbilical prevesical fascia
Transversalis fascia
Rectus abd. m.
Perivesical space

Skin
Superficial fasciae
Camper's
Scarpa's
Ant. rectus sheath
Retropubic space

Prostato-peritoneal membrane

I.

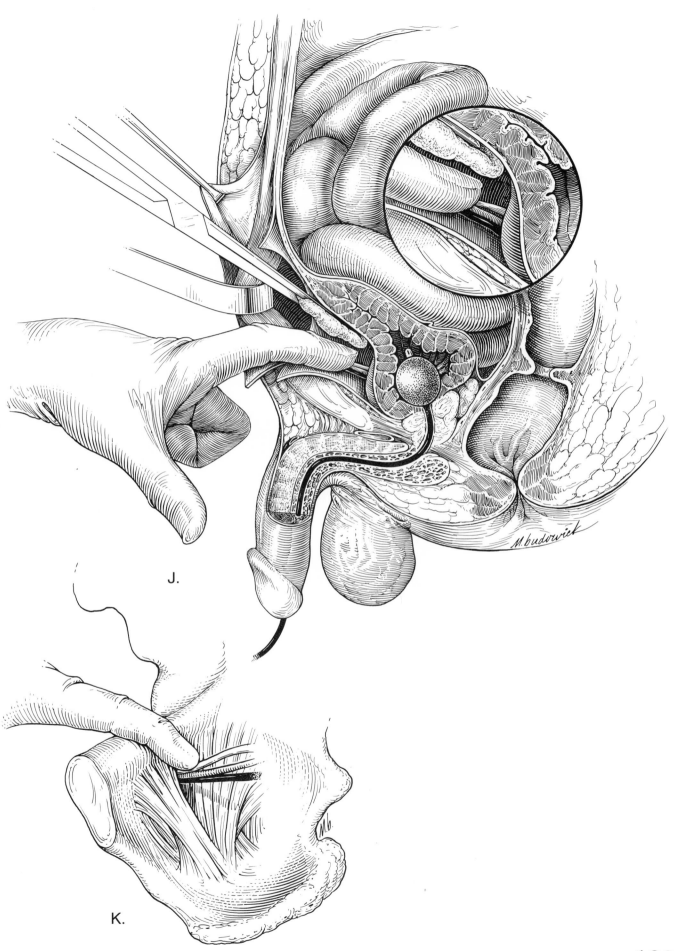

J.

K.

183

PLATE 51 (*Continued*)

Repair of Obturator Hernia

L. *Step 10*

> **a.** Close a small obturator defect with one or more simple sutures.

M.

> **b.** Use a patch of Prolene mesh and 000 or 0000 Prolene sutures to close a larger defect.

If the obturator hernia is unrecognized and "intestinal obstruction" is the only diagnosis, an exploratory laparotomy through a lower midline incision is necessary. If the herniated intestinal loop is strangulated or necrotic, resect the intestine and make an end-to-end anastomosis. *Complications:* There are the usual complications of inguinal hernia repair, the most important being injury of the obturator nerve, obturator vessels, vas deferens, and ureter.

N,O. *Step 11.* Excise the sac and close the obturator foramen with Prolene mesh as in a sciatic hernia.

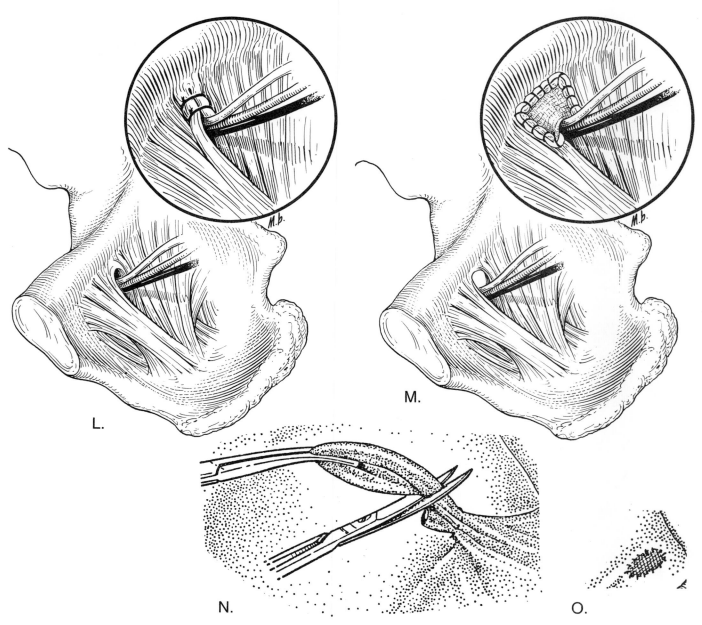

L.

M.

N.

O.

Perineal Hernia

Definition

A perineal hernia is the protrusion of a viscus through the floor of the pelvis (pelvic diaphragm) into the perineum. A hernial sac is present. The hernia may be primary, or it may be secondary to pelvic surgery. Only primary hernias are of concern here.

Perineal hernia is among the rarest of human hernias. Unlike inguinal hernia, which appears to be related to the erect posture of humans, perineal hernia is more common in quadrupeds than in humans. Recently, 85 affected dogs were treated in 5 years at one veterinary clinic.

By definition the pelvic diaphragm is the floor of the pelvic basin and the roof of the perineum. The hernial sac passing through any abnormal opening of the pelvic diaphragm will eventually appear in the perineal area. It may be anterior or posterior to the superficial transverse perineus muscle.

Sites of Perineal Hernia

A primary perineal hernia may occur anterior or posterior to the superficial transverse perineus muscle.

An anterior perineal hernia passes through the pelvic and urogenital diaphragms, lateral to the urinary bladder and vagina, and anterior to the urethra. It has been variously called pudendal, labial, lateral, or vaginal-labial. It is found only in women. It is hard to see how this kind of perineal hernia could occur in males.

A posterior perineal hernia passes between components of the pelvic diaphragm or through the hiatus of Schwalbe, when present, lateral to the urethra, vagina, and rectum. The hiatus is formed by the nonunion of the obturator internus and levator ani muscles. There are two possible locations: (1) an upper posterior hernia between the pubococcygeus and iliococcygeus muscles; and (2) a lower posterior hernia between iliococcygeus and coccygeus muscles, below the lower margin of the gluteus maximus muscle.

In males the perineal hernia enters the ischiorectal fossa. In females it may enter the fossa or the labium majus, or it may lie close to the vaginal wall or below the lower margin of the gluteus maximus muscle.

Surgical Anatomy of the Perineum and the Pelvic Floor

The Perineum

The perineum is the region extending from the coccyx to the pubis; it occupies the space between the thighs externally. It is bounded anteriorly by the pubic symphysis, anterolaterally by the ischiopubic rami, inferolaterally by the ischial tuberosities, posterolaterally by the sacrotuberous ligaments, and posteriorly by the coccyx. Its floor is the skin; its roof is the pelvic diaphragm and the urogenital diaphragm.

This diamond-shaped area may be divided into an anterior or urogenital triangle and a posterior or anal triangle by a line connecting the ischial tuberosities.

The superficial transverse perineus muscle passes from the ischial tuberosity to the central tendon of the perineum. It may be well developed, hypotrophic, or absent. Its action is obscure, but it may serve to assist in fixation of the perineal body. Do not confuse this muscle with the deep transverse perineus muscle, which belongs to the urogenital diaphragm.

The Urogenital Diaphragm (Deep Pouch)

The urogenital diaphragm forms a fibromuscular bridge between the two sides of the pubic arch. It consists of two fascial layers with two muscles between them, the deep transverse perineus muscle and the sphincter urethrae membranosum. Anteriorly the two fascial layers join to form the transverse perineal ligament. Posteriorly they join and fuse with Colles' fascia. Remember, the inferior fascial layer is also known as the perineal membrane and the posterior part of the diaphragm is attached to the perineal body.

The urogenital diaphragm of the male contains the muscular sphincter of the membranous urethra and the deep transverse perineus muscle. The diaphragm also contains the dorsal nerve, the arteries and veins of the penis, the arteries and nerves of the penile bulb, the bulbourethral glands and their ducts, a venous plexus, and the internal pudendal vessels.

In the female, the urogenital diaphragm is perforated by the vagina, in addition to the female counterparts of the muscles, vessels, and nerves listed above. The main artery is the artery of the clitoris, and the main nerve is the deep perineal or pudendal nerve.

The Superficial Pouch

The superficial pouch of the perineum consists of inferior and superior fasciae, three paired muscles, erectile tissue elements, and, in the female, paired vestibular glands. The laterally placed ischiocavernosus muscles cover the corpora cavernosa penis or clitoris. The medially situated bulbospongiosus muscles cover the corpus spongiosum penis or vestibular bulbs (and vestibular glands). The superficial transverse perineus muscles pass from the ischial tuberosities laterally to the perineal body. The pouch is sealed inferiorly by the fascia of the musculature (external perineal fascia; Gallaudet). The roof of the pouch is provided by the perineal membrane (inferior fascia of urogenital diaphragm).

The Perineal Body

In the male the perineal body is a fibromuscular fatty mass lying between the bulb of the penis and the anus. The interlacing fibers form a central tendinous point or "perineal center." This structure provides a central point of attachment for the superficial and deep transverse perineus, bulbospongiosus, external sphincter, and levator ani muscles.

In the female, a similar and proportionately larger structure lies between the anus and vagina. It lies below the pelvic floor, and injury to it may jeopardize the stability of the pelvic organs. This is the "perineum" of the obstetrician and gynecologist. Cranially, the perineal fibers blend into those of the rectovaginal septum.

Perineal Fascia

SUPERFICIAL FASCIA (TABLE 4)

Camper's fascia is subcutaneous tissue, largely fat, of the anterior inferior body wall. Deep to this is Scarpa's fascia, the membranous layer of superficial

186

TABLE 4
Corresponding Connective Tissue Layers of the Abdominal Wall and Perineum

Abdominal Wall Fasciae	Genital Fasciae	Perineal Fasciae
Fatty layer of superficial fascia (Camper).	Fatty and membranous layers fuse to form the superficial fascia of penis, clitoris; this is infiltrated with smooth muscle to form dartos tunic of scrotum and labia minora tissue.	Fatty layer of superficial fascia of urogenital triangle (Camper).
Membranous layer of superficial fascia (Scarpa).		Membranous layer of superficial fascia of the urogenital triangle (Colles).
External muscle fascia of external oblique and rectus sheath (Gallaudet).	Deep fascia of penis and clitoris (Buck's) —also external spermatic fascia of spermatic cord.	External perineal fascia or muscular fascia of superficial perineal muscles (Gallaudet).

fascia. These two fasciae intermingle inferiorly, forming the superficial fascia of the penis and clitoris. Infiltrated with smooth muscle, they form the dartos tunic of the scrotum or the substance of the labia minora. Scarpa's fascia continues into the perineum as Colles' fascia, whereas Camper's fascia continues as the adiposal layer there.

The deep layer of the superficial fascia is attached to the fascia lata of the thigh (the fascia of Elliot Smith), the pubic arch, and the posterior border of the perineal membrane (inferior or superficial layer of the urogenital diaphragm). The most characteristic fascial attachment in the peritoneum, from a surgical standpoint, is the union of the Colles' fascia with the posterior portion of the urogenital diaphragm, forming a potential space closed behind but open anteriorly. This is the superficial perineal cleft or pouch.

The infraanal fascia covers the inferior or superficial surface of the levator ani and coccygeus muscles and is continuous with the deep (superior) fascia of the urogenital diaphragm in the region of the anterior recess of the ischiorectal fossa.

DEEP FASCIA
The deep muscle fascia (of Gallaudet) of the anterior abdominal wall is continuous with the penile or clitoral deep fascia and, in the perineum, is represented by the muscular fascia there (external perineal fascia of Gallaudet). On the penis, this fascial layer is referred to as Buck's fascia; however, some anatomists believe that Buck's fascia is a continuation of Scarpa's fascia.

Deep fascia covers the extrapelvic portion of the obturator internus muscle as the obturator fascia, fusing with the fascia lunata to form the pudendal canal (Alcock), which contains the pudendal nerve and the internal pudendal artery and vein. Medially the fascia forms the superior and inferior fascia of the levator ani muscle. There is confusion in the literature about the deep fascia, which is nothing but the pelvic fascia—parietal and visceral.

The Pelvic Diaphragm
The pelvic diaphragm is composed of two paired muscles, the levator ani and coccygeus. They form the floor of the pelvis and the roof of the perineum.

The levator ani is itself formed by the iliococcygeus and pubococcygeus muscles. A subdivision of the pubococcygeus, the puborectalis muscle, is the most important in maintaining rectal continence.

The puborectalis muscle originates from the body of the pubic bone and the superior layer of the deep perineal pouch (urogenital diaphragm). Fibers from the two puborectalis muscles pass posteriorly and then join posterior to the rectum, forming a well-defined sling. The puborectalis, with the superficial and deep parts of the external sphincter and the proximal part of the internal sphincter, form the so-called anorectal ring. This ring can be palpated, and, because cutting through it will produce incontinence, it must be identified and protected during surgical procedures. It is at the approximation of these divisions of levator ani that weak areas may permit a posterior perineal hernia to bulge. Remember, the pelvic floor does not prolapse; the defect is through splitting of the muscle along fascial planes.

Peritoneal Relations of the Pelvis

Peritoneum envelops the front and sides of the upper third of the rectum. As the rectum passes deeper into the pelvis, however, progressively more fat is interposed between the peritoneum and the rectal musculature.

Finally, the peritoneum separates completely from the rectum and passes anteriorly and superiorly over the uterus or, in males, over the bladder. This creates a depression called either the rectouterine or rectovesical pouch. With infection or trauma, it may fill with pus.

Spaces of the Pelvis

1. Definition and Boundaries of the Six Unpaired Spaces

    a. *Prevesical or Retropubic Space (of Retzius)*

      This is a triangular cleft at the front and sides of the urinary bladder and behind the pubis.

      Boundaries

      MEDIAL: Anteroinferior lateral surface of the urinary bladder.

      LATERAL: From above downward: Pubic bone, obturator internus fascia, levator ani muscle.

      INFERIOR: Reflection of levator ani fascia onto the bladder, extending to the cardinal ligament.

      SUPERIOR: Peritoneum.

    b. *Vesicovaginal Space*

      Space between bladder and vagina.

      Boundaries

      ANTERIOR: Adventitia of the urinary bladder.

      POSTERIOR: Adventitia of the vagina.

      SUPERIOR: The fusion of the above two adventitia (vesicocervical ligament).

      INFERIOR: The fusion of the vaginal and urethral adventitia.

    c. *Rectovaginal Space*

      Midline space between rectum and vagina.

      Boundaries

      ANTERIOR: Rectovaginal septum (fibromuscular entity at the posterior vaginal wall).

LATERAL: Rectouterine or descending rectal septum.
SUPERIOR: Peritoneum lining space of Douglas.
INFERIOR: Perineal body.

d. *Retrorectal Space*

Midline space between the inner surface of the sacrum and the posterior fascia of the rectum.

e. *Rectouterine Space of Douglas*

The female pelvis is subdivided by the uterus and broad ligament of the uterus into an anterior, shallow vesicouterine space and a posterior, deep rectouterine space. In the male pelvis the peritoneum forms a rectovesical fossa or pouch.

f. *Superficial Perineal Cleft*

A cleft or potential space between the external perineal fascia or muscle fascia of Gallaudet above and Colles' fascia below.

Boundaries

INFERIOR: Colles' fascia.

SUPERIOR: The external fascia of the superficial muscles of the perineum, the external perineal fascia (of Gallaudet).

POSTEROLATERAL: Closed by the fusion of its superior and inferior fasciae.

ANTERIOR: Communicates freely around the labia majora or scrotum with the interval between the membranous layer of superficial fascia (Scarpa's fascia) and the external investing fascia of the musculature of the abdominal wall (fascia of Gallaudet or innominate fascia). The external investing fascia is the outer fascial layer of the external oblique, its aponeurosis, and the anterior layer of the rectus sheath.

2. Definition and Boundaries of the Four Paired Spaces

a. *Pararectal Spaces*

These peculiar potential spaces below the cardinal ligament may be divided into proximal and distal portions forming an L. The proximal part communicates with the retrorectal space to surround the upper rectum completely.

Boundaries of the Proximal Spaces

ANTERIOR: Cardinal ligament.

POSTERIOR: Lateral part of sacrum.

LATERAL: Internal iliac vessels.

MEDIAL: Ureter.

Boundaries of the Distal Spaces (the horizontal part of the L)

SUPERIOR: Cardinal ligament.

INFERIOR: Levator ani muscle.

MEDIAL: Rectal septum.

b. *Paravesical Spaces*

Fat-filled, preformed spaces lie above the cardinal ligament.

Boundaries

SUPERIOR: Medial umbilical ligament.

LATERAL: Pelvic wall, fascia of obturator internus muscle, superior fascia of levator ani muscle.

MEDIAL: Urinary bladder.

189

c. *Suprategmental Spaces*

These are the upper, or deep, portions of the ischiorectal fossae.

Boundaries

MEDIAL: Inferior fascia of levator ani muscle.

LATERAL: Fascia of obturator internus muscle.

INFERIOR: Fascia lunata—the fascia that bridges the interval between the levator ani and the obturator internus and that contributes to the formation of the pudendal canal.

d. *Ischiorectal Fossae*

These spaces are pyramidal in shape, filled with fat, and lined by fascia. They are located, one on each side, close to the surgical anal canal, a little apart from the lower rectum.

Boundaries

INFERIOR: Skin without underlying fascial layer.

LATERAL: Thick fascia of the obturator internus muscle and the ischial tuberosities with overlying falciform processes of the sacrotuberous ligaments.

MEDIAL: External anal sphincter, thin infraanal fascia covering the perineal surface of levator ani muscle.

POSTERIOR: Fascia covering the sacrotuberous ligament and gluteus maximus muscle.

ANTERIOR: Deep or superior fascia of the urogenital diaphragm in the region of the anterior recess of the isciorectal fossa.

There are three areas of weakness in the wall of the ischiorectal fossa through which an abscess of the fossa may pass (Plate 57). Of these three areas, the weakest is medial, through the anal wall. Slightly stronger is the inferior boundary of skin, and strongest is a medial pathway through the levator ani muscle or between its components. This last pathway can be taken in the opposite direction by a perineal hernia of the ischiorectal type.

Connective Tissue Septa of the Perineum

Septa are planes of loose connective tissue which support other structures; separate potential spaces; and provide pathways for nerves, blood vessels, and lymphatics. Most septa do not have the strength of true anatomical ligaments. Only a few can be mentioned here.

The supravaginal septum is the connective tissue between the bladder and the upper vagina and cervix.

The ascending septa of the bladder connect the upper surface of the cardinal ligaments to the bladder.

The descending rectal septum passes from the inferior surface of the cardinal ligament to the lateral surface of the rectum and sacrum.

The rectovaginal septum extends from the deepest aspect of the pouch of Douglas to the superior surface of the perineal body. It represents the early developmental fusion of the peritoneum of the caudal extension of the pouch of Douglas to the pelvic floor. It is the anterior layer of the rectovesical fascia (Denonvilliers). Stouter than the other septa, it contains elastic and smooth muscle fibers.

TABLE 5
The Layers and Contents of Pouches and Spaces of the Urogenital Triangle

1. Superficial fasciae
   A. Adipose layer of Camper
   B. Membranous layer of Colles
2. Superficial perineal cleft
   A. Floor: membranous fascia of Colles
   B. Roof: external muscular fascia of Gallaudet
   C. Posterior boundary: attachment to perineal membrane
   D. Lateral boundary: attachment to ischiopubic rami
3. Superficial perineal pouch or compartment
   A. Boundaries
      (1) Inferior: external muscular fascia of Gallaudet
      (2) Superior: perineal membrane (inferior UGD fascia)
   B. Contents
      (1) Ischiocavernosus muscles and underlying corpora cavernosa penis, clitoris
      (2) Bulbospongiosus muscles and underlying penile bulb or vestibular bulb
      (3) Superficial transverse perineus muscles
      (4) Vestibular glands in female
      (5) Transverse perineal vessels and nerves
4. Deep perineal pouch or compartment: urogenital diaphragm
   A. Boundaries
      (1) Inferior: perineal membrane (inferior fascia of urogenital diaphragm)
      (2) Superior: superior fascia of urogenital diaphragm—continuous with supraanal fascia and infraanal fascia at urogenital hiatus of the pelvic diaphragm; also related superiorly in part to anterior recess of ischiorectal fossa bilaterally
   B. Contents
      (1) Deep transverse perineus muscles
      (2) Sphincter urethralis in male
      (3) Sphincter urethrovaginalis in female
      (4) Bulbourethral glands in male
      (5) Internal pudendal artery and veins
         a. artery of the bulb (and veins)
         b. artery of the crus penis or clitoris (and veins)
         c. dorsal artery (and veins)
         d. dorsal nerve of penis or clitoris

PLATE 52

The Female Perineum

A. The female perineum seen from below showing possible sites of perineal hernias. A primary perineal hernia may occur anterior or posterior to the superficial transverse perineus muscle.

An anterior hernia protrudes through the urogenital diaphragm into the triangle formed by the bulbocavernosus muscle medially, the ischiocavernosus muscle laterally, and the superficial transverse perineus muscle inferiorly. Anterior hernias occur only in females.

A posterior perineal hernia may emerge between component muscle bundles of levator ani muscle or between that muscle and coccygeus muscle midway between the rectum and the ischial tuberosity.

B. Boundaries of the perineum seen from above. This diamond-shaped area may be divided by a line connecting the ischial tuberosities into an anterior or urogenital triangle and a posterior or anal triangle.

PLATE 52 (*Continued*)
The Female Perineum

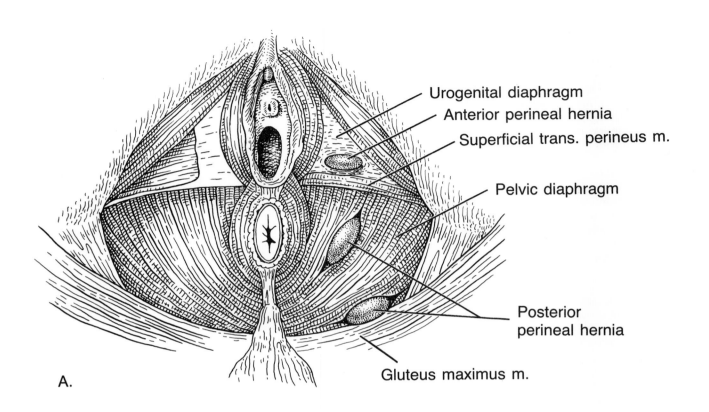

Urogenital diaphragm
Anterior perineal hernia
Superficial trans. perineus m.

Pelvic diaphragm

Posterior
perineal hernia

Gluteus maximus m.

A.

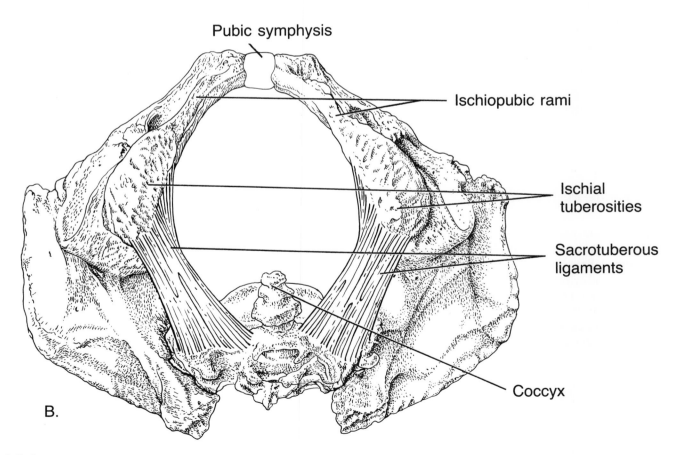

Pubic symphysis

Ischiopubic rami

Ischial
tuberosities

Sacrotuberous
ligaments

Coccyx

B.

192

PLATE 53

The Course of Anterior and Posterior Perineal Hernia in the Female—Sagittal Section of the Female Pelvis

A. Course of an anterior perineal hernia. The sac passes between the urinary bladder and the vagina to reach the surface of the perineum.

B. Course of a posterior perineal hernia. The sac passes between the vagina and rectum to reach the surface of the perineum.

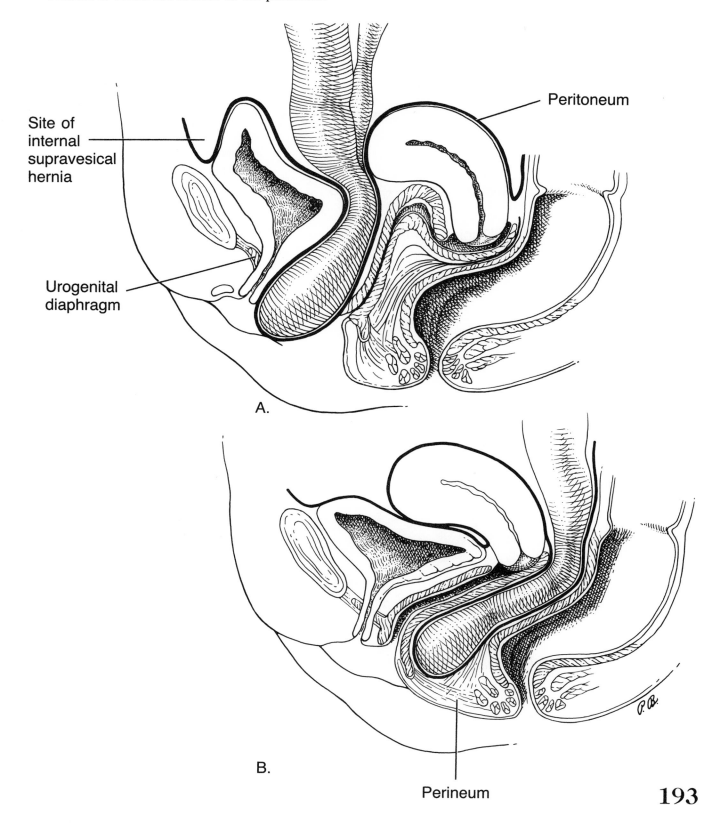

Site of internal supravesical hernia

Urogenital diaphragm

Peritoneum

A.

B.

Perineum

193

PLATE 54

The Male Pelvis—Sagittal and Coronal Sections

A. The male pelvis seen in diagrammatic sagittal section.

Inset: Diagram of the relations of the superficial fasciae of the inguinal area showing the formation of the superficial perineal pouch.

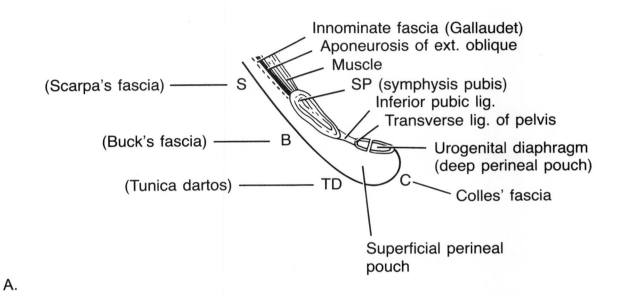

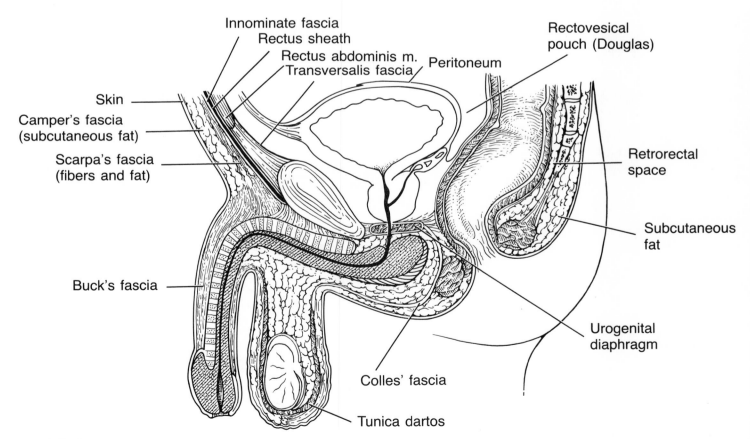

A.

194

B. Diagrammatic coronal section of the pelvis through the anal canal showing the relation of the fascia to the levator ani muscle. The broken lines indicate the superficial and deep fasciae. The deep fascia is the parietal and visceral pelvic fascia, including the fascia lunata of Elliot Smith.

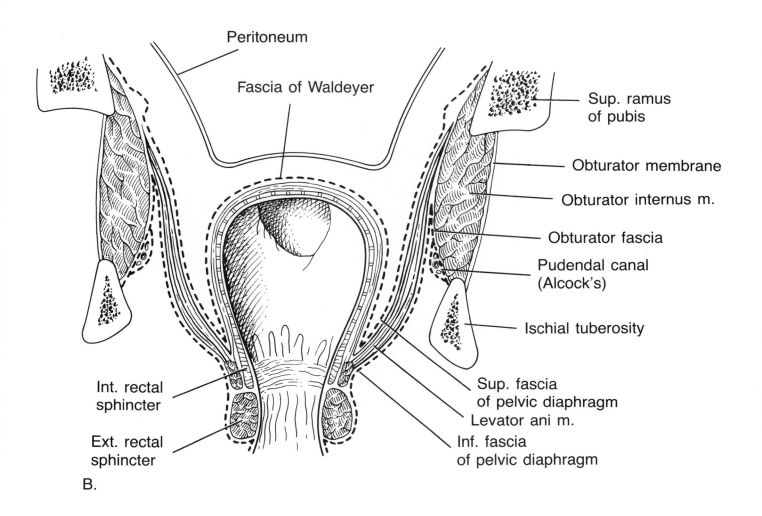

Peritoneum

Fascia of Waldeyer

Sup. ramus of pubis

Obturator membrane

Obturator internus m.

Obturator fascia

Pudendal canal (Alcock's)

Ischial tuberosity

Int. rectal sphincter

Ext. rectal sphincter

Sup. fascia of pelvic diaphragm

Levator ani m.

Inf. fascia of pelvic diaphragm

B.

195

PLATE 55
The Urogenital Diaphragm

A. The urogenital diaphragm in the male. Two fascial layers contain the deep transverse perineus muscle, and the sphincter of the membranous urethra and the bulbourethral glands. On the viewer's left the perineal membrane (inferior fascia of the urogenital diaphragm) has been removed.

B. The urogenital diaphragm in the female. The vagina passes through the diaphragm posterior to the urethra. On the viewer's left, the perineal membrane has been removed to show the deep transverse perineus muscle and the urethrovaginal sphincter.

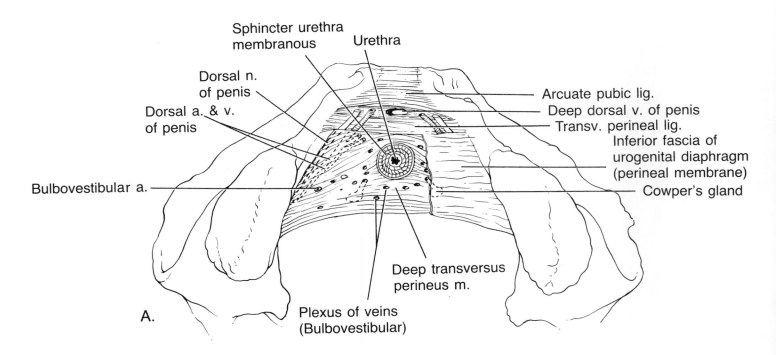

Sphincter urethra membranous
Urethra
Dorsal n. of penis
Dorsal a. & v. of penis
Arcuate pubic lig.
Deep dorsal v. of penis
Transv. perineal lig.
Inferior fascia of urogenital diaphragm (perineal membrane)
Bulbovestibular a.
Cowper's gland
Deep transversus perineus m.
Plexus of veins (Bulbovestibular)

A.

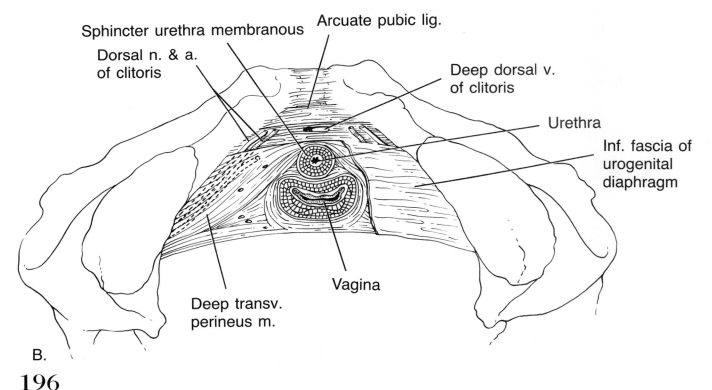

Sphincter urethra membranous
Arcuate pubic lig.
Dorsal n. & a. of clitoris
Deep dorsal v. of clitoris
Urethra
Inf. fascia of urogenital diaphragm
Deep transv. perineus m.
Vagina

B.

196

C. Diagrammatic sagittal section of the female urogenital diaphragm showing its relation to the urethra and vagina.

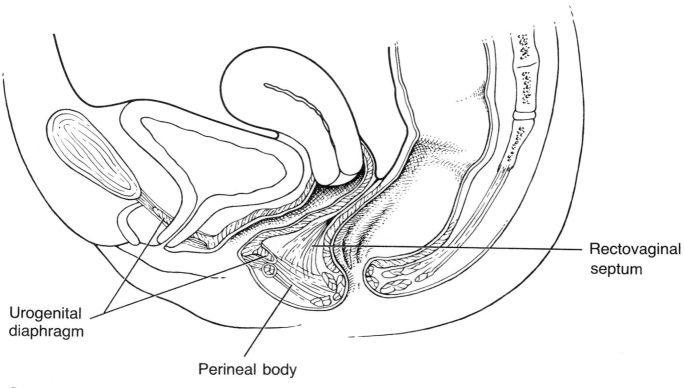

Urogenital diaphragm

Perineal body

Rectovaginal septum

C.

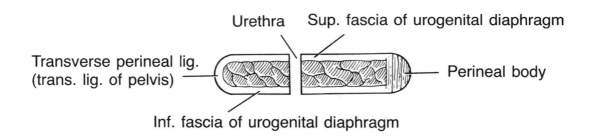

Urethra   Sup. fascia of urogenital diaphragm

Transverse perineal lig.
(trans. lig. of pelvis)

Perineal body

Inf. fascia of urogenital diaphragm

PLATE 56
The Pelvic Diaphragm and Related Muscles

The pelvic diaphragm forms the roof of the perineum and the floor of the pelvic basin. Two muscles, the levator ani and coccygeus, compose the diaphragm. The levator ani may be considered to be divided into the pubococcygeus and iliococcygeus. The pubococcygeus can be further subdivided into a puborectalis component, in addition to pubovaginalis in the female or levator prostatae in the male.

A. The female pelvic diaphragm seen from above.

B. The female pelvic diaphragm seen from below.

Source: Plate 56A,B from Gray SW, Skandalakis JE: *Atlas of Surgical Anatomy for General Surgeons.* Williams & Wilkins, Baltimore, 1985, p. 257, Fig. 10-13.

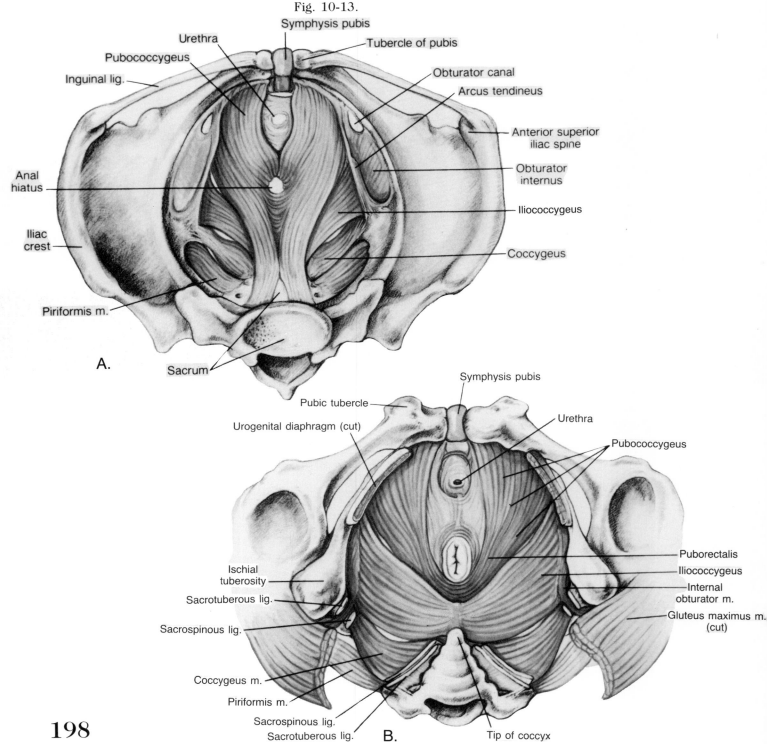

198

C. The pelvic diaphragm of the male seen from below. The perineal membrane has been removed from the right side of the urogenital triangle.

D. The pelvic diaphragm of the female seen from below.

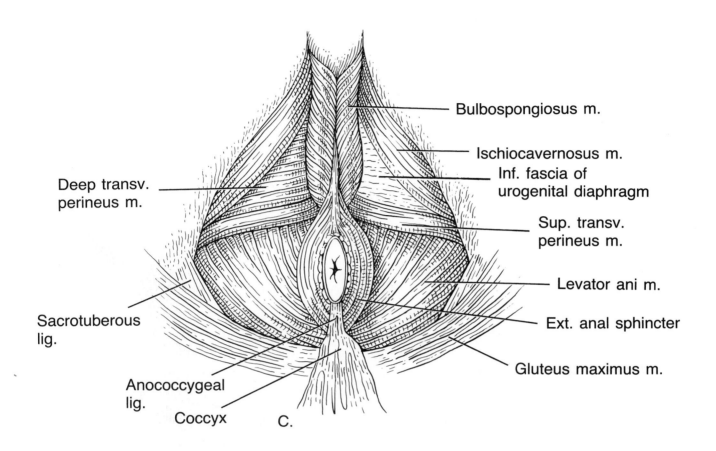

Bulbospongiosus m.

Ischiocavernosus m.

Inf. fascia of urogenital diaphragm

Deep transv. perineus m.

Sup. transv. perineus m.

Levator ani m.

Ext. anal sphincter

Sacrotuberous lig.

Gluteus maximus m.

Anococcygeal lig.

Coccyx

C.

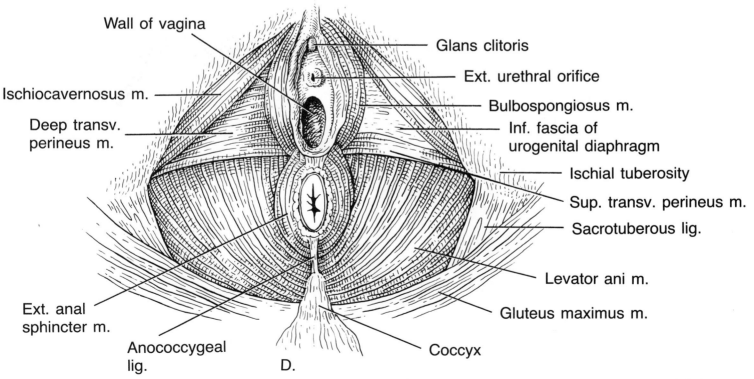

Wall of vagina

Glans clitoris

Ext. urethral orifice

Ischiocavernosus m.

Bulbospongiosus m.

Deep transv. perineus m.

Inf. fascia of urogenital diaphragm

Ischial tuberosity

Sup. transv. perineus m.

Sacrotuberous lig.

Levator ani m.

Ext. anal sphincter m.

Gluteus maximus m.

Anococcygeal lig.

Coccyx

D.

199

PLATE 57
Spaces of the Pelvis

A. Diagrammatic sagittal section of the pelvis showing the six unpaired spaces of the pelvis. All are potential spaces except the rectouterine space of Douglas in the female (rectovesical space in the male) which is a true space lined with peritoneum.

B. Diagrammatic coronal section of the pelvis through the anal canal showing three of the four paired spaces of the pelvis. The fourth pair, the paravesical spaces, lie anterior to the plane of section, separated from the pararectal spaces by the cardinal ligaments.

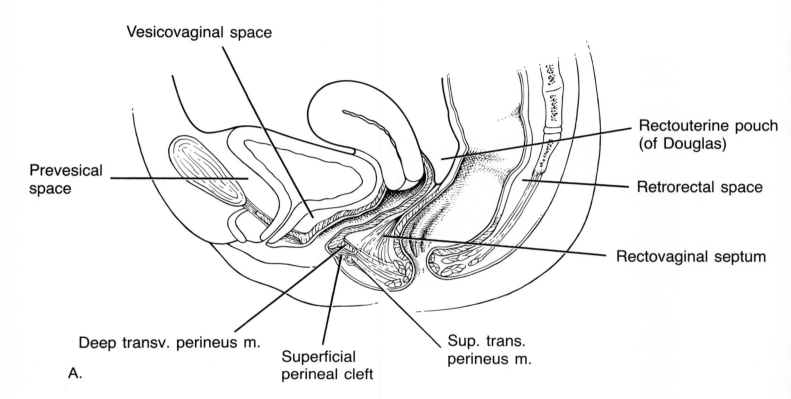

Vesicovaginal space

Prevesical space

Rectouterine pouch (of Douglas)

Retrorectal space

Rectovaginal septum

Deep transv. perineus m.

Superficial perineal cleft

Sup. trans. perineus m.

A.

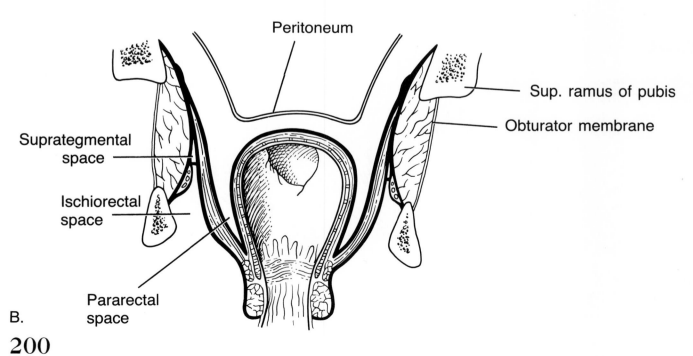

Peritoneum

Suprategmental space

Ischiorectal space

Pararectal space

Sup. ramus of pubis

Obturator membrane

B.

200

Schemata of the Pelvic Spaces

C.,D. Schematic cross sections of the female pelvis below the level of the uterine cervix showing the relations of the spaces, septa, and viscera of the female pelvis. The unpaired rectouterine space and the superficial perineal pouch are not shown.

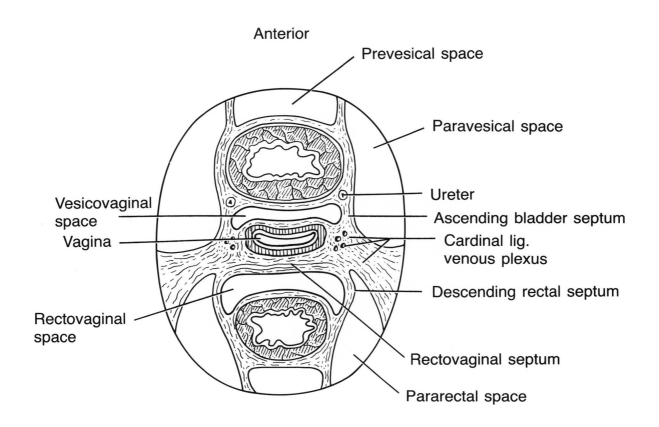

Anterior

Prevesical space

Paravesical space

Ureter

Ascending bladder septum

Vesicovaginal space

Cardinal lig. venous plexus

Vagina

Descending rectal septum

Rectovaginal space

Rectovaginal septum

Pararectal space

C.   Posterior

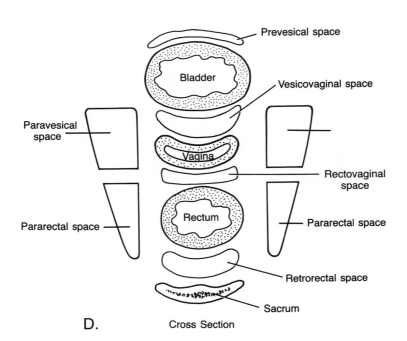

Prevesical space

Bladder

Vesicovaginal space

Paravesical space

Vagina

Rectovaginal space

Pararectal space

Rectum

Pararectal space

Retrorectal space

Sacrum

D.   Cross Section

201

PLATE **57** (*Continued*)

Schemata of the Pelvic Spaces

E. Schematic coronal section of the pelvis. Three of the paired spaces are shown in this section; the remaining pair is shown in part D.

F. The pudendal canal (Alcock's canal). The canal is formed by the internal obturator fascia and the fascia lunata of Elliot Smith. This is the deepest fascia of the ischiorectal fossa; this fascia is separated from the skin by the fat filling the fossa. The canal carries the dorsal nerve of the penis, the internal pudendal artery, and the perineal division of the pudendal nerve.

G. The hiatus of Schwalbe. If the internal fascia of the obturator internus muscle and the inferior fascia of the levator ani muscle fail to fuse, there is an opening between the suprategmental and pararectal spaces. This is the hiatus of Schwalbe. It is a potential place for a posterior perineal hernia.

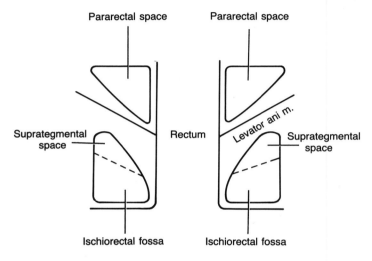

E.   Coronal Section

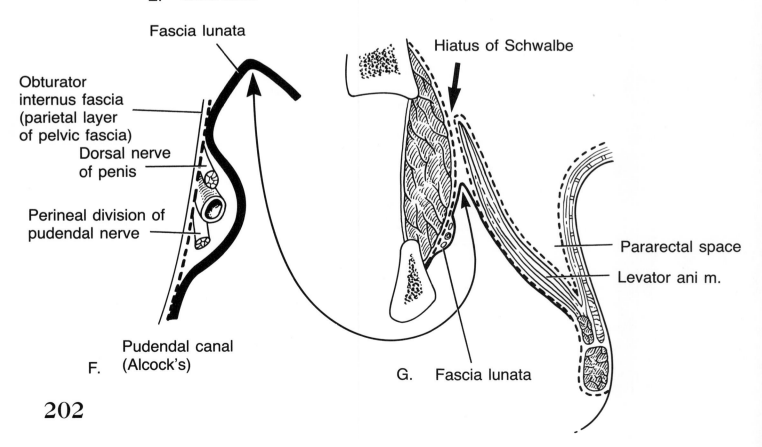

H. Weak areas of the ischiorectal fossa. The sizes of the arrows indicate the degrees of weakness. The weakest point is medial, through the area in contact with the fascia of the external anal sphincter.

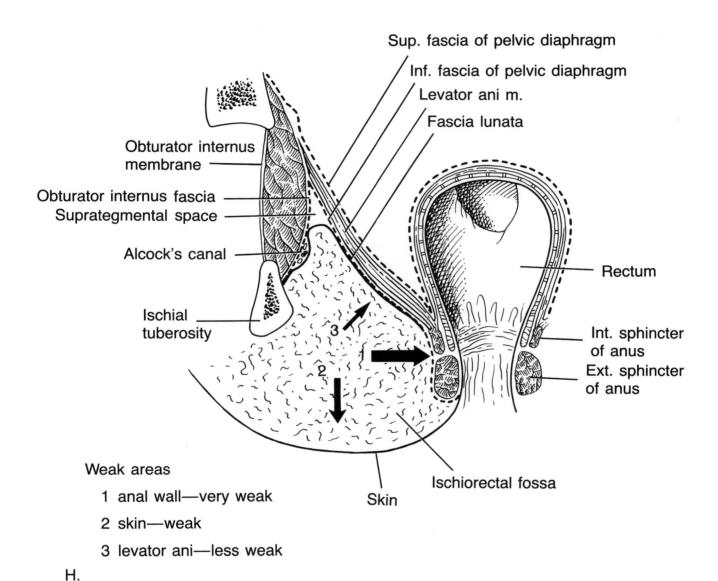

Sup. fascia of pelvic diaphragm

Inf. fascia of pelvic diaphragm

Levator ani m.

Fascia lunata

Obturator internus membrane

Obturator internus fascia

Suprategmental space

Alcock's canal

Ischial tuberosity

Rectum

Int. sphincter of anus

Ext. sphincter of anus

Ischiorectal fossa

Skin

Weak areas

1 anal wall—very weak

2 skin—weak

3 levator ani—less weak

H.

Repair of Perineal Hernia

Perineal Approach

The patient is placed in the lithotomy or the Trendelenburg position, depending on the location of the perineal bulge. A transverse or longitudinal skin incision over the swelling exposes the sac. The sac is opened and its contents reduced. The sac is excised and the ring is closed with nonabsorbable sutures. The muscles are approximated. This approach is not recommended except in rare instances.

Abdominal Approach

A lower midline incision is made with the patient in the Trendelenburg position. If incarceration or strangulation has occurred, free the intestinal loop from the sac. The viability of the intestinal loop must be evaluated. Any necrotic intestine must be resected and an end-to-end anastomosis performed.

The hernial sac is withdrawn, ligated, and excised, as in the case of other internal abdominal hernias. The surgeon may excise the sac or obliterate it. The hernial ring can be closed by sutures in the musculature if the ring is small, by suturing to the uterus or the broad ligament, or by using synthetic mesh.

Iatrogenic Perineal Hernia

A perineal hernia that occurs as the result of a radical perineal operation such as abdominoperineal resection or perineal prostatectomy is very rare. It is usually secondary to the loss of the levator ani muscle or pelvic fascia and the inability of the surgeon to close the defect.

Repair, whether by abdominal or perineal approach, is aimed at closing the hernial ring with any type of mesh, using anatomic entities such as the uterus, uterosacral ligaments, urogenital diaphragm, or any remnant of the pelvic floor. Other firm structures in the vicinity, such as periosteum or ligamentous tissue (from the sacrotuberous ligaments) of the ischial tuberosities or the inferior ischial ramus, can be used.

PLATE 58
Repair of Perineal Hernia—Perineal Approach

A. *Step 1.* Incise the skin over the swelling.

B. *Step 2.* Open the hernial sac and reduce the contents.

C. *Step 3.* Ligate and trim the sac.

D. *Step 4.* Suture the defect with nonabsorbable, interrupted sutures.

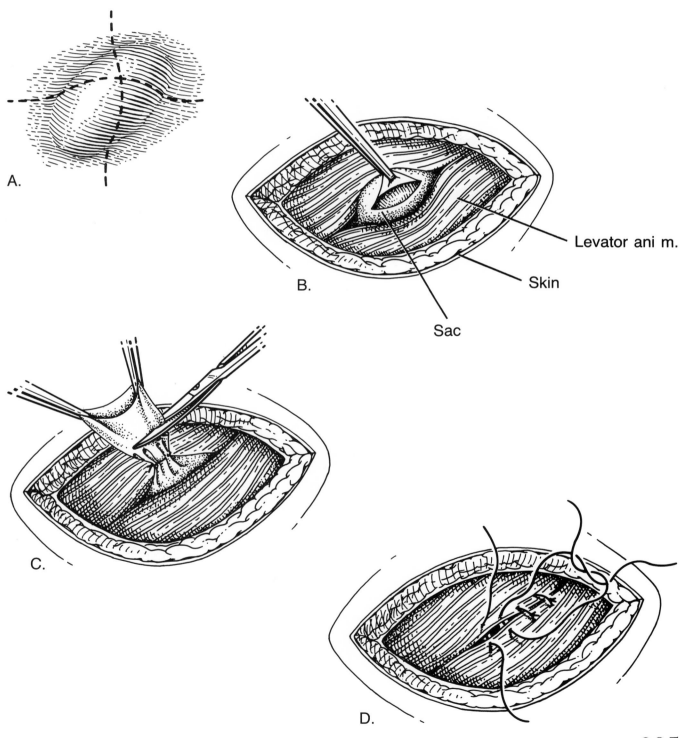

A.

B.

Levator ani m.

Skin

Sac

C.

D.

PLATE 59
Repair of Perineal Hernia—Abdominal Approach

A. *Step 3*

    a. Ligate the sac and approximate the uterosacral ligaments.

    b. Alternative procedure. Obliterate the sac with continuous sutures through the cervix and the rectal wall.

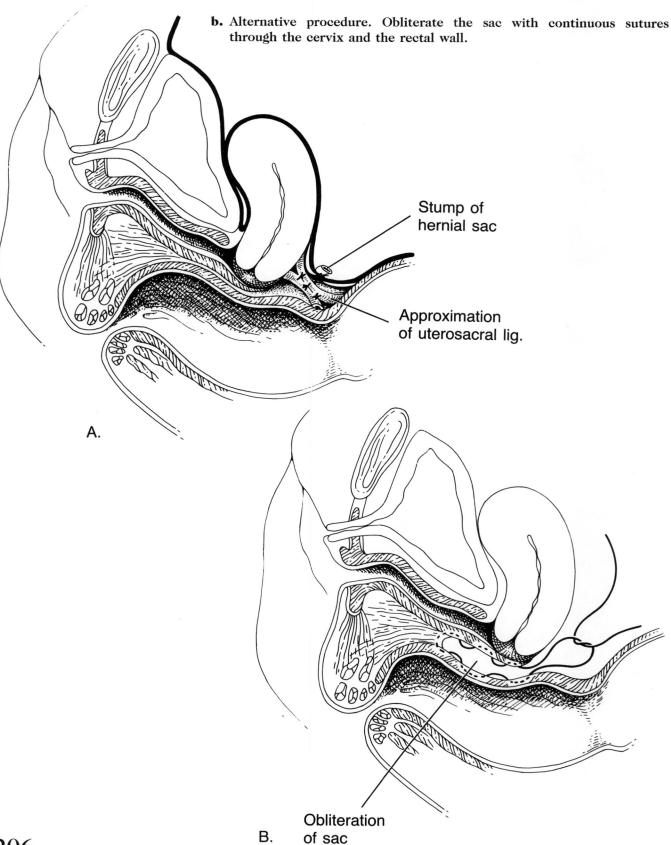

Stump of
hernial sac

Approximation
of uterosacral lig.

A.

B.   Obliteration
of sac

206

Rectal Prolapse

*Ye that will not apply new remedies must expect new
evils, for time is the great innovator.*

FRANCIS BACON

Definition

Rectal prolapse is a pathologic entity in which part or all layers of the rectum
are protruded mucosal side out through the surgical anal canal.

It is beyond the scope of this chapter to evaluate the concept of a sliding
hernia of the rectovaginal or rectovesical pouch, as opposed to the concept of
intussusception of the rectum. At the present time, the concept of intussusception is the most acceptable.

Anorectal Support

The anorectum is held in position by the following anatomical entities:

1. The rectal fascia (of Waldeyer) is a thin areolar tissue lateral, medial, and
   anterior to the rectum, becoming thicker posteriorly and anchoring the
   posterior surface of the rectum to the presacral fascia in the hollow of the
   sacrum. The superior rectal artery, the beginning of the internal iliac vein,
   the inferior mesenteric vein, and lymphatics are enveloped by the rectal
   fascia.
2. The lateral ligament of the rectum (rectal stalk) 2 to 3 cm above the pelvic
   diaphragm is thickened fascia anchoring the rectum to the third sacral
   vertebra. It contains the middle rectal artery as well as the pelvic splanchnic nerves (nervi erigentes) of the second and third or the third and fourth
   sacral nerves.
3. The pelvic diaphragm with its superior and inferior fasciae.
4. The urogenital diaphragm.
5. The anococcygeal ligament (posterior) and the perineal body (anterior).
6. Perianal and perirectal fat.
7. Sphincters of the anal canal.

Surgical Anatomy of the Anorectum

The Surgical Anal Canal
The surgeon and the anatomist are not always in agreement about the termi-
nology of the lower end of the rectum and the anal canal. To some anatomists,
the anal canal is the region distal to the pectinate line, whereas to the surgeon, the region distal to the insertion of the levator ani muscle on the rectum
is the anal canal.

We consider the *surgical anal canal,* the "anorectum" of Harkins, to
include the anatomic anal canal and the distal 2 cm or so of the rectum above
the pectinate line. Although this line marks a histologic junction, a vascular
divide, and an embryologic boundary, there are pathologic changes unique to
the 2 cm on either side of the line that define the surgical anal canal.

The Musculature of the Wall of the Anal Canal

Two layers of smooth muscle surround the anal canal. The outer, longitudinal coat lies between the internal and external sphincters. Above, it is continuous with the longitudinal muscularis externa of the rectal wall. Below, it terminates in the vicinity of the subcutaneous external sphincter.

Some longitudinal muscle fibers have been described as penetrating the internal sphincter to form the muscularis submucosae or the mucosal suspensory ligament of Parks. Parks described this ligament as a fibromuscular thickening around the anal crypts, attached both to mucosa and to the internal sphincter. Anatomically, the longitudinal muscle fibers appear to prevent separation of the sphincteric elements from each other; they also permit a slight telescopic movement between internal and external sphincters. We witness this in the operating room when the external sphincters roll back and the internal sphincter rolls forward.

The circular smooth muscle layer lies beneath the longitudinal layer. It becomes greatly thickened at the point where it forms the internal anal sphincter.

The External Sphincter

Unlike the longitudinal and circular muscles of the anal canal, which are composed of smooth muscle and arise from splanchnic mesoderm around the gut, the external sphincter consists of striated muscle and arises from somatic mesoderm. The external sphincter as a unit forms a sleeve around the distal two-thirds of the anal canal. At the middle one-third it lies over the internal sphincter and is separated from it by the longitudinal muscle.

The external sphincter has long been described as having three separate fiber bundles: subcutaneous, superficial, and deep. In normal, healthy individuals these bundles are continuous, with no gross or histologic evidence of separation, but it is useful to consider the three parts of the muscle separately.

The subcutaneous portion surrounds the outlet of the anus, with no apparent anterior or posterior attachments.

The superficial portion surrounds the anus and joins the anococcygeal ligament, which attaches posteriorly to the coccyx. This creates the triangular space of Minor behind the anus. Anteriorly, some fibers intermingle with the transverse perineal muscles at the perineal body, creating a potential space toward which anterior midline fistulae may point.

The deep portion, like the subcutaneous one, surrounds the canal, with no obvious anterior or posterior attachments.

The degree to which these portions, together with their anterior and posterior attachments, are separated from one another has been a source of controversy. We agree that no real separation exists between deep and superficial portions of the sphincter. We question, however, some of the anterior and posterior attachments shown in drawings. Our views are shown in Plate 63.

The Lining of the Surgical Anal Canal

The lining of the anal canal may be divided into three regions. The *cutaneous zone,* at the anal verge, is covered by pigmented skin with hair follicles and sebaceous glands. Within it lies the intersphincteric groove produced, according to Parks, by the mucosal suspensory ligament mentioned above. More certainly the groove merely indicates the division between the external sphincter below and the internal sphincter above.

208

Beyond the cutaneous zone lies the *transitional zone,* separated from the cutaneous zone by the anocutaneous line. It is about 1 cm wide and is covered by smooth skin having sebaceous glands but no hair. Its upper margin is the pectinate line (also called the dentate line), above which begins the true mucosa of the anal canal.

The *pectinate line* is the most important landmark in the anal canal. It marks the transition between the visceral area above and the somatic area below. The arterial supply, the venous and lymphatic drainage, the nerve supply, and the character of the lining all change at, or very near to the pectinate line.

The pectinate line is formed by the margins of the anal valves, small mucosal pockets between the 5 to 10 vertical folds of mucosa known as the anal columns of Morgagni. These columns extend upward from the pectinate line to the upper end of the surgical anal canal, at the level of the puborectalis sling. They are formed by underlying parallel bundles of the muscularis mucosae. The actual junction of stratified squamous and columnar epithelia is usually just above the pectinate line; hence, the mucocutaneous line is not always precisely equivalent to the pectinate line.

Anal Glands and Anal Papillae

The pockets formed by the anal valves are termed *anal sinuses.* From some of these, especially those on the posterior rectal wall, ducts lead downward and outward, reaching the intersphincteric longitudinal muscle and occasionally penetrating the internal sphincter. These glands appear to be vestigial structures; many lack mucus-secreting cells. Anal glands can become infected and provide pathways for anal fistulae.

Where the margins of the anal valves join the anal columns, some individuals have small projections, the anal papillae. In a few patients, one or more of these may become hypertrophied and, when large enough, may prolapse as a fibrous polyp as much as 2 cm long.

Arteries and Veins of the Rectum and Anal Canal

These are shown in Tables 6 and 7.

Lymphatics of the Rectum and Anal Canal

The lymphatics of the anal canal and lower rectum form plexuses in both the mucosal and submucosal layers. Those above the pectinate line drain into lymph nodes lying on the posterior surface of the rectal wall. Their efferent vessels ascend along the superior rectal artery to the sacral and lumbar nodes. Lymph vessels originating below the pectinate line drain to the medial group of subinguinal nodes.

Nerves of the Rectum and Anal Canal

The internal anal sphincter's motor innervation is supplied by parasympathetic fibers that cause contraction of the conjoined longitudinal muscle. These parasympathetic fibers are carried by the pelvic splanchnic nerves, branches of the ventral rami of S_2, S_3, and S_4. These nerves also carry visceral sensory fibers which mediate sensations of rectal distension. The external anal sphincter is innervated by the inferior rectal (hemorrhoidal) branch of the pudendal nerve and by the perineal branch of the fourth sacral nerve.

TABLE 6
Arteries of the Rectum and Anal Canal

Artery	Origin	Course	Supplies
Superior rectal (hemorrhoidal) artery	From inferior mesenteric artery	Descends to posterior wall of upper rectum	Bifurcates to supply posterior wall of upper rectum and lateral wall of mid-rectum down to pectinate line
Middle rectal (hemorrhoidal) artery	From internal iliac or branch thereof	Passes forward medially in lateral ligament of rectum	Anastomoses with inferior and superior rectal arteries
Inferior rectal (hemorrhoidal) artery	From internal pudendal artery	Passes ventrally and medially	Anal canal below the pectinate line
Median sacral artery	From aorta just above bifurcation	Descends beneath the peritoneum on lower lumbar vertebrae, sacrum, and coccyx	Posterior wall of rectum

TABLE 7
Veins of Rectum and Anal Canal

Vein	Origin	Drainage to
Superior rectal (hemorrhoidal) vein	Internal rectal venous plexus	Inferior mesenteric vein; portal nervous system
Middle rectal (hemorrhoidal) vein	External rectal venous plexus, bladder, prostate, and seminal vesicle	Internal iliac vein; systemic venous system
Inferior rectal (hemorrhoidal) vein	Lower portion of external rectal venous plexus	Internal pudendal vein; systemic venous system

The pelvic splanchnic nerves (parasympathetic) and the sympathetic fibers of the left and right pelvic plexuses supply the lower rectal wall. Together these nerves form the rectal plexus. The levator ani muscles receive skeletal motor supply from the third and the fourth sacral nerves.

The inferior rectal (hemorrhoidal) branches of the pudendal nerve mediate the sensory innervation of the perineal skin around the anus.

The Pelvic Diaphragm

The pelvic diaphragm forms the floor of the pelvis or the roof of the perineum and is composed of two paired muscles, the levator ani and the coccygeus.

The levator ani is itself formed by three muscles: the iliococcygeus, the pubococcygeus, and the puborectalis. Only the puborectalis muscle is important in maintaining rectal continence. This muscle originates from the posterior surface of the symphysis pubis and the superior layer of the deep perineal pouch (urogenital diaphragm). Fibers from each side of the muscle pass posteriorly and then join behind the rectum, forming a well-defined sling. The puborectalis muscle, together with the superficial and deep parts of the external sphincter and the proximal part of the internal sphincter, forms the so-called anorectal ring, which is responsible for the closing of the anorectal canal.

The pubococcygeus muscle is responsible for the integrity of the pelvic floor.

Peritoneum

The upper one-third of the rectum is almost completely enveloped by the peritoneum. As the rectum passes deeper into the pelvis, however, progressively more fat is interposed between the peritoneum and the rectal musculature. The peritoneum finally separates completely from the rectum and passes anteriorly and superiorly over the uterus or, in males, over the bladder. The mnemonic "rule of 4" (Plate 60C) will help the surgeon to remember the topographical anatomy of the peritoneum in relation to the rectum.

Spaces of the Pelvis

These are described in the chapter "Perineal Hernia."

Complications

The complications of the surgical treatment of rectal prolapse depend on the procedure chosen by the surgeon.

1. Anastomotic complications:
   Leakage
   Disruption of anastomosis
   Obstruction
2. Vascular injury. The following vessels should be protected to prevent bleeding:
   Left gastrohepatic artery and vein
   Left splenic polar artery
   Renocolic vessels
   Left gonadal vein
   Marginal artery
   Middle colic artery
   Vein of the left pelvic wall
   Presacral venous plexus
   Superior, middle, and inferior rectal veins
3. Organ injury:
   Ureters
   Spleen
   Pancreas
   Prostate
   Seminal vesicles
   Vagina
   Urinary bladder
4. Nerve injury:
   Autonomic nerve injury with bladder dysfunction and impotence
5. Inadequate procedures
   Failure to close mesenteric defect

PLATE 60
The Rectum and the Surgical Anal Canal

A. Diagram of the structures of the anus and rectum. The surgical anal canal is defined as 2 cm above and below the pectinate line. IRA = inferior rectal artery; MRA = middle rectal artery; SRA = superior rectal artery; LRV = lower rectal valve; MRV = middle rectal valve; SRV = superior rectal valve. Arrows indicate direction of lymphatic drainage.

Source: Plate 60A,B from Gray SW, Skandalakis JE: *Atlas of Surgical Anatomy for General Surgeons.* Williams & Wilkins, Baltimore, 1985, p. 248, Plate 10-9.

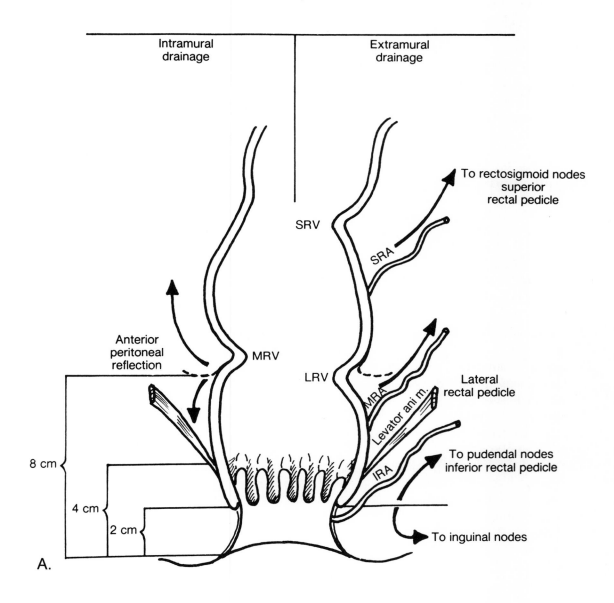

B. Functional and anatomical changes at the pectinate line.

C. The segments of the rectum and the anal canal and peritoneal relations.

Source: Plate 60C from Skandalakis JE, Gray SW, Olafson RP: Surgical embryology, anatomy and physiology of the anal canal with some clinical applications, in ΤΙΜΗΤΙΚΟΣ ΤΟΜΟΣ (Honorary Volume), volume in honor of CN Alvisatos. Privately published, Athens, Greece, 1976, p. 449.

Change	Above the Pectinate Line	Below the Pectinate Line
Embryonic origin	Endoderm	Ectoderm
Anatomy:		
Epithelial lining	Simple columnar	Stratified squamous
Arterial supply	Superior rectal artery	Inferior rectal artery
Venous drainage	Portal, by way of superior rectal vein	Systemic, by way of inferior rectal vein
External lymphatic drainage	To pelvic and lumbar nodes	To inguinal nodes
Nerve supply	Autonomic fibers (visceral)	Inferior rectal nerves (somatic)
Physiology	Sensation quickly diminishes	Excellent sensation
Pathology:		
Cancer	Adenocarcinoma	Squamous cell carcinoma
Varices	Internal hemorrhoids	External hemorrhoids

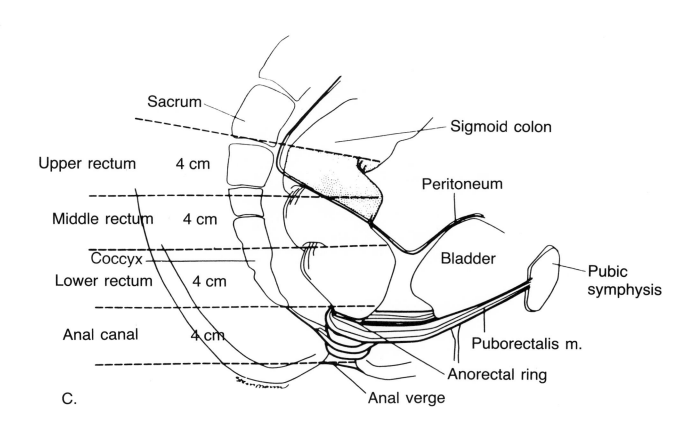

C.

213

PLATE 61

Normal Structures Holding the Anorectum in Place

A. Sagittal section through the female pelvis. The fascia of Waldeyer surrounds the rectum, anchoring the posterior surface of the rectum to the presacral fascia of the sacrum.

B. Diagrammatic coronal section of the pelvis and the surgical anal canal. The levator ani muscle, with its superior and inferior fascial sheaths, probably supplies the greatest support.

The lateral rectal pedicle or rectal stalk, shown diagrammatically in Plate 60A, is a thick fascia anchoring the rectum to the third sacral vertebra. It contains the parasympathetic pelvic splanchnic nerve fibers from the second and third or the third and fourth sacral nerves, as well as from the middle rectal artery.

For other structures contributing to the support of the rectum, see page 207.

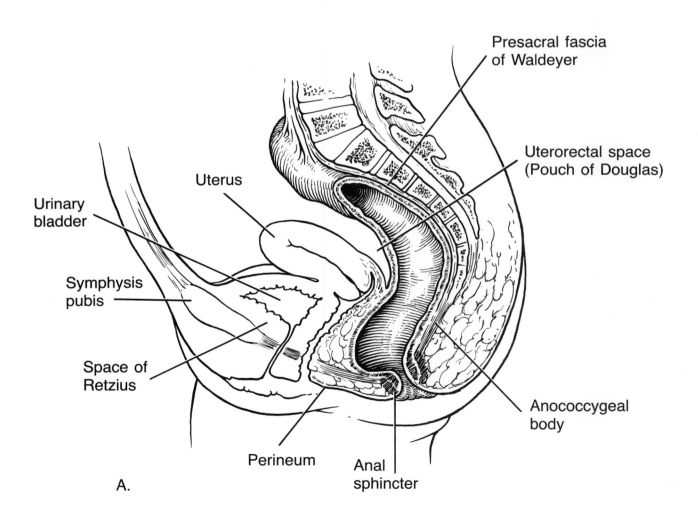

Presacral fascia
of Waldeyer

Uterorectal space
(Pouch of Douglas)

Uterus

Urinary
bladder

Symphysis
pubis

Space of
Retzius

Anococcygeal
body

Perineum

Anal
sphincter

A.

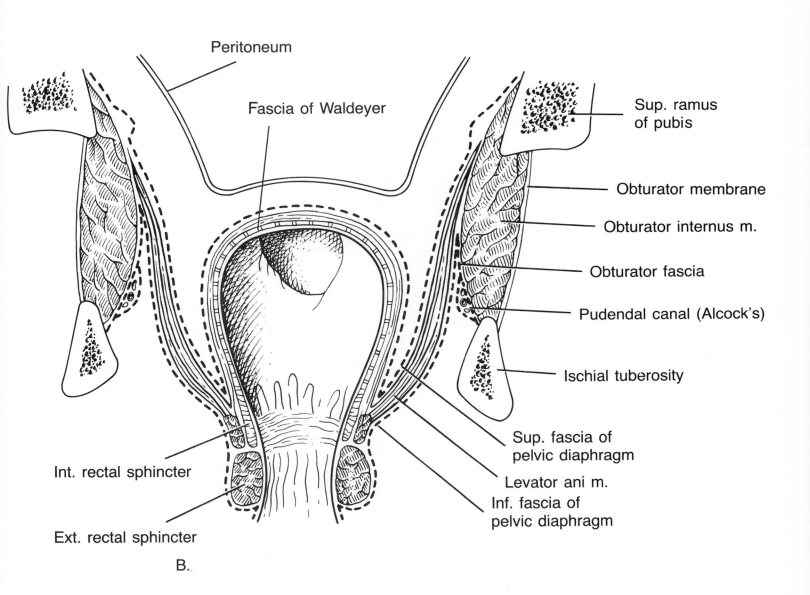

Peritoneum

Fascia of Waldeyer

Sup. ramus
of pubis

Obturator membrane

Obturator internus m.

Obturator fascia

Pudendal canal (Alcock's)

Ischial tuberosity

Sup. fascia of
pelvic diaphragm

Levator ani m.

Inf. fascia of
pelvic diaphragm

Int. rectal sphincter

Ext. rectal sphincter

B.

215

PLATE 62

The Female Pelvic Diaphragm and Related Structures

A. Seen from above.

B. Seen from below.

Remember: Relaxation of the pelvic diaphragm may result in enterocele, but not in rectal prolapse, which is a true intussusception.

Source: Plate 62A,B from Gray SW, Skandalakis JE: *Atlas of Surgical Anatomy for General Surgeons.* Williams & Wilkins, Baltimore, 1985, p. 257, Fig. 10-13.

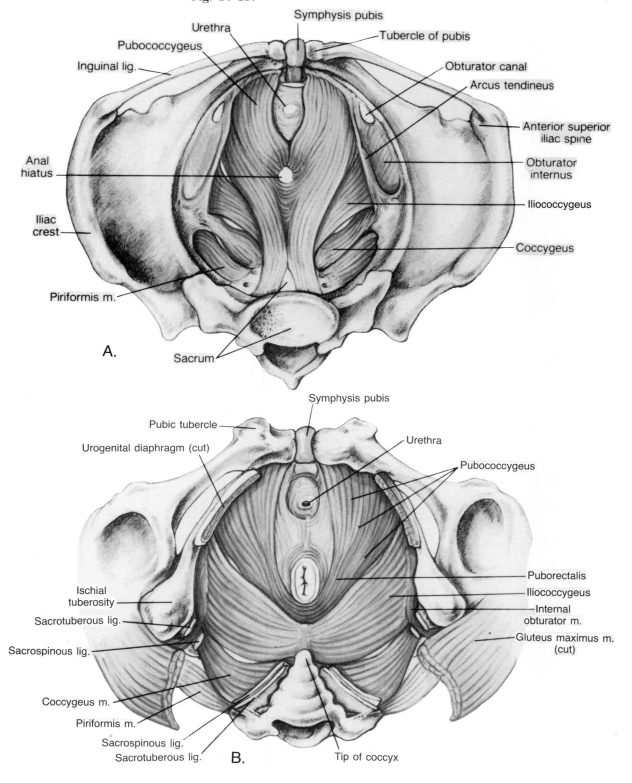

PLATE 63

The Anal Sphincter

A. Coronal section through the anal canal showing the relations of the internal and external sphincters and levator ani muscles to the wall of the anal canal.

B. Diagram of the triple loop system of Shafik. The deep portion and puborectalis are considered to act as a unit.

Source: Plate 63A,B from Gray SW, Skandalakis JE: *Atlas of Surgical Anatomy for General Surgeons.* Williams & Wilkins, Baltimore, 1985, A: p. 236, Fig. 10-13; B: p. 260.

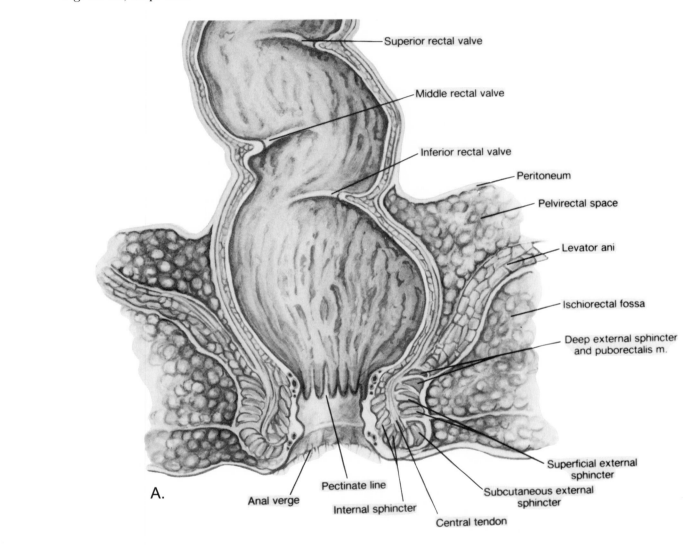

A.

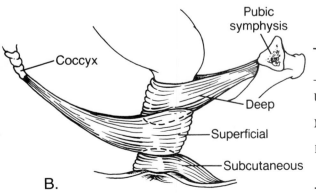

B.

	Composition	Nerve Supply
Upper loop	Puborectalis muscle and deep external sphincter.	Inferior rectal branch of the pudendal nerve
Middle loop	Superficial external sphincter.	Perineal branch of the fourth sacral nerve
Base loop	Subcutaneous external sphincter; those fibers insert on the perianal skin.	Inferior rectal nerve

PLATE 64
Nerve Supply of the Anal Sphincters

The functional autonomic nerve supply to the anal canal and lower rectum. Note that the striated muscle of the external sphincter and the levatores ani are innervated by the somatic fibers of the pudendal nerve.

Source: Plate 64 from Skandalakis JE, Gray SW, Olafson RP: Surgical embryology, anatomy and physiology of the anal canal with some clinical applications, in ΤΙΜΗΤΙΚΟΣ ΤΟΜΟΣ (Honorary Volume), volume in honor of CN Alvisatos. Privately published, Athens, Greece, 1976.

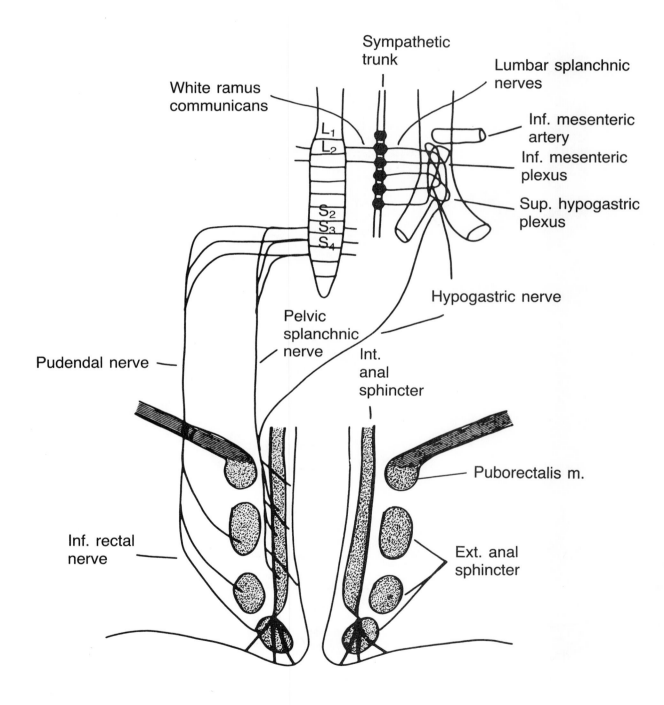

PLATE 65
Development of Rectal Prolapse

A. Sagittal section through the normal pelvis.

B. Start of rectal prolapse. The proximal segment (intussusceptum) is telescoping into the distal segment (intussuscipiens).

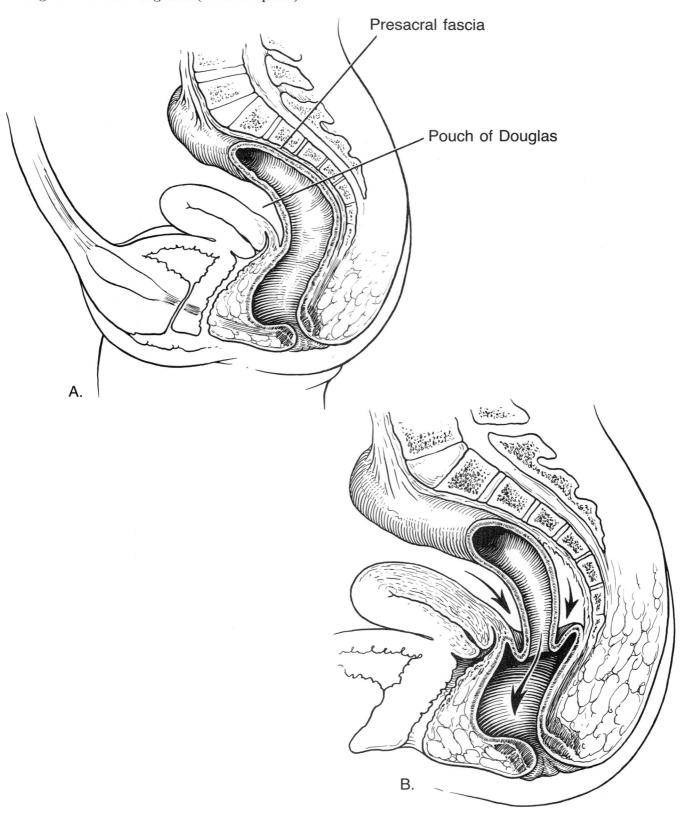

Presacral fascia

Pouch of Douglas

A.

B.

PLATE 65 (*Continued*)
Development of Rectal Prolapse

C. Intussusceptum at the pectinate line.

D. Intussusceptum protrudes through the anus.

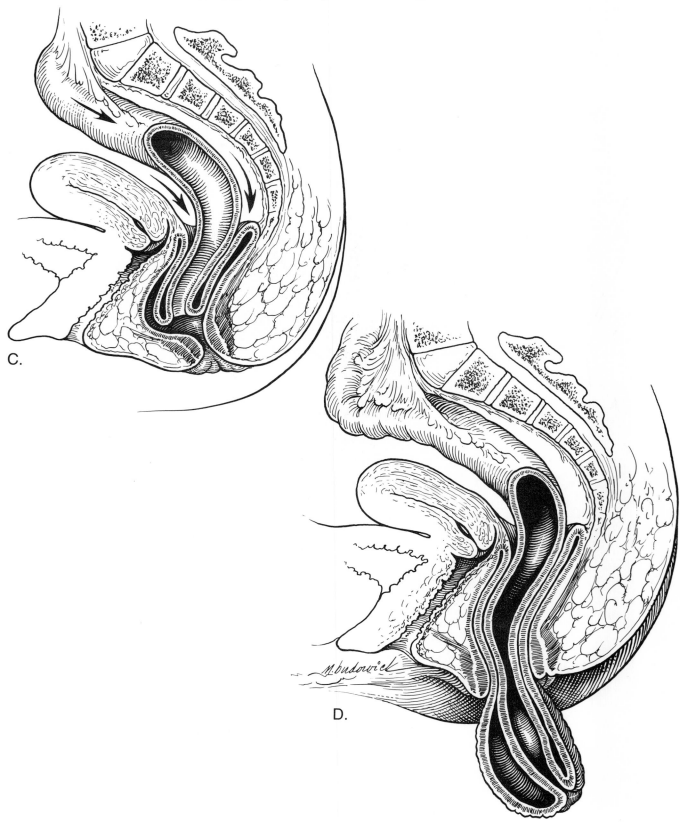

C.

D.

E. Coronal section through the anal canal showing prolapse beginning. Compare with sagittal section (Plate 65B).

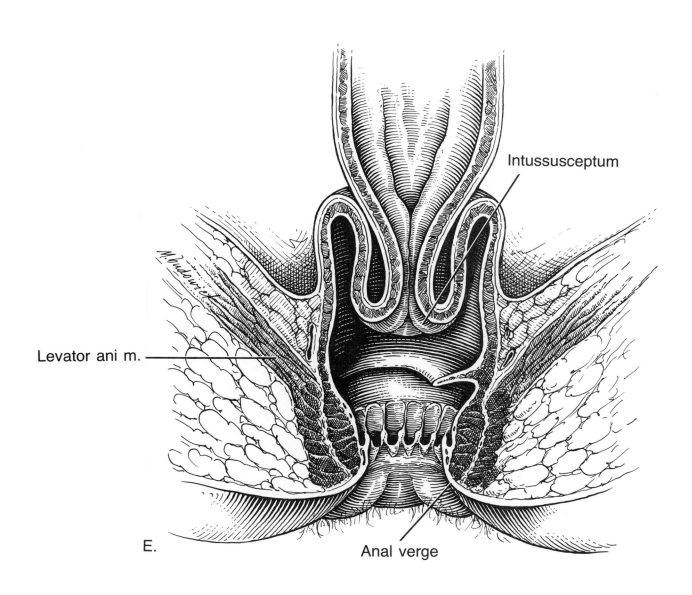

Intussusceptum

Levator ani m.

E.

Anal verge

PLATE 66
Treatment of Rectal Prolapse—Perineal Approach

A. *Step 1.* Place the patient in the lithotomy position with the prolapsed rectum protruding from the anus. The mucosa forms the external surface.

B. *Step 2.* With the patient in the lithotomy position, pull down the prolapsed rectum. Place stay sutures at the pectinate line.

C. *Step 3.* Make a circumferential incision through the rectal wall, above the pectinate line to preserve the sphincter muscles. Retract the incised rectal wall downward.

D. *Step 4.* Put traction on the exterior coats (intussuscipiens) to identify the lowest point of the rectouterine pouch (of Douglas).

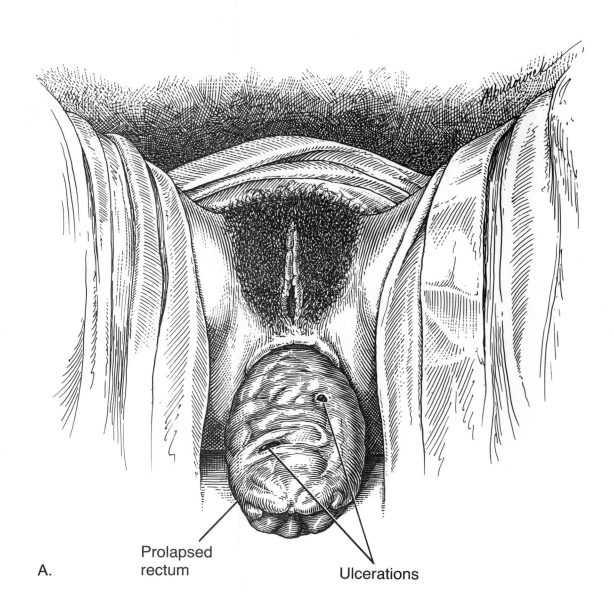

Prolapsed
rectum

A.

Ulcerations

222

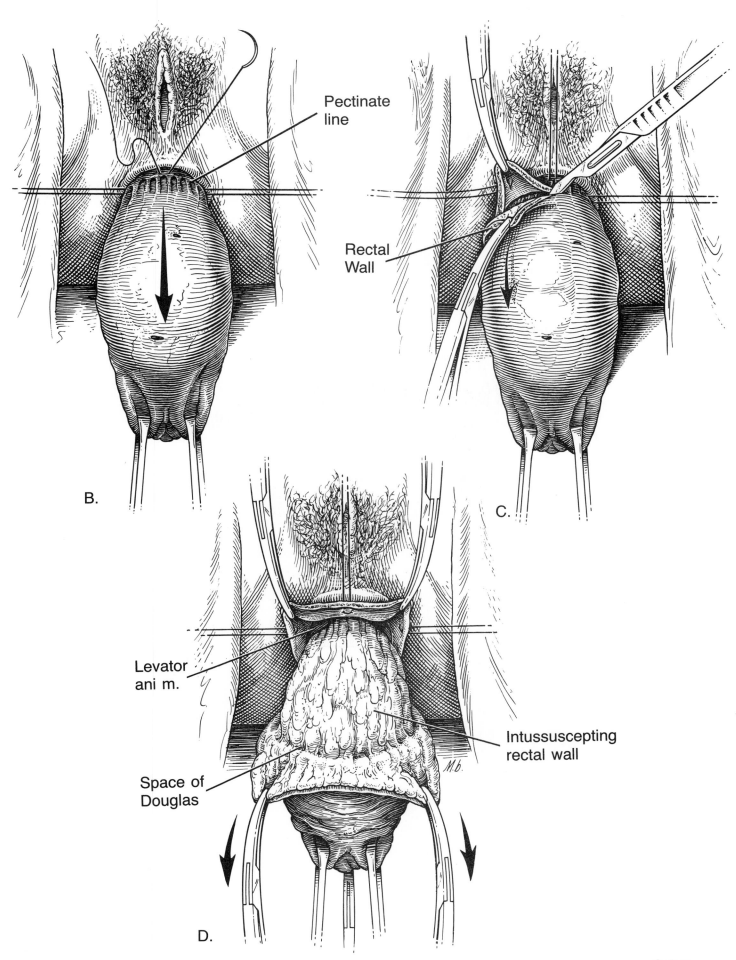

Pectinate line

Rectal Wall

B.

C.

Levator ani m.

Space of Douglas

Intussuscepting rectal wall

D.

223

PLATE 66 (*Continued*)

Treatment of Rectal Prolapse—Perineal Approach

E. *Step 5.* Incise the peritoneum at the rectouterine pouch. Visualize the pelvic diaphragm.

F. The peritoneum is opened and the sigmoid colon exposed.

G. *Step 6.* Excise the redundant peritoneal sac.

H. *Step 7.* Mobilize and apply traction to pull down the redundant sigmoid colon as far as possible.

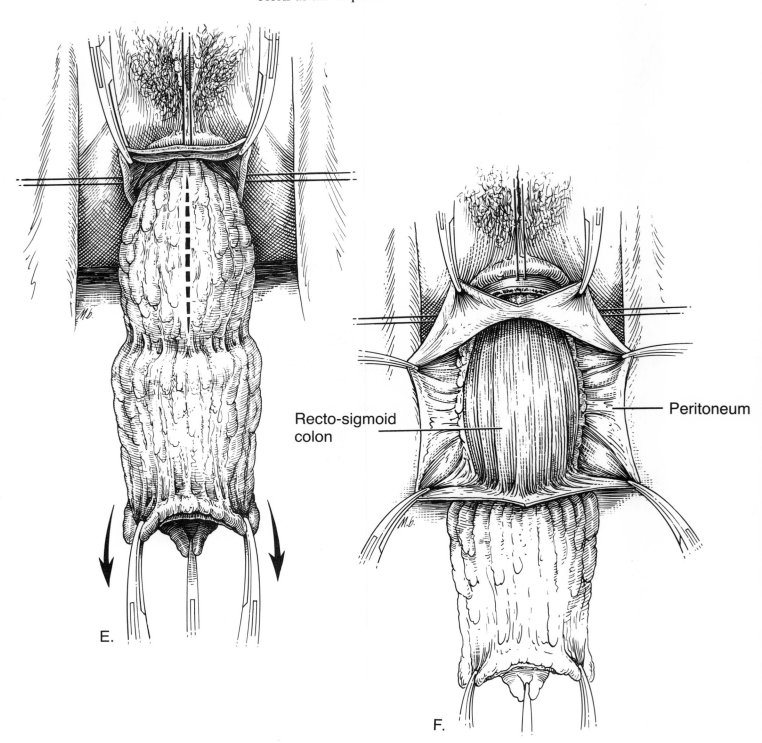

Recto-sigmoid colon

Peritoneum

E.

F.

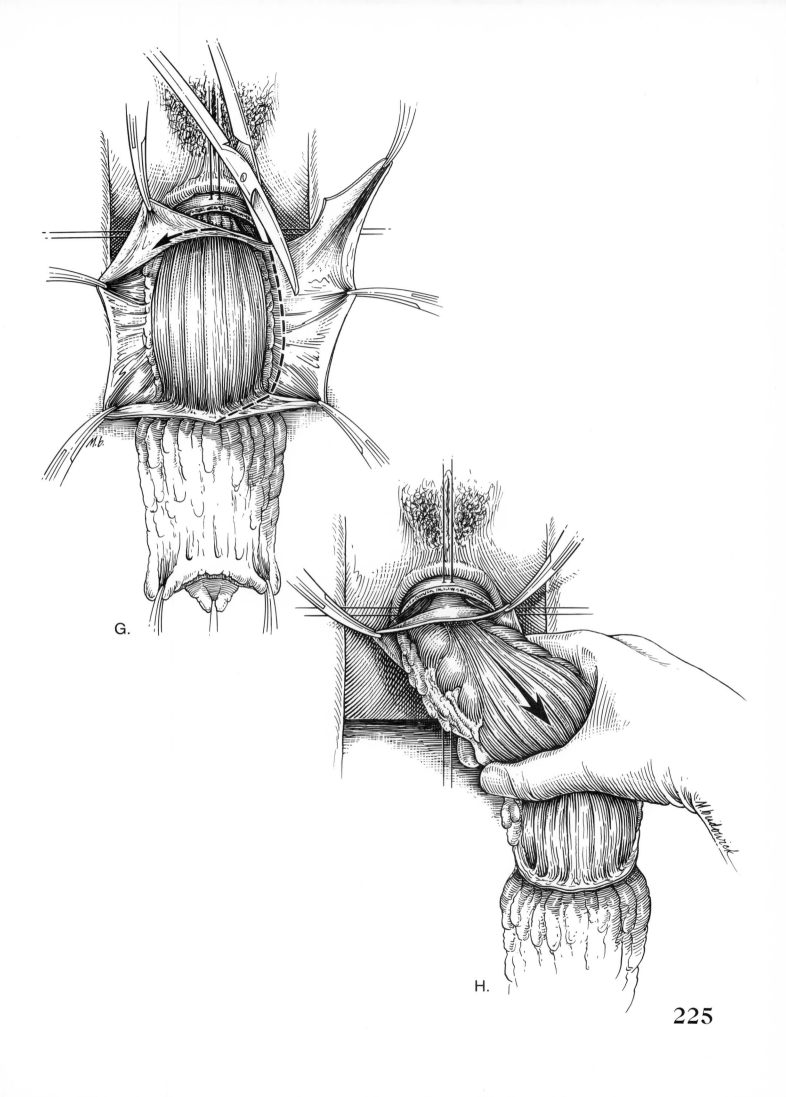

G.

H.

225

PLATE 66 (*Continued*)

Treatment of Rectal Prolapse—Perineal Approach

I. *Step 8.* Divide the rectosigmoid vessels between proximal and distal ligation.

J. *Step 9.* Suture the peritoneum to the upper proximal colon, obliterating the rectouterine pouch.

K. *Step 10.* Suture the levator ani muscles anterior to the peritoneal suture line.

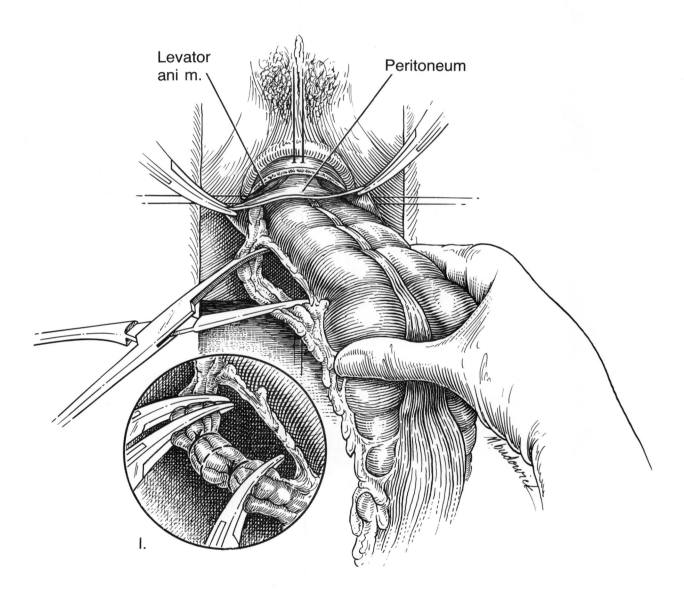

Levator ani m.

Peritoneum

I.

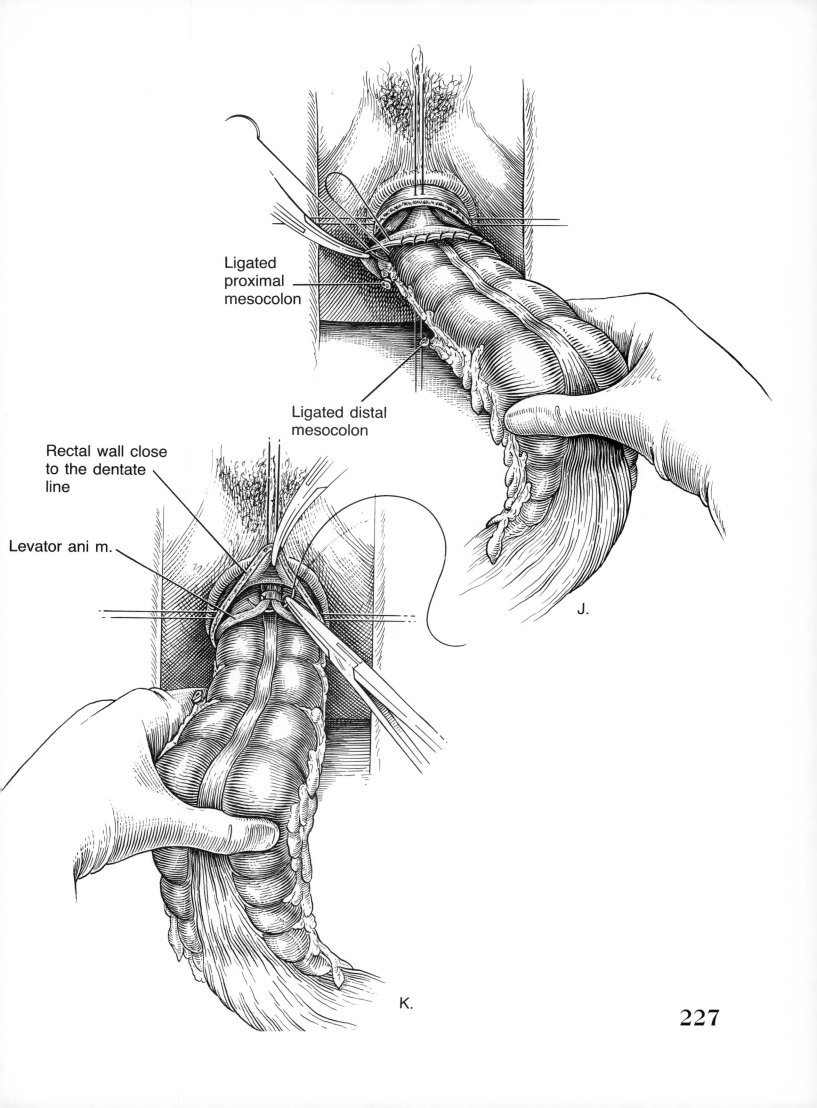

Ligated
proximal
mesocolon

Ligated distal
mesocolon

Rectal wall close
to the dentate
line

Levator ani m.

J.

K.

227

PLATE 66 (*Continued*)

Treatment of Rectal Prolapse—Perineal Approach

L. *Step 11.* Begin amputation of the sigmoid colon.

M. *Step 12.* Begin anastomosis of the sigmoid colon to the anus in two layers in the area of the dentate line.

N. *Step 13.* Complete the amputation of the sigmoid colon.

O. *Step 14.* Complete the anastomosis.

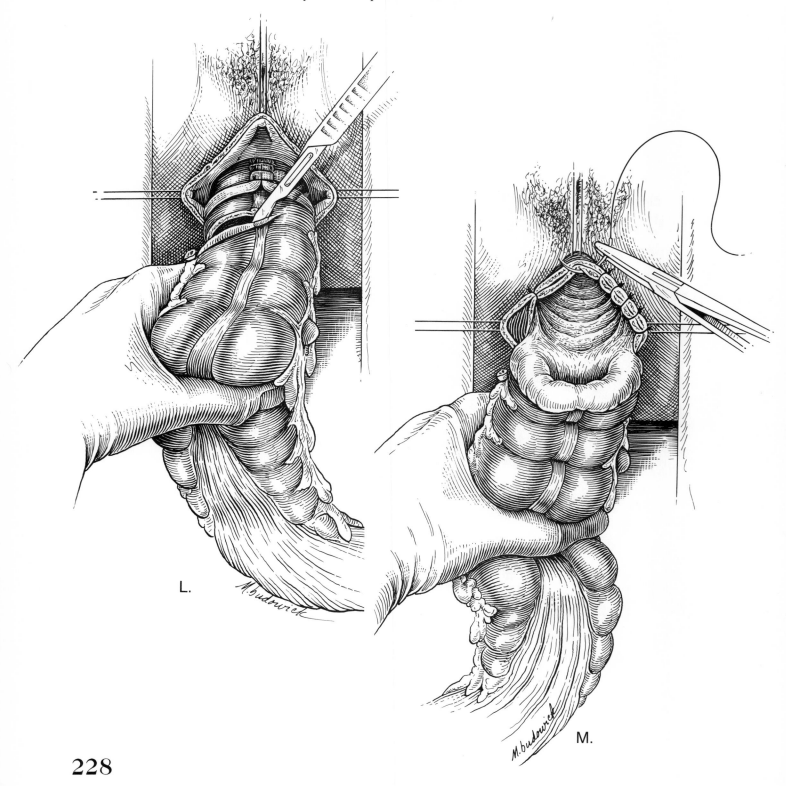

L.

M.

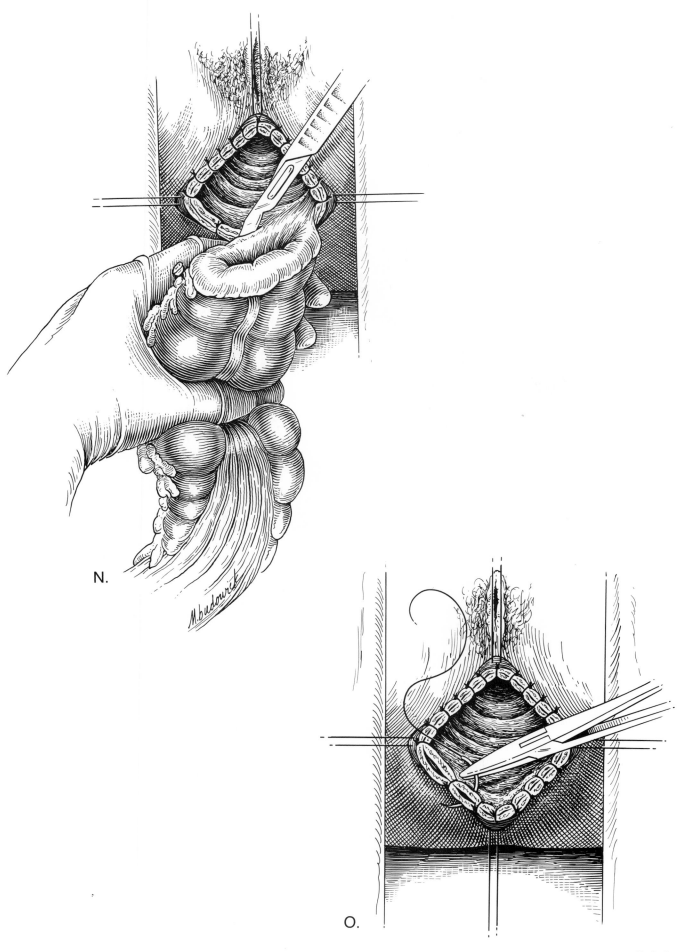

N.

O.

PLATE 66 (*Continued*)

Treatment of Rectal Prolapse—Perineal Approach

P.–S. Steps in completion of the two-layered anastomosis.

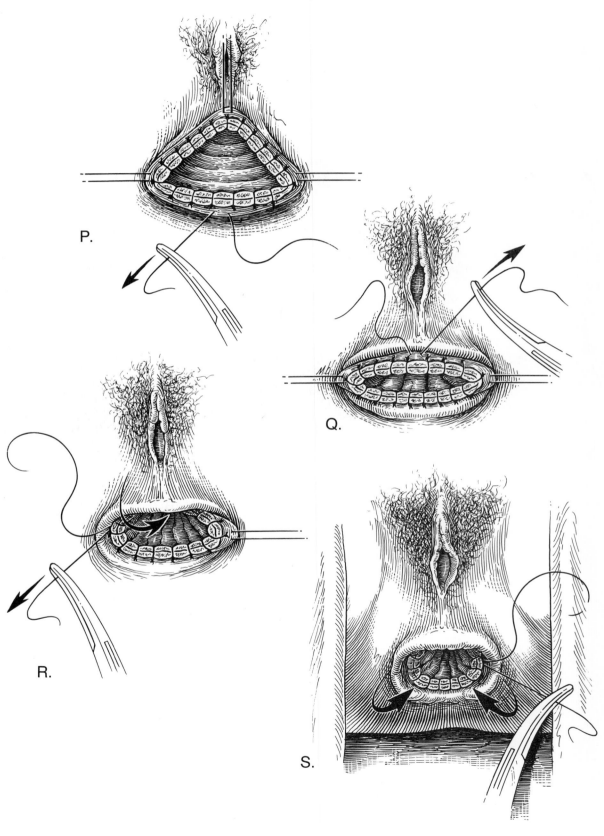

P.

Q.

R.

S.

T. Finished operation: The anastomosis is pushed into the anus.

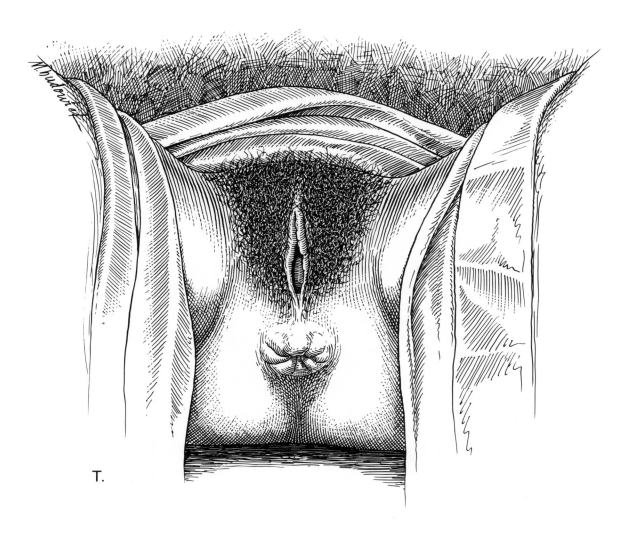

T.

PLATE 67

Perineal Approach—Thiersch Procedure and Some Modifications

These procedures are suitable for elderly or debilitated patients.

A. *1.* Insert two 20-gauge silver wires through short anterior and posterior incisions. The wires should pass 1.5 cm lateral to the anal verge. The wire should be tightened over the surgeon's finger.

B. *2.* Insert long hypodermic needles lateral to the anus, which is stretched into an anteroposterior straight line. The silver wires may be passed through the needles, which are then redrawn.

C. The wire should be tightened to fit snugly around the assistant's finger, which is inserted as deeply as possible into the anal canal.

D. *3.* Insert a Mersilene or Prolene suture through bilateral incisions into the perianal tissues. Pull the suture so that the anus fits snugly over the first joint of the surgeon's index finger.

E. *4.* Pass a Silastic sling through bilateral incisions and a perianal tunnel as in D above.

Source: Plate 68A,B,C from Welch CE, Ottinger LW, Welch J: *Manual of Lower Gastrointestinal Surgery.* Springer-Verlag, New York, 1980; Plate 68D,E from Roberts PL, Veidenheimer M: Rectal prolapse. *Surgical Rounds,* December 1987, p. 24, Figs. 4, 5.

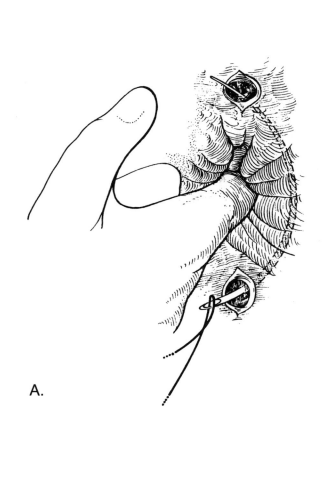

A.

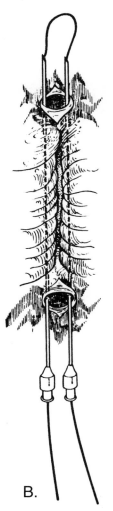

B.

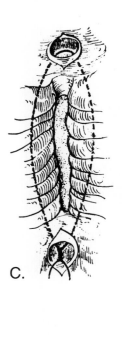

C.

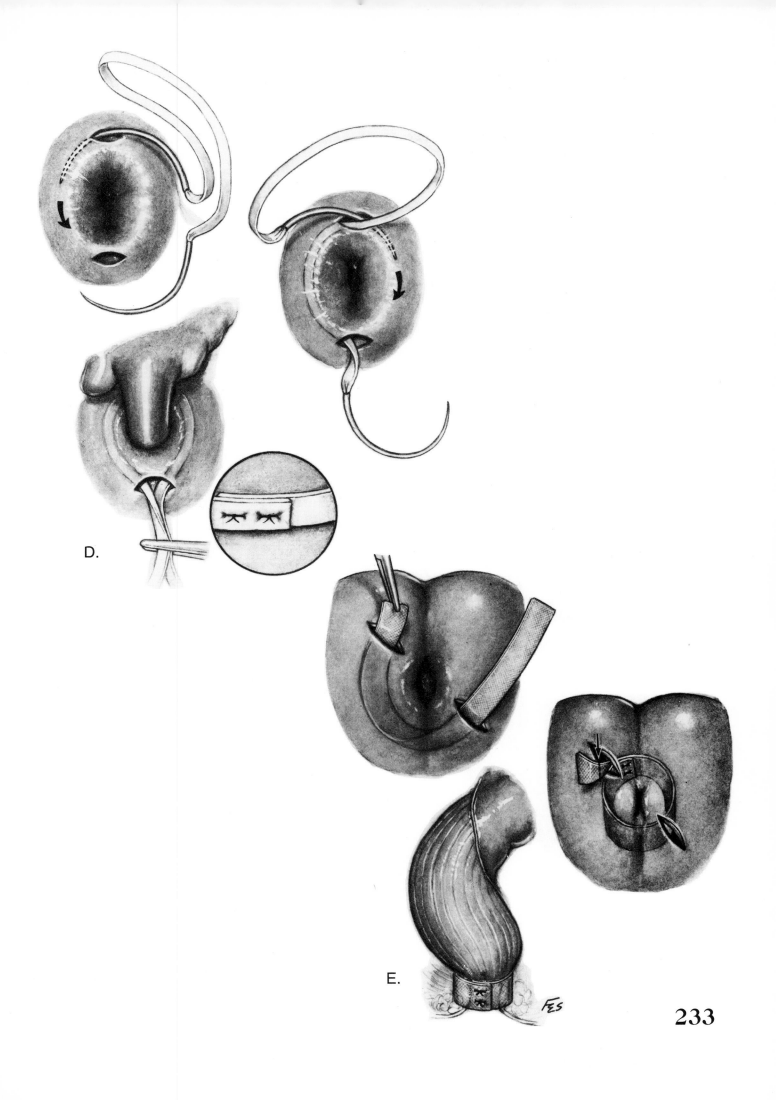

D.

E.

233

PLATE 68
Abdominal Approach—Rectopexy of Frykman-Goldberg

Several abdominal procedures for repair of rectal prolapse have been developed.

A. Completely mobilize the rectum down to the pelvic diaphragm, preserving the lateral ligaments (rectal stalks). Pull taut the rectum, peritoneum, rectal fascia, and rectal wall.

B. Suture these structures to the presacral fascia just below the promontory of the sacrum with 000 silk.

Remember: The surgeon must stay close to the posterior rectal wall to prevent impotence, neurogenic bladder, or bleeding from the venous plexus under the presacral fascia.

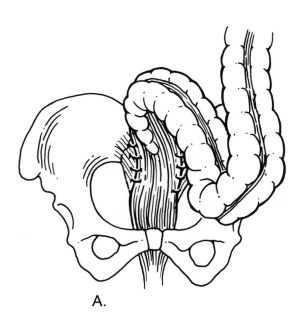

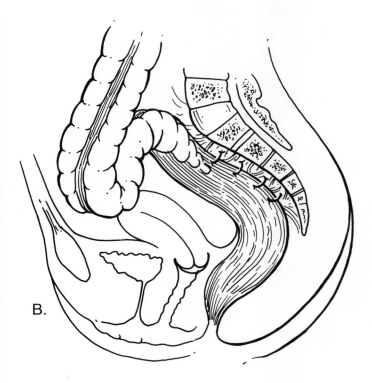

A.

B.

PLATE 69

Abdominal Approach—Low Anterior Resection

A. Completely mobilize the rectum.

B. Perform a low anterior resection of the rectum.

C. Perform an end-to-end anastomosis.

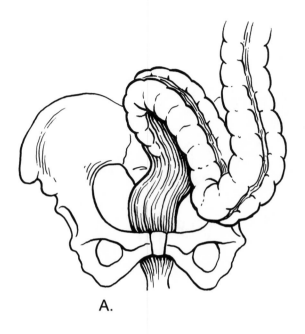

A.

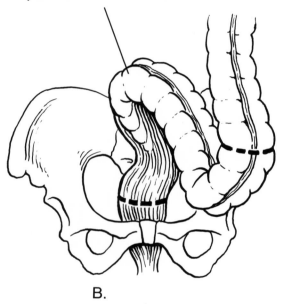

Specimen of low anterior resection

B.

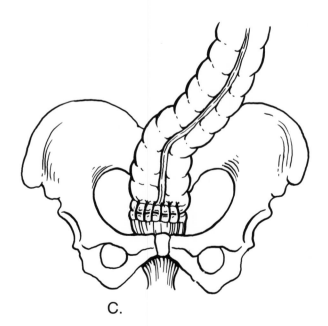

C.

PLATE 70
Abdominal Approach—Combination Procedure

A. Combine the first two procedures.

B. *Roscoe Graham Procedure* (not illustrated)
Mobilize the rectum. Expose and suture the levator muscles anterior to the rectum. Excise the rectouterine pouch.

C. Combine the first four procedures above (not illustrated).

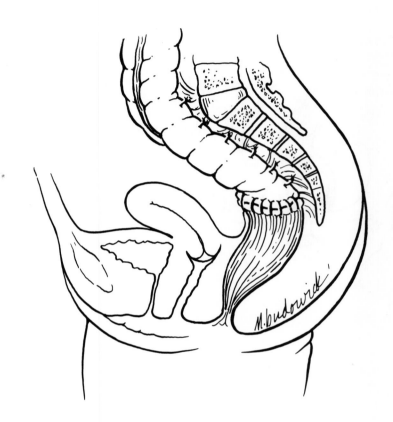

236

PLATE 71
Rectal Sling Procedure of Ripstein

Mobilize the rectum and pull it taut. Place a 5-cm band of Teflon or Marlex mesh around the rectum 5 cm below the promontory of the sacrum, suturing the free ends to the presacral fascia with 000 interrupted silk sutures.

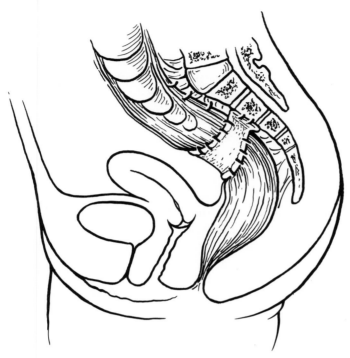

PLATE 72
Ivalon sponge wrap operation of Wells

Mobilize the rectum and pull it taut. Suture a rectangular sheet of Ivalon sponge to the presacral fascia; wrap the sponge over the rectum and suture it to the lateral, but not the anterior, surfaces of the rectum.

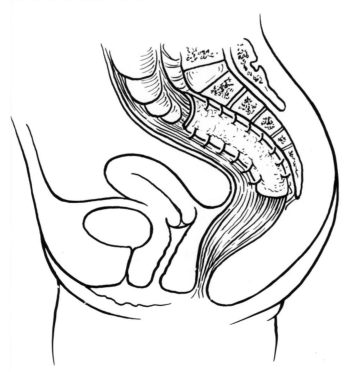

Pelvic Support Defects in Women (Urethrocele, Cystocele, Uterine Prolapse, Enterocele, and Rectocele)

For those who have dissected or inspected many, have at least learn'd to doubt when the others, who are ignorant of anatomy, and do not take the trouble to attend to it, are in no doubt at all.

GIOVANNI BATTISTA MORGAGNI (1682–1771)
De Sedibus et Causis Morborium, Vol I, Book 2, Letter 16 (tr. by
B. Alexander)

Definition

Urethrocele, cystocele, uterine prolapse, enterocele, and rectocele all occur as a result of some weakness of the tissue supporting the floor of the female pelvis. When a loss of the integrity of the supporting tissue occurs, one or more extraperitoneal viscera are pushed outward; the defect is then named according to the viscus so displaced.

Thus, to understand pelvic support defects in the female, one must remember that the pathologic anatomy is a weakness in the pelvic portion of the wall of the cavity, not a problem of the displaced organs. Although some texts speak of "uterine supports" or "bladder supports" as though these organs were suspended in some way from above, in fact all of the visceral structures rest upon or are contained within the floor of the abdominopelvic cavity. They will not fall out; they are always pushed out by pressure from within.

Our attention, therefore, should be directed to that portion of the wall of the cavity that extends down into the bony pelvis, its strength and structure, and the pathologic anatomy present when there is a urethrocele, cystocele, enterocele, rectocele, or uterine prolapse.

Anatomy of the Pelvic Portion of the Abdominopelvic Cavity

The walls of the pelvic portion of the abdominopelvic cavity are a combination of active and passive supporting tissues. Active supports are the striated muscles that are attached to the bones. They are capable of contracting and strengthening the wall in response to sudden load changes. Passive supports are those incapable of changing in response to sudden pressure changes. They consist of (1) bones of the pelvis (ilium, ischium, pubis, sacrum, and coccyx) and (2) connective tissue. Lining the abdominopelvic cavity and covering the retroperitoneal organs is the peritoneum, which contributes little to the support of the pelvic wall.

Connective tissue covers the muscles and some of the viscera and surrounds and accompanies the major blood vessels. Depending upon such characteristics as orientation, organization, and strength of connective tissue bundles or layers, in places it is referred to as "ligaments" and in other areas it is called "fasciae." In areas where it contains a large amount of smooth muscle, it may be referred to as muscle or muscularis.

238

In the pelvis, connective tissue plays an important role in maintaining the strength of the bottom of the cavity containing the viscera, for these passive supports maintain the structures in their normal position at rest. The active supports reinforce the walls in response to transitory changes in intra-abdominal pressure.

The female pelvic cavity—containing the lower sigmoid colon, rectum, uterus, and bladder—is not spherical. It is rounded posteriorly at the sacrum, with slightly converging sidewalls that come forward to the back of the pubic symphysis anteriorly, and has an irregularly convex inferior surface. The pelvic side walls are provided by the sacrum posteriorly; the piriformis, coccygeus, obturator internus, and levator muscles laterally; and the symphysis anteriorly.

The bottom of this space is closed by those soft tissues that close the space between bones and is usually referred to as the *pelvic floor*. Resting upon or contained within this floor are the urethra, bladder, vagina, uterus, and rectum.

The pelvis contains essentially three layers of supporting tissue. From above downward, these layers are (1) a network of connective tissue surrounding the viscera and major vessels and overlying the striated muscles (described by Curtis, Anson, and McVay[1] as the endopelvic fascia); (2) the fairly strong striated muscles (levator ani and coccygeus); and (3) the urogenital diaphragm with its attached underlying perineal muscles and fascia. The three layers do not parallel each other. Each varies in thickness from place to place. Together they form the floor of the cavity containing the abdominal and pelvic viscera.

In the female, the pelvic floor is perforated by the vagina and cervix, the urethra, and the rectum. It is this pelvic floor that must stretch or dilate sufficiently for the birth of an infant. This stretching or dilatation of the pelvic floor in the birth process is often responsible for tears and subsequent failure.

Support Defects

All support defects involve some break in the continuity of support from one or more layers of the pelvic floor.

In the uppermost layer (connective tissue), a break can contribute to the occurrence of a urethrocele, cystocele, uterine prolapse, or enterocele. There may or may not be defects in the other two layers. These hernias can occur with intact levator ani muscles and a good urogenital diaphragm.

In the bottom layer (urogenital diaphragm and perineum), an isolated break can result in a rectocele and a deformed perineum. Again, the other two layers may remain intact.

In the middle layer (levator ani and coccygeus muscles) alone, a weakness or tear does not result in a specific hernia or prolapse. However, because these muscles support the layer above, any major weakness or tear will predispose to the development of urethrocele, cystocele, uterine prolapse, or enterocele.

[1]Curtis AH, Anson BJ, McVay CB: The anatomy of the pelvic and urogenital diaphragms in relation to urethrocele and cystocele. *Surg Gynecol Obstet* 68:161, 1939.

Since the gynecologist tends to view the world from below and through a vaginal speculum, it has been traditional to group the pelvic support defects according to whether they bulge the anterior vaginal wall, the upper portion of the vagina, or the posterior vaginal wall, and to speak of these as anterior segment, central segment, or posterior segment defects. In turn, when viewed from above, the pelvic floor can also be arbitrarily divided into three segments: anterior, central, and posterior. Defects that begin in the anterior segment will bulge the anterior vaginal wall, those in the central segment will displace the upper vagina, and those in the posterior segment will bulge the posterior vaginal wall.

This division is artificial because the pelvic floor is an entity in itself. It provides a continuity of support from symphysis to sacrum and from ischial spine to ischial spine at its uppermost layer and from the under edge of the symphysis to the coccyx and from ischial tuberosity to ischial tuberosity at its lowest layer.

When the continuity of support gives way, it tends to do so from a single break, not from generalized stretching or attenuation. Although there may be more than one break, the breaks tend to be isolated and identifiable. Once such a break occurs, it tends to spread further without additional breaks in the immediate area.

Thus, before attempting to repair any support defect, it is necessary to locate the break or breaks and repair them directly by restoration of normal anatomy. Only in extreme circumstances will the procedure of choice be the creation of a compensatory abnormality, leaving the patient with distorted and abnormal anatomy.

Some Anatomical Entities Related to Pelvic Support Defects in Women

In general: Pelvic peritoneum
Endopelvic fascia
Levator ani muscle (pelvic floor)
Urogenital diaphragm
Superficial perineal pouch
Perineal muscles and fascia

Specifically: Ligaments of the urethra
Ligaments of the bladder
Ligaments of the uterus
Fascial covering of obturator internus and levator muscles
Arcus tendineous fascia pelvis (white line)
Arcus tendineous levator ani
Muscles, vessels, nerves

Pelvic Peritoneum
In the pelvis, the peritoneum forms some folds and fossae caused by reflection over the several pelvic structures. They will be discussed with the specific organs.

Endopelvic Fascia
Fascia of the lateral pelvic wall:
This fascia is strong and almost like an aponeurosis. It forms a covering on

240

the obturator internus, piriformis, and upper portion of puborectalis muscles.

Fascia of the pelvic floor:
This is loose connective tissue covering both surfaces of the pelvic diaphragm (levator ani muscle).

Fascia of Waldeyer:
This fascia anchors the posterior rectal wall to the presacral fascia. It is strong and similar to the fascia of the lateral pelvic wall.

Loose areolar connective tissue:
This fills the space between the pelvic peritoneum and the pelvic floor. Through this loose tissue pass blood vessels and nerves.

White line or arcus tendineus:
This marks the origin and not the insertion of the levator ani muscles. This origin is from the fascia of the obturator internus muscle.

Pelvic diaphragm, urogenital diaphragm, and superficial perineal pouch:
These are described in the chapter "Perineal Hernia."

Pelvic Organs

Female urethra:
The urethra is anchored to the anterior vaginal wall, to the pubic arch by the pubovesical ligament, and to the pubis by a thickening of the superior fascia of the urogenital diaphragm.

Urinary bladder:
The "ligaments" of the bladder are listed and discussed in the chapter "Internal Supravesical Hernias."

Muscles, vessels, and nerves are described in the chapter "Sciatic Hernia."

Uterus:
The corpus of the uterus is supported by the round and broad ligaments. The cervix perforates the endopelvic fascia and is supported laterally and posteriorly by the cardinal and uterosacral ligaments and anteriorly by the pubocervical fascia.

PLATE 73
Surgical Anatomy of the Abdominopelvic Cavity

A. The anterior abdominopelvic wall is formed by active (muscular) and passive (connective tissue) elements. All hernias represent a break in the supporting tissue, allowing abdominal pressure to push the peritoneum outward creating a blind pouch. The pouch may or may not contain an abdominal or pelvic viscus.

B. Diagrammatic drawing of the right half of the female pelvic cavity.

C. Diagram of the three chief active supporting elements of the pelvic floor.

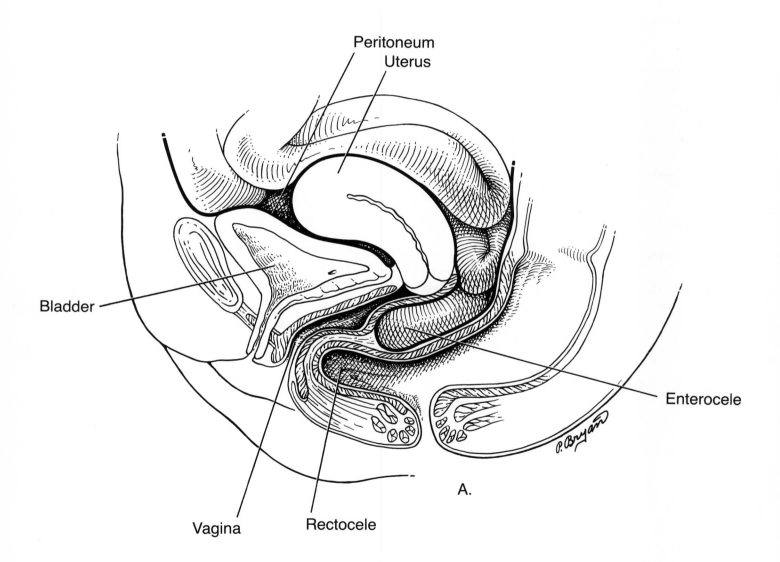

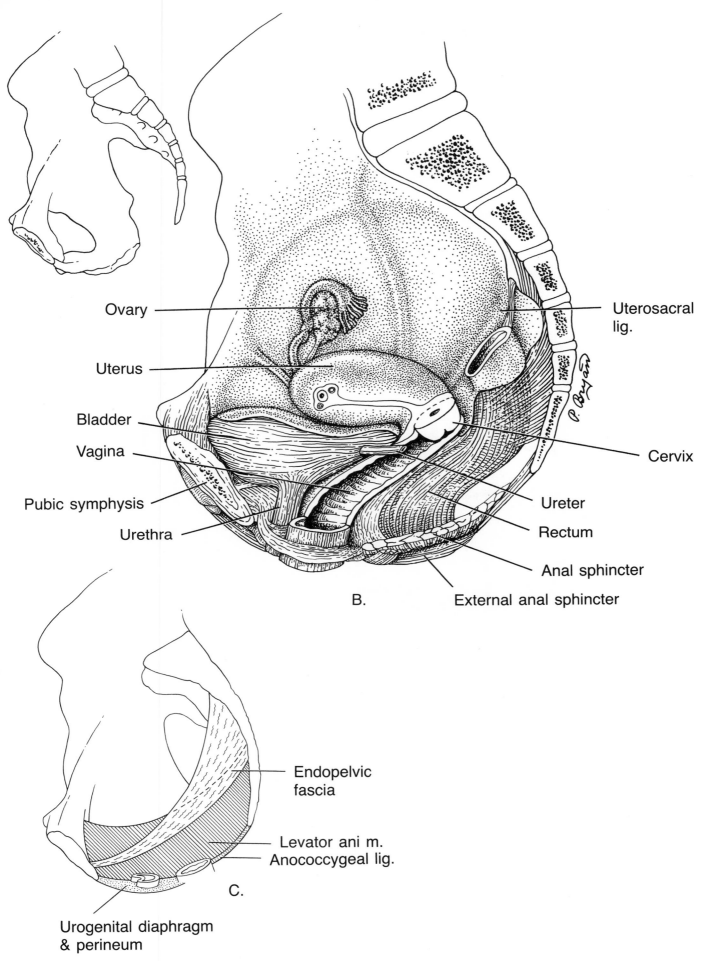

Ovary

Uterus

Bladder

Vagina

Pubic symphysis

Urethra

Uterosacral
lig.

Cervix

Ureter

Rectum

Anal sphincter

External anal sphincter

B.

Endopelvic
fascia

Levator ani m.
Anococcygeal lig.

C.

Urogenital diaphragm
& perineum

PLATE 73 (*Continued*)
Surgical Anatomy of the Abdominopelvic Cavity

D. Endopelvic fascia viewed from above.

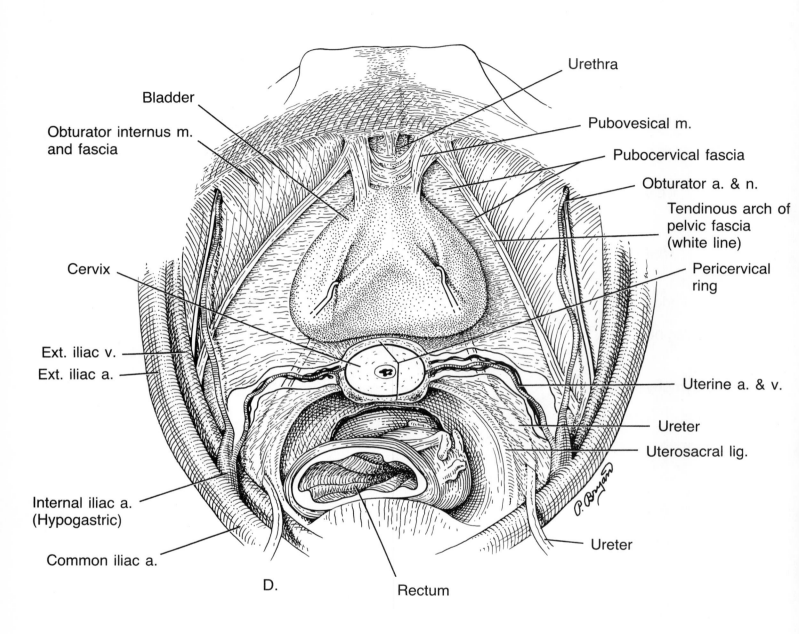

Urethra

Bladder

Obturator internus m. and fascia

Pubovesical m.

Pubocervical fascia

Obturator a. & n.

Tendinous arch of pelvic fascia (white line)

Cervix

Pericervical ring

Ext. iliac v.
Ext. iliac a.

Uterine a. & v.

Ureter

Uterosacral lig.

Internal iliac a. (Hypogastric)

Ureter

Common iliac a.

D.

Rectum

E. Lateral view of the female pelvis showing the upward extension of the fascia overlying the obturator internus and levator ani muscles.

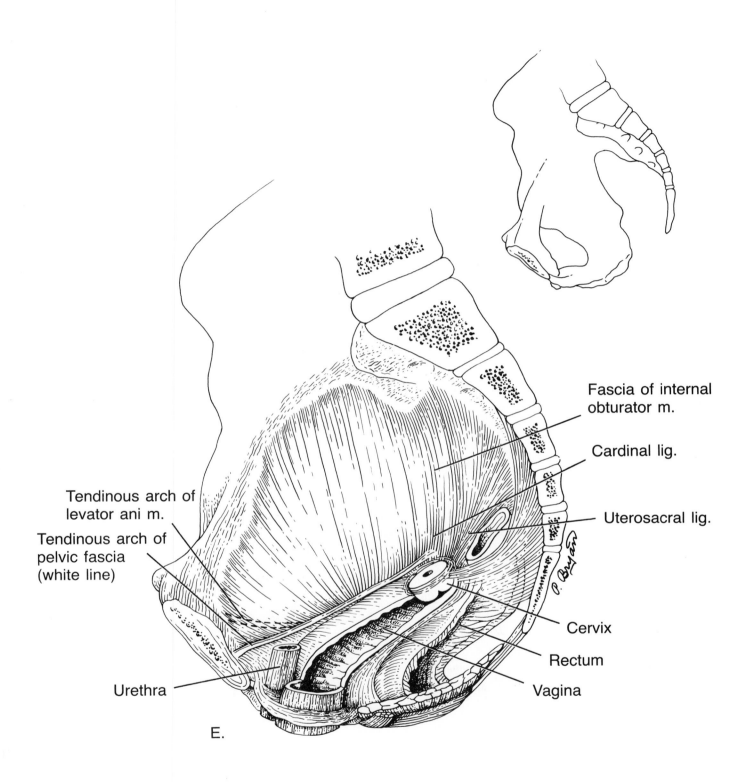

Fascia of internal obturator m.

Cardinal lig.

Uterosacral lig.

Tendinous arch of levator ani m.

Tendinous arch of pelvic fascia (white line)

Cervix

Rectum

Urethra

Vagina

E.

PLATE 73 (*Continued*)

Surgical Anatomy of the Abdominopelvic Cavity

F. Striated muscles of the pelvic sidewall and floor in the female.

G. The urogenital diaphragm and perineal muscles and fascia in the female, seen from below.

H. Pubocervical part of the endopelvic fascia. The base of the bladder (trigone) is densely adherent to its fascial support with no clear cleavage plane.

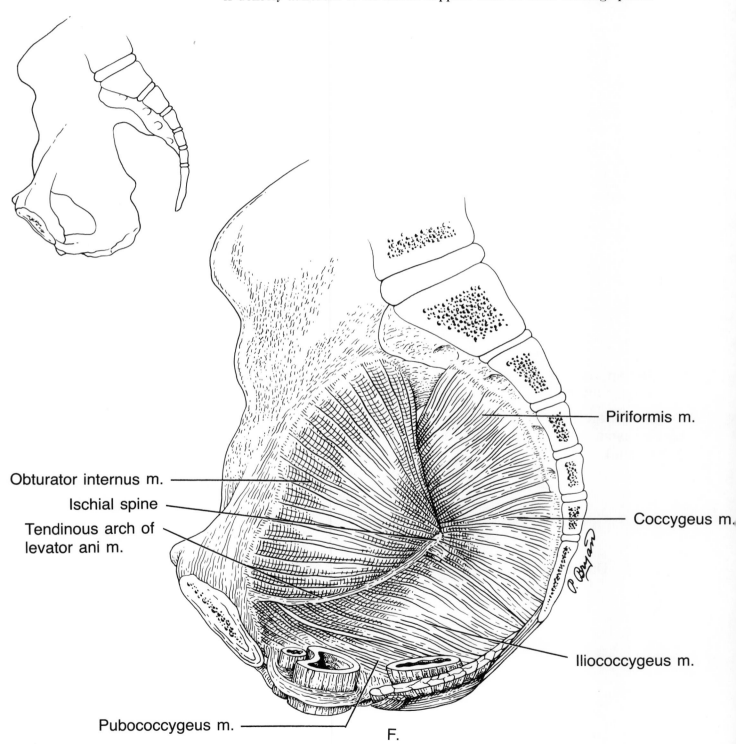

Piriformis m.

Obturator internus m.

Ischial spine

Tendinous arch of levator ani m.

Coccygeus m.

Iliococcygeus m.

Pubococcygeus m.

F.

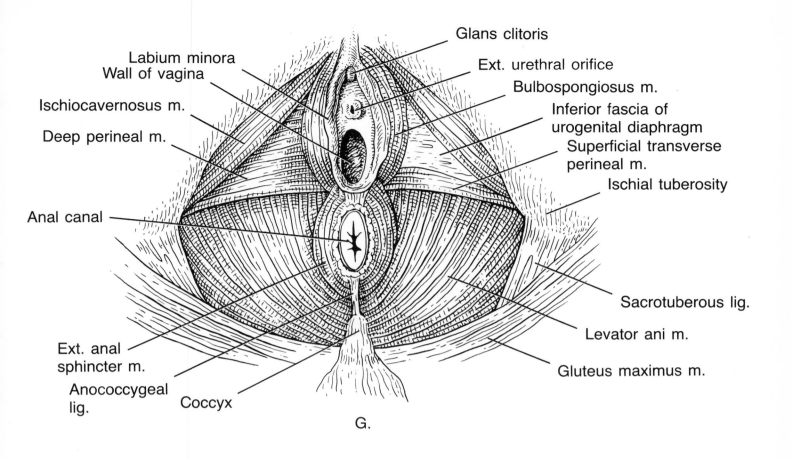

Labium minora
Wall of vagina
Ischiocavernosus m.
Deep perineal m.
Anal canal
Ext. anal sphincter m.
Anococcygeal lig.
Coccyx
Glans clitoris
Ext. urethral orifice
Bulbospongiosus m.
Inferior fascia of urogenital diaphragm
Superficial transverse perineal m.
Ischial tuberosity
Sacrotuberous lig.
Levator ani m.
Gluteus maximus m.

G.

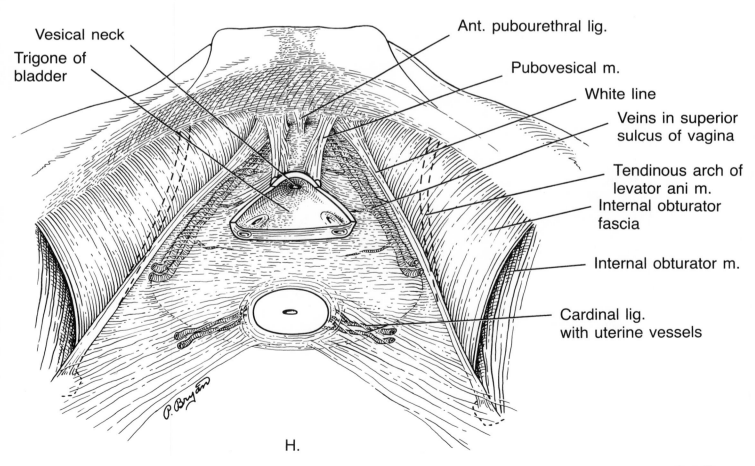

Vesical neck
Trigone of bladder
Ant. pubourethral lig.
Pubovesical m.
White line
Veins in superior sulcus of vagina
Tendinous arch of levator ani m.
Internal obturator fascia
Internal obturator m.
Cardinal lig. with uterine vessels

H.

247

PLATE 73 (*Continued*)
Surgical Anatomy of the Abdominopelvic Cavity

I. Cross section of the pelvis through the vagina. Note the difference between the tendinous arch of the pelvic fascia (white line) and the tendinous arch of levator ani muscle. The former is readily palpated at pelvic examination.

J. Diagrammatic cross section through the neck of the bladder.

K. Diagrammatic section through the vagina. Anterior wall of vagina and bladder removed. The vagina is trapezoidal and its lateral walls parallel the white line.

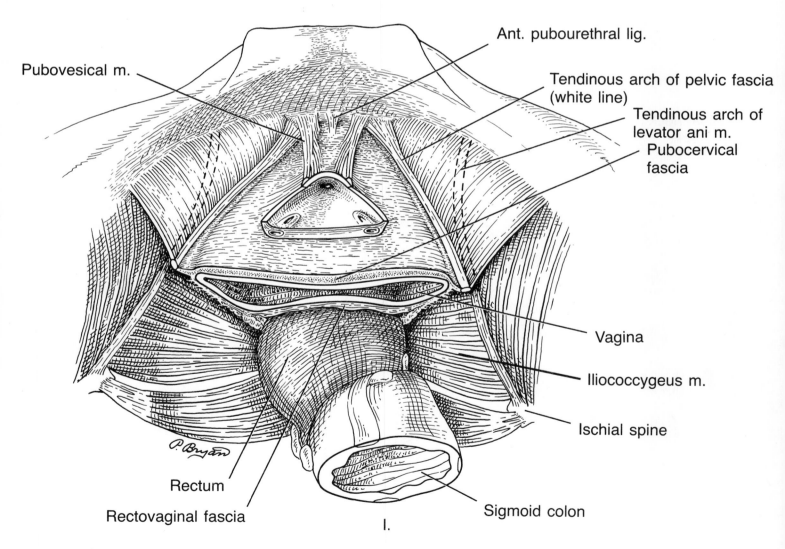

Pubovesical m.

Ant. pubourethral lig.

Tendinous arch of pelvic fascia (white line)

Tendinous arch of levator ani m.

Pubocervical fascia

Vagina

Iliococcygeus m.

Ischial spine

Rectum

Rectovaginal fascia

Sigmoid colon

I.

248

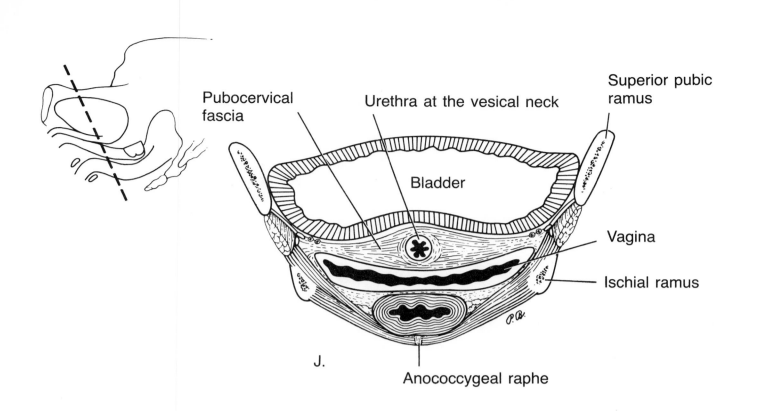

Pubocervical fascia

Urethra at the vesical neck

Superior pubic ramus

Bladder

Vagina

Ischial ramus

J.

Anococcygeal raphe

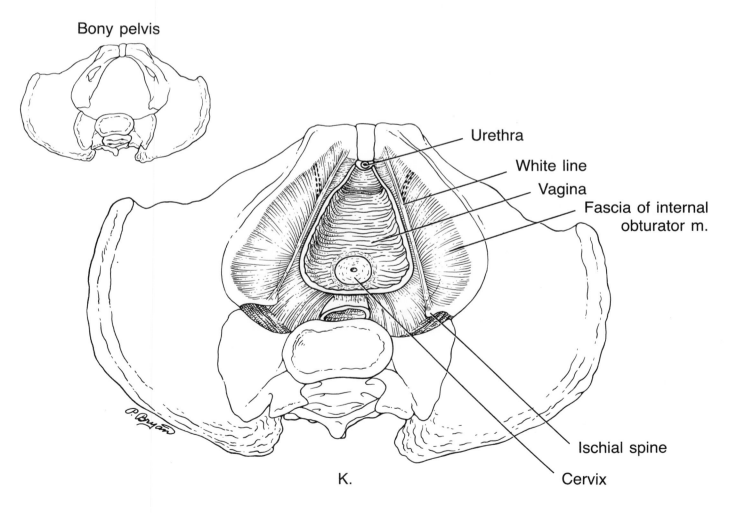

Bony pelvis

Urethra

White line

Vagina

Fascia of internal obturator m.

Ischial spine

Cervix

K.

249

PLATE 74
Sites of Pelvic Support Defects

A. Defects in the pelvic supports may occur in three different segments of the pelvic floor: anterior, central, and posterior.

B. A cystocele can result from any break in the continuity of the pubocervical fascial, hammocklike supports of the bladder. The three sites of possible defects are indicated. The paravaginal break is the most common, accounting for about 85 percent of all cystoceles and urethroceles.

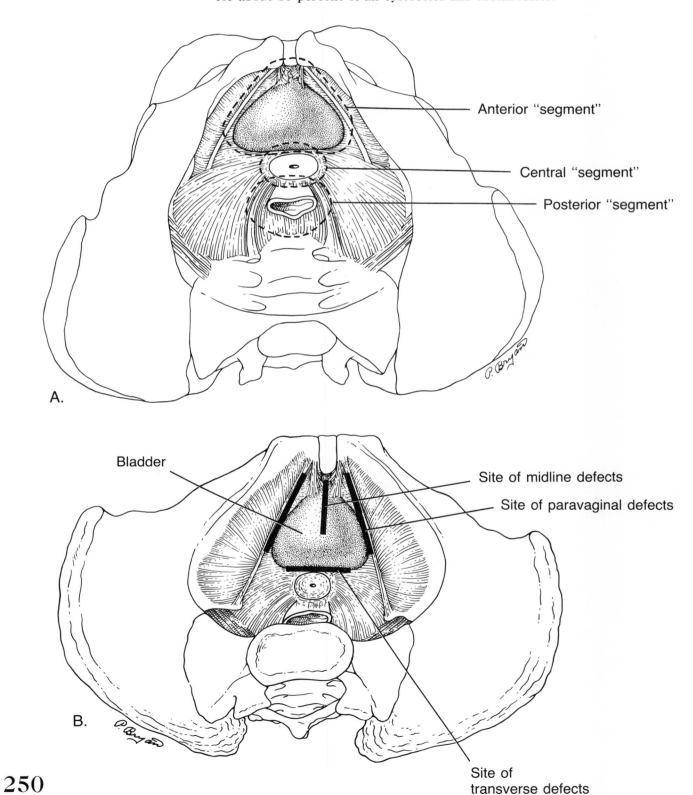

Anterior "segment"

Central "segment"

Posterior "segment"

A.

Bladder

Site of midline defects

Site of paravaginal defects

B.

Site of
transverse defects

PLATE 75
Pathology of Paravaginal Defect

A. Note the separation of the pubocervical fascia over the lateral wall of the vagina from the fascia overlying the obturator internus muscle at the white line. The break may occur lateral to the white line, down its central portion, or, as shown here, medial to the white line.

B. Diagrammatic cross section through a right paravaginal defect.

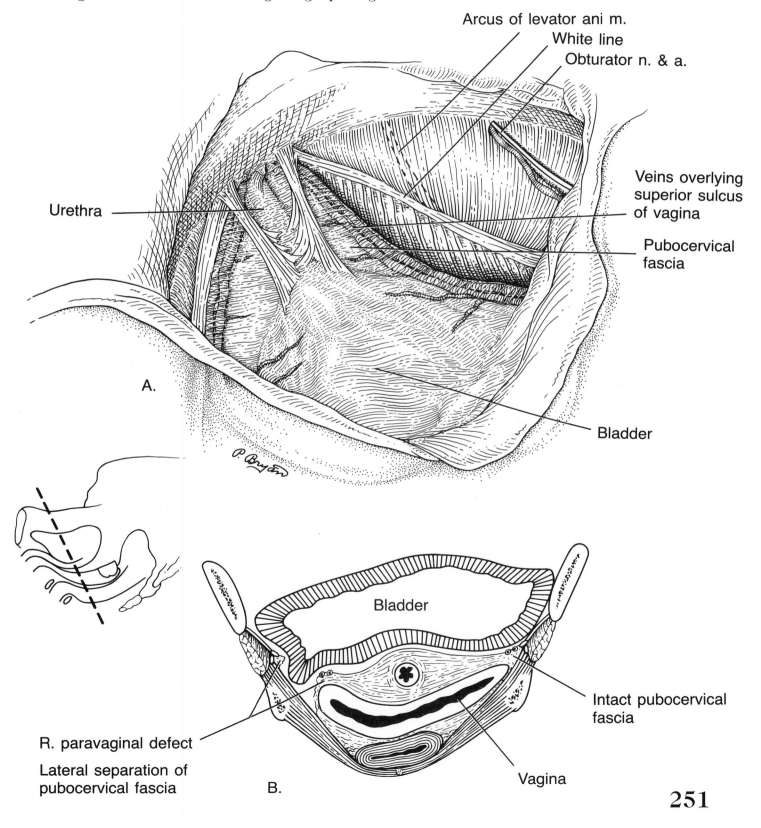

Arcus of levator ani m.

White line

Obturator n. & a.

Veins overlying superior sulcus of vagina

Pubocervical fascia

Urethra

Bladder

A.

Bladder

Intact pubocervical fascia

R. paravaginal defect

Lateral separation of pubocervical fascia

B.

Vagina

251

PLATE 76
Repair of Paravaginal Defect

A. *Step 1.* To enter the retropubic space, incise the transversalis fascia at its insertion into the superior pubic ramus.

B. *Step 2.* Blunt separation of the transversalis fascia lateral to the symphysis. This is carried laterally until the obturator notch can be palpated on the lower edge of the superior pubic ramus.

C. *Step 3.* Insert the left index finger in the vagina and elevate the superior lateral sulcus of the vagina opposite the vesical neck.

D. *Step 4.* The first stitch is placed full thickness through the fascia over the superior sulcus of the vagina. This is carried laterally so as to bring the urethra back into the pelvis.

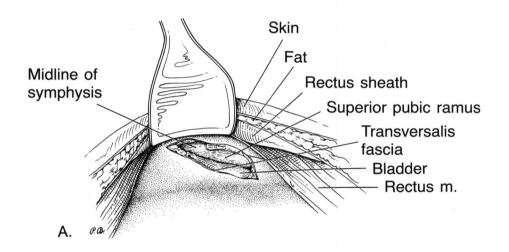

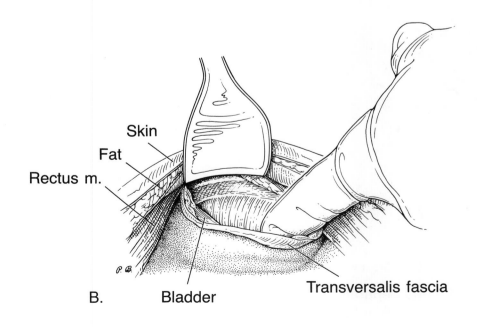

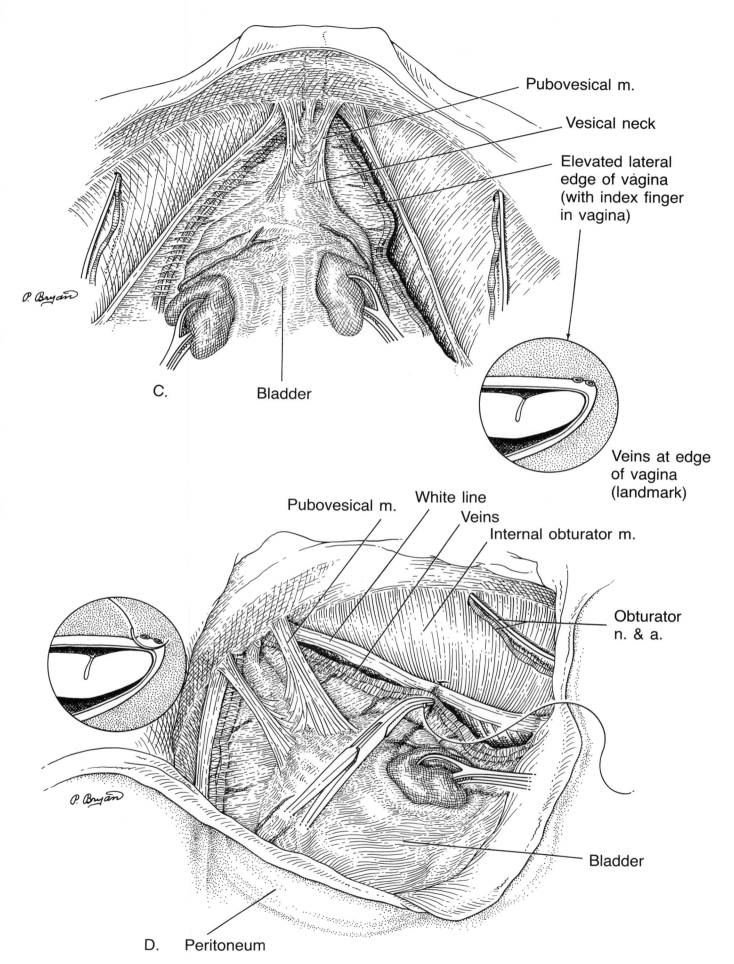

Pubovesical m.

Vesical neck

Elevated lateral
edge of vagina
(with index finger
in vagina)

C. Bladder

Veins at edge
of vagina
(landmark)

Pubovesical m.   White line
Veins
Internal obturator m.

Obturator
n. & a.

Bladder

D. Peritoneum

PLATE 76 (*Continued*)
Repair of Paravaginal Defect

E. *Step 5.* Completed procedure. It is advisable to repeat this on the opposite side even if there is no obvious separation or defect.

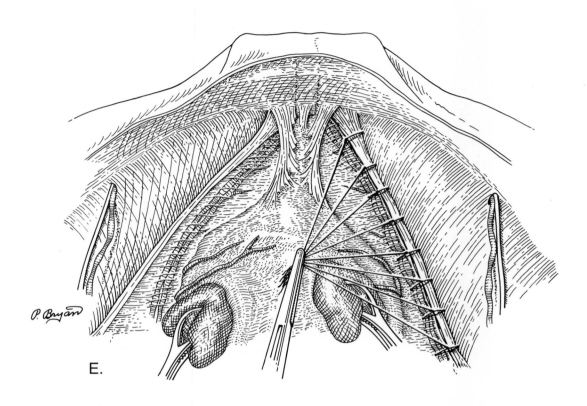

E.

254

PLATE 77

Pathology of Transverse Defect in Pubocervical Fascia

Diagrammatic sketch showing the pubocervical fascia separated from its attachment into the pericervical ring. Note that the bladder is covered only by vaginal mucosa over the cystocele.

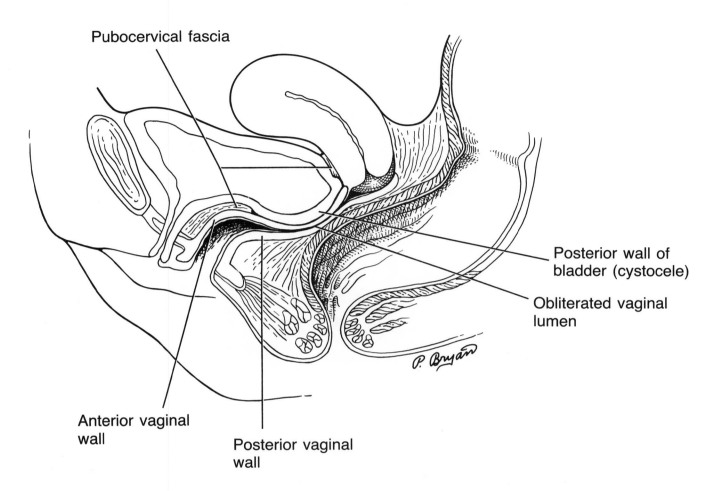

Pubocervical fascia

Posterior wall of bladder (cystocele)

Obliterated vaginal lumen

Anterior vaginal wall

Posterior vaginal wall

PLATE 78
Repair of Transverse Defect

A. *Step 1.* After completion of vaginal hysterectomy, close the peritoneum. The anterior vaginal mucosa (epithelium and lamina propria) is reflected off the underlying bladder and pubocervical fascia. By palpation the demarcation of the edge of the fascia can be determined.

B. *Step 2.* Place anteroposterior sutures bringing the edge of the pubocervical fascia anteriorly to the pericervical ring of fascia posteriorly. Laterally these sutures bring the cut ends of the cardinal and uterosacral ligaments and the cut ends of the uterine vessels into this fascial closure.

C. *Step 3.* Close the vaginal mucosa.

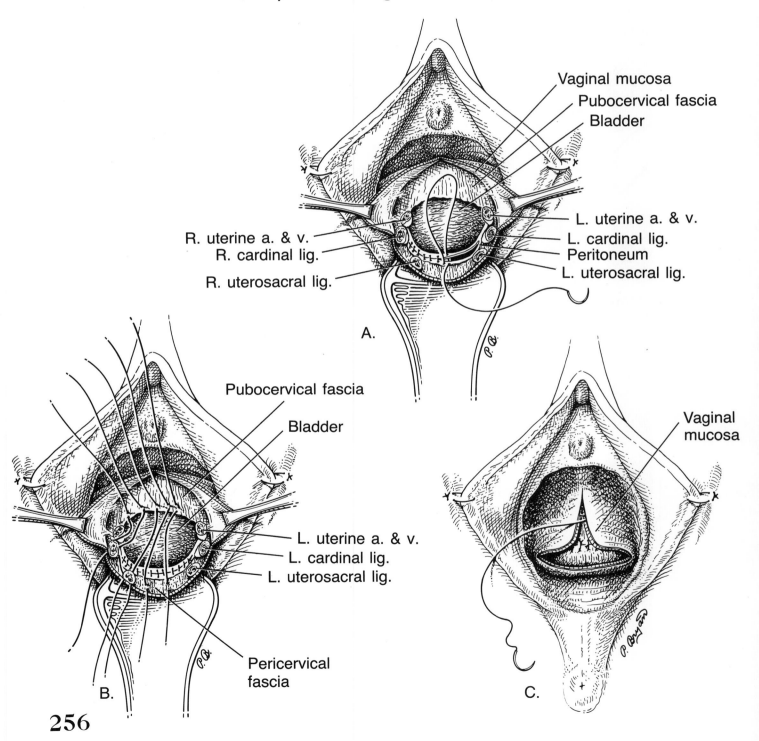

256

PLATE 79
Repair of Midline Anterior Segment Defect

A. *Step 1.* Vaginal mucosa reflected off the underlying bladder and pubocervical fascia. The defect can be detected by careful observation and palpation. Place sutures so as to bring the separated edges of the fascia together.

B. *Step 2.* Complete closure of the pubocervical fascia. Closure of vaginal mucosa will complete the procedure.

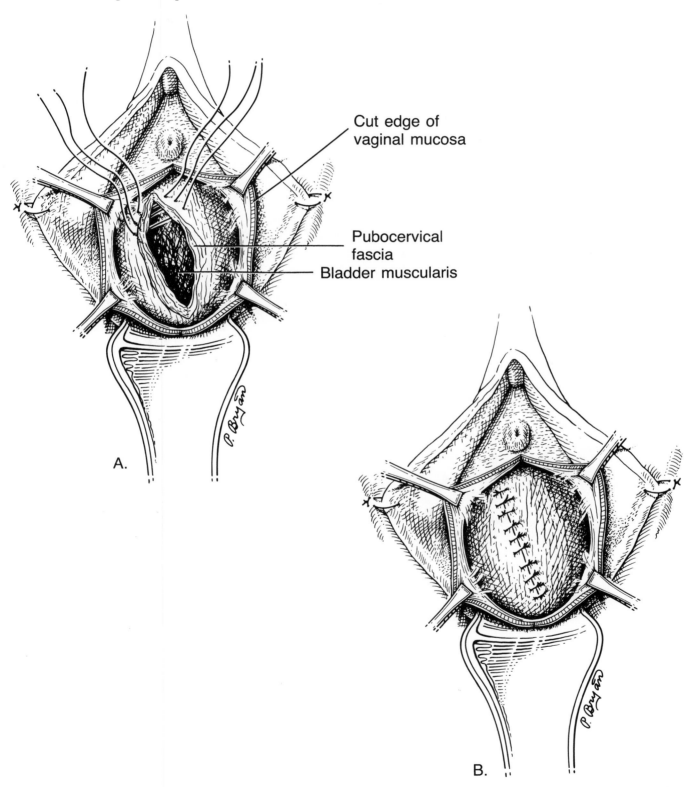

Cut edge of
vaginal mucosa

Pubocervical
fascia

Bladder muscularis

A.

B.

PLATE 80
Surgical Anatomy of Central Pelvic Support

The normal supports of the cervix radiate anteriorly, laterally, and posteriorly from the pericervical ring of fibromuscular tissue that attaches to the predominantly collagenous cervix.

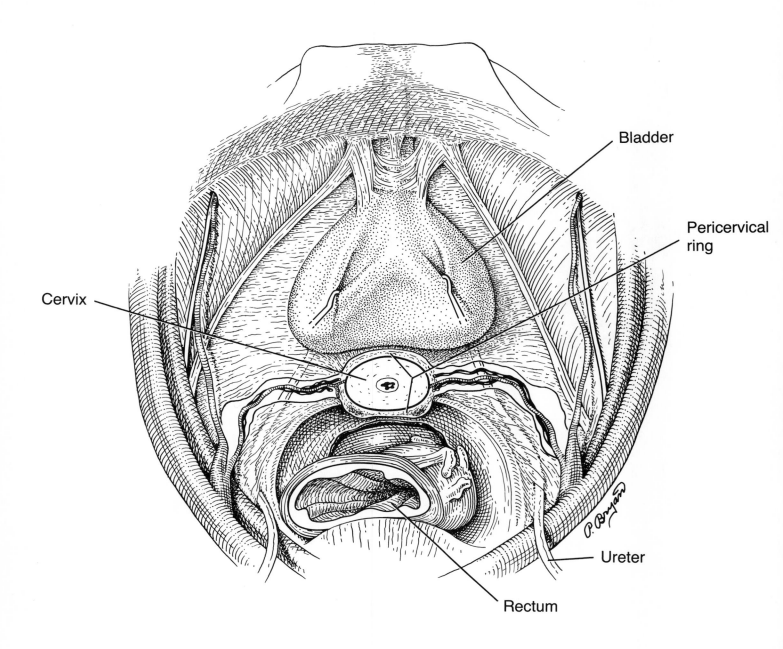

Bladder

Pericervical ring

Cervix

Ureter

Rectum

PLATE 81

Repair of Uterine Prolapse

A. Uterine prolapse. The uterosacral ligaments are separated from the pericervical ring posteriorly.

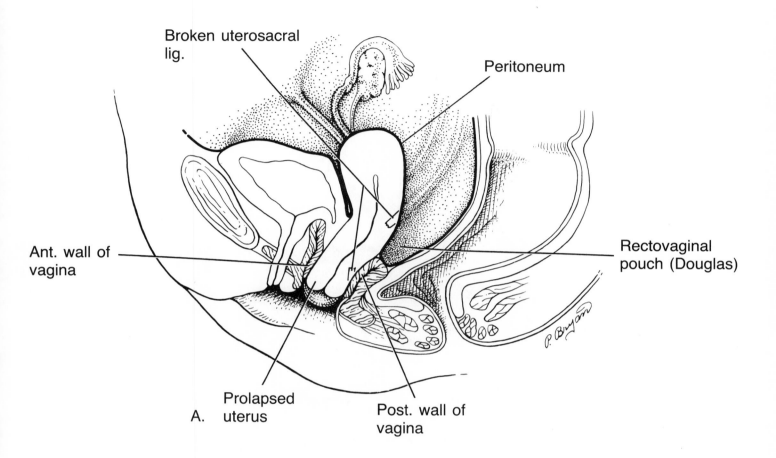

Broken uterosacral lig.

Peritoneum

Ant. wall of vagina

Rectovaginal pouch (Douglas)

Prolapsed uterus

A.

Post. wall of vagina

PLATE 81 (*Continued*)

Repair of Uterine Prolapse

B. *Step 1.* Vaginal closure after vaginal hysterectomy for prolapse. Place sutures anteroposteriorly to reestablish the continuity of support from the pubocervical fascia anteriorly to the pericervical fascia and uterosacral ligaments posteriorly.

Step 2. Attach the cut ends of the cardinal ligaments and uterine vessels to the pericervical ring.

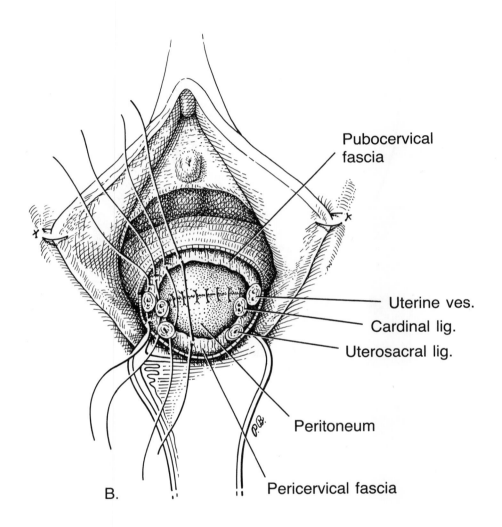

Pubocervical fascia

Uterine ves.

Cardinal lig.

Uterosacral lig.

Peritoneum

Pericervical fascia

B.

PLATE 82
Pathology of Posterior Segment Support Defects

Pulsion type entrocele in sagittal section.

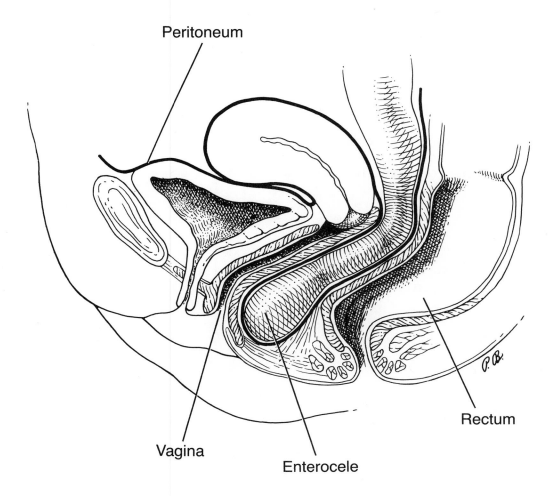

Peritoneum

Rectum

Vagina

Enterocele

PLATE 83
Repair of Posterior Support Defects

A. *Step 1.* Open the posterior enterocele sac from below.

B. *Step 2.* Bring together the uterosacral ligaments in the midline to reinforce the cul-de-sac. The rectovaginal fascia is plicated to obliterate a coexistent rectocele.

C. *Step 3.* Perineorrhaphy. Bring together the edges of the medial portions of the pubococcygeus muscles in the midline to narrow the levator hiatus.

D. *Step 4.* Approximate the levator muscles and reconstruct the perineal body.

E. *Step 5.* Close the vaginal mucosa to complete posterior repair.

F. *Step 6.* Completed rectocele and enterocele repairs.

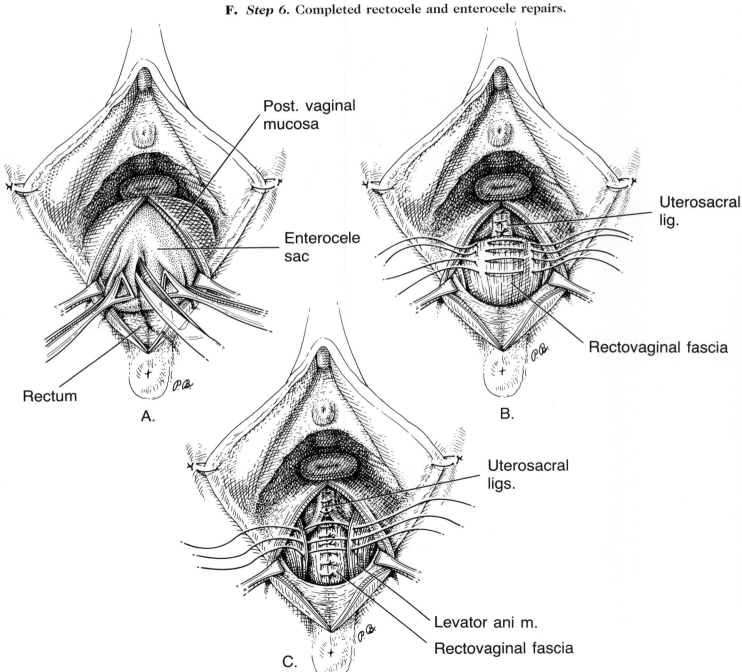

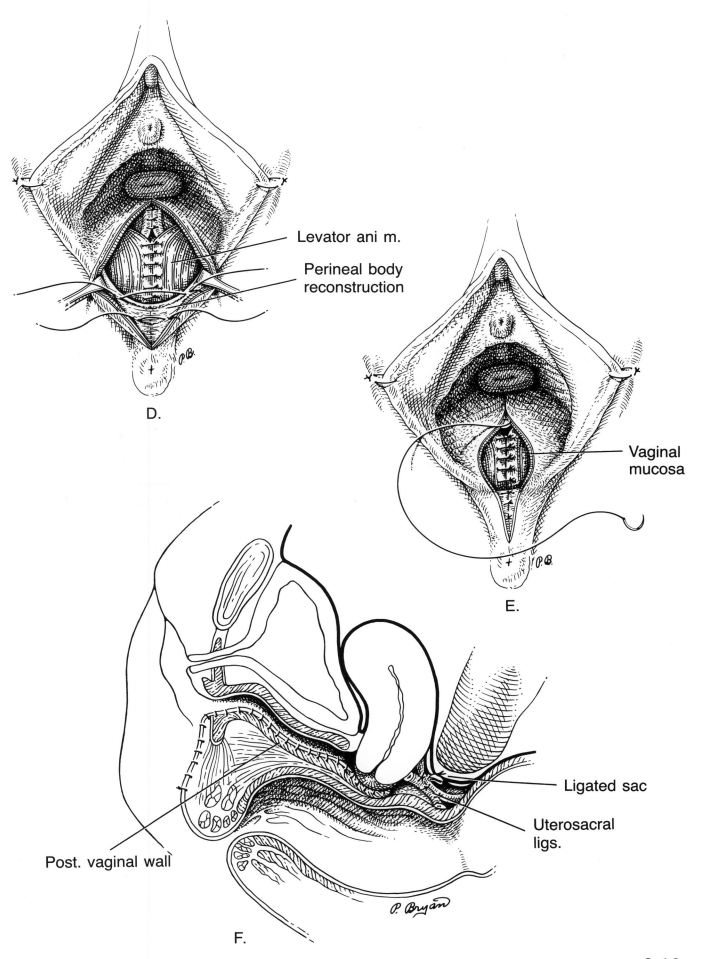

Levator ani m.

Perineal body reconstruction

D.

Vaginal mucosa

E.

Ligated sac

Uterosacral ligs.

Post. vaginal wall

F.

263

SECTION THREE
INTERNAL ABDOMINAL HERNIAS

Definition

Two types of internal hernias may be distinguished:

1. The passage of a viscus through a defect in a mesentery or the omentum.
2. Protrusion of a viscus through an opening formed by a fold of peritoneum.

None of these hernias is common. They are difficult to detect and frequently asymptomatic, with confusing anatomy and obscure etiology. They account for about 1 percent of intestinal obstruction.

Hernias through an Omental Defect

Surgical Anatomy

Omenta

From a surgical standpoint, the greater omentum can be divided into two parts: (1) the proximal portion between the greater curvature and the first inch of the first portion of the duodenum to the transverse colon, the gastrocolic ligament; and (2) the portion from the transverse colon that is hanging free in the peritoneal cavity, the greater omentum per se (fat apron). The splenocolic, the gastrosplenic, and the gastrohepatic ligaments are also part of the greater omentum.

In typical locations, the greater omentum is very thin and, therefore, subject to defects. The "thin" areas are between the arch of Barkow and/or the anterior and posterior epiploic branches.

The four layers of the greater omentum, two anterior and two posterior, are fused, and the omentum itself is fused with the wall and the mesentery of the transverse colon.

Derivatives of the Ventral Mesentery

Only the cranial portion of the embryonic ventral mesentery persists in the adult. The anterior part is represented by the falciform ligament between the liver and the anterior body wall. The posterior part becomes the gastrohepatic and hepatoduodenal mesenteries that form the lesser omentum.

THE FALCIFORM, TRIANGULAR, AND CORONARY LIGAMENTS (NONOMENTAL)
The falciform ligament, a remnant of the embryonic ventral mesentery, extends from the anterior abdominal wall to the diaphragm and the anterior surface of the liver. The free edge contains the round ligament, which is the obliterated left umbilical vein.

The leaves of the falciform ligament separate as they reach the liver to form the anterior, superior, and posterior (inferior) layers of the coronary ligament. Laterally these layers reunite to form the right and left triangular ligaments. From a surgical standpoint, the division of the left triangular and coronary ligament as a unit is anatomically justified for the exposure of the gastroesophageal junction.

GASTROHEPATIC LIGAMENT (LESSER OMENTUM)
The gastrohepatic ligament is the proximal part of the lesser omentum; it extends from the porta hepatis to the lesser curvature of the stomach and upward as the mesentery of the abdominal esophagus. The ligament contains the left gastric artery and vein, hepatic division of the anterior vagal trunk, anterior and posterior gastric divisions of the vagus nerve (nerves of Latarjet), and an aberrant left hepatic artery, where present.

THE HEPATODUODENAL LIGAMENT

The hepatoduodenal ligament is the distal part of the lesser omentum. The free edge envelops the hepatic triad of hepatic artery, portal vein, and extrahepatic bile ducts.

Derivatives of the Dorsal Mesentery

In the upper part of the abdomen, the primitive dorsal mesentery gives rise to three structures: the gastrocolic ligament, the gastrosplenic ligament, and the gastrophrenic ligament.

GASTROCOLIC LIGAMENT

The gastrocolic ligament is a portion of the greater omentum passing from the greater curvature of the stomach and the first part of the duodenum to the transverse colon. It contains the right and left gastroepiploic arteries and veins.

GASTROSPLENIC LIGAMENT

The gastrosplenic ligament attaches to the greater curvature of the stomach and is a downward continuation of the gastrophrenic ligament. The contents are

Upper part: Short gastric arteries and veins and lymph nodes
Lower part: Left gastroepiploic artery and vein, terminal branches of the splenic artery, and lymph nodes

GASTROPHRENIC LIGAMENT

The gastrophrenic ligament is a continuation of the gastrohepatic ligament to the left of the esophagus. It has an avascular area through which the surgeon's finger may pass and through which may be inserted a Penrose drain around the cardia to pull down the esophagus. The contents of the ligament are

Upper part: Avascular
Lower part: Short gastric arteries and veins and lymph nodes

Blood Supply to the Greater Omentum

This is shown in Plate 86A.

Blood Supply to the Small Intestine

ARTERIAL SUPPLY

The superior mesenteric artery arises from the aorta below the origin of the celiac trunk. In about 1 percent of individuals, there is a combined celiacomesenteric trunk.[1] The superior mesenteric artery continues beyond the ileal border to supply Meckel's diverticulum, if one is present.

On average, the left side of the superior mesenteric artery gives rise to five intestinal arteries above the origin of the ileocolic atery and 11 arteries below that level. Eight more arteries arise from the ileal branch of the ileocolic artery.[1]

[1]Michels NA, Siddharth P, Kornblith PI, Parke WW: The variant blood supply to the small and large intestines: Its import on regional resections. *J Int Coll Surg* 39:127, 1963.

268

These intestinal vessels branch a few centimeters from the border of the intestine to form a series of arterial arcades connecting the intestinal arteries with one another. These arches form the primary anastomoses of the arterial supply.

From the arches of the arcades, numerous arteries, the vasa recta, arise and pass (without cross communication) to the intestinal wall. They may bifurcate to supply each side, or they may pass singly to alternate sides of the intestine. They branch but do not anastomose beneath the serosa before piercing the muscularis externa. This configuration provides the best supply of oxygenated blood to the mesenteric side of the intestine and the poorest supply to the antimesenteric border.

Within the wall, the arteries form a large plexus in the submucosa. From this, short vessels reach the lamina propria to supply a network of capillaries around the intestinal crypts, while longer arteries supply the cores of the intestinal villi. There are thus two regions of anastomosis of intestinal arteries: the extramural arches between intestinal arteries and the intramural submucosal plexus.

VENOUS DRAINAGE

One or more small veins originate near the tip of each intestinal villus and travel outward, receiving contributions from a plexus of veins around the intestinal glands. They enter the submucosal plexus. This is drained through the muscular layer by larger veins traveling with the arteries in the mesentery to reach the superior mesenteric vein. These intestinal veins are interconnected by venous arcades similar to, but less complex than, the accompanying arterial arcades.

Mesentery of the Small Bowel

This mesentery extends from the left upper quadrant at the level of the first or second lumbar vertebra to the right iliac fossa at the sacroiliac joint. It has a length of 6 in. at its base, which is fused with the retroperitoneal space. The failure of fusion results in a defect which can permit loops of small bowel to enter with incarceration or strangulation. This is the hernia of Waldeyer. However, other defects can take place in any part of the mesentery.

The danger in these types of hernias is vascular. The surgeon should remember the vascular arrangements in this area.

Remember that there is no collateral circulation of the vasa recta in the wall of the small bowel.

Pelvic Mesocolon

The pelvic mesocolon forms the Greek letter Λ with one leg at the left pelvic wall and the other in the vicinity of S_3 with the left colic and sigmoid arteries from the inferior mesenteric artery.

A defect may be located at the fossa intersigmoida or at any part of the sigmoid mesocolon. The danger in this area lies in injury to the left ureter and vascular injury.

269

Transverse Mesocolon

This mesentery is attached to the second part of the duodenum, lower pole of the right kidney, anterior border of the pancreas, and lower pole of the left kidney. The middle colic artery is the most important anatomical entity within the transverse mesocolon.

Broad Ligament

This triangular mesentery of the uterus, tubes, and ovaries is extended from each lateral uterine side to the lateral pelvic wall. Medially, the broad ligament envelops the uterus. The upper free part is related to the tubes (mesosalpinx) and ovaries (mesovarium), and the lower fixed part is attached to the levator ani muscle through a special formation, the cardinal ligament. The broad ligament has thin vascular areas through which a viscus may pass.

Falciform Ligament

The falciform ligament begins at the umbilicus and passes obliquely to the superior surface of the left lobe of the liver, where it forms an excellent landmark that separates the lateral and medial segments of the left lobe. The free edge of the falciform ligament contains the cordlike round ligament (ligamentum teres) of the liver. This is the remnant of the left umbilical vein. The right umbilical vein disappears early in development; the left vein carries placental blood to the fetus and closes at birth. This vascular remnant is often patent for much of its length.[1] Its intrahepatic portion becomes the ligamentum venosum, which connects the left branch of the portal vein with the left hepatic vein. The falciform ligament is thus the mesentery of the umbilical vein.

Hernias in this first group (mesenteric or omental defect) have been called *false hernias* by Bertelsen because there is no hernial sac.

All mesenteries in the abdominal cavity are subject to defects through which herniation may take place. The origin of the defects is unknown. Some are developmental, and some may be the result of trauma. The chief locations are

through the mesentery (Plate 86),
through the greater omentum (Plate 86),
through the sigmoid mesocolon (Plate 87),
through the broad ligament of the uterus (Plate 88), and
through the falciform ligament (Plate 89).

These hernias are asymptomatic unless incarcerated; their frequency is unknown. Omental and mesenteric types are the most common.

Starting in a relatively avascular area of the mesentery, the defect enlarges until at least one free edge is formed by an artery, usually a branch of the superior or inferior mesenteric artery. In many cases, an intestinal loop may pass freely through the defect without strangulation, but adhesions between the hernial ring and the herniated intestinal loop are not unusual. If strangulation has occurred, it may be necessary to resect a gangrenous loop of intestine.

[1]Silva YJ: In vivo use of human umbilical vessels and the ductus venosus Arantii. *Surg Gynecol Obstet* 148:595, 1979.

TABLE 8
Derivatives of the Mesentery

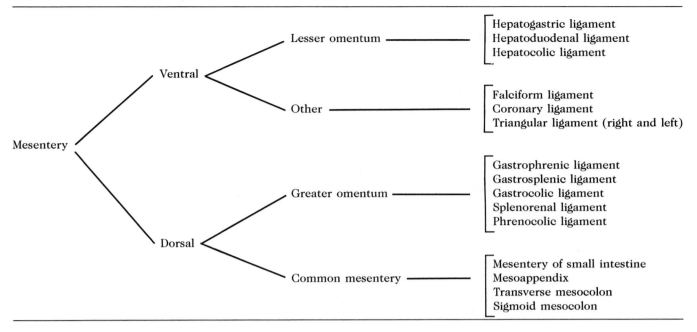

Mesentery
- Ventral
  - Lesser omentum
    - Hepatogastric ligament
    - Hepatoduodenal ligament
    - Hepatocolic ligament
  - Other
    - Falciform ligament
    - Coronary ligament
    - Triangular ligament (right and left)
- Dorsal
  - Greater omentum
    - Gastrophrenic ligament
    - Gastrosplenic ligament
    - Gastrocolic ligament
    - Splenorenal ligament
    - Phrenocolic ligament
  - Common mesentery
    - Mesentery of small intestine
    - Mesoappendix
    - Transverse mesocolon
    - Sigmoid mesocolon

PLATE 84

Some Derivatives of the Dorsal and Ventral Mesentery

The colon and the hepatocolic and phrenocolic ligaments are not shown.

Source: Plate 84 from Skandalakis JE, Gray SW, Rowe JS Jr: *Anatomical Complications in General Surgery*. McGraw-Hill, New York, 1983, p. 304, Fig. 16-2.

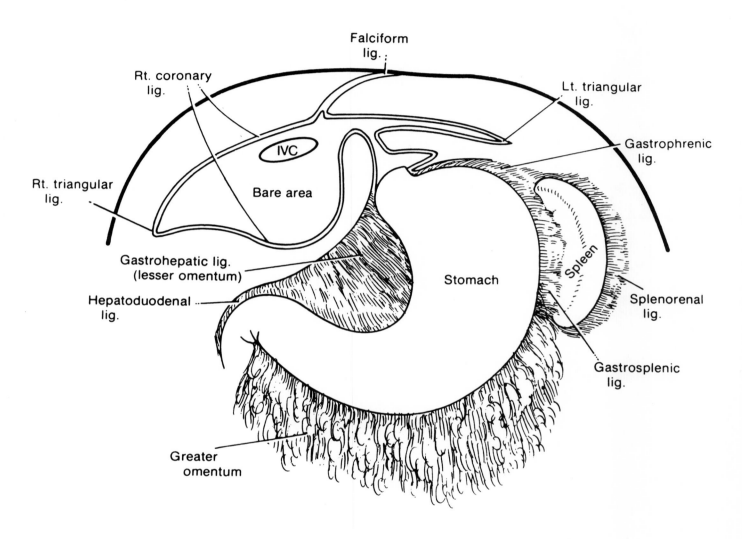

PLATE 85
Arterial Supply to the Small Bowel

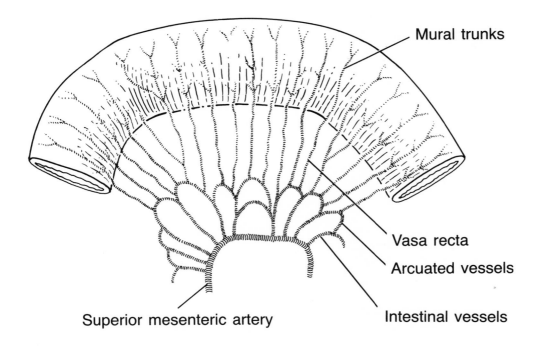

Mural trunks

Vasa recta

Arcuated vessels

Intestinal vessels

Superior mesenteric artery

PLATE 86
Repair of Omental and Mesenteric Hernia

Omental Hernia

A. Arterial supply to the greater omentum. REG = right gastroepiploic a.; LGE = left gastroepiploic a.; RE = right epiploic a.; LE = left epiploic a.; AB = arc of Barkow; G = gastric branches; AE = anterior epiploic branches; PE = posterior epiploic branches; P = pancreatic a.; VR = vasa recta of midcolic a. Herniation can occur between any of these descending arteries.

Source: Griffith CA: Anatomy, in *Surgery of the Stomach and Duodenum,* 4th ed, Nyhus LM, Wastell C (eds). Little, Brown, Boston, 1986, Fig. 2-18.

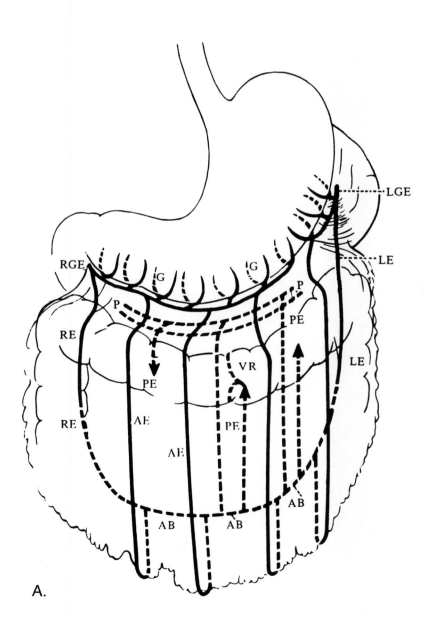

A.

B. A loop of small intestine has entered a defect in the greater omentum.

C. *Step 1.* Incise the omentum and free the bowel.

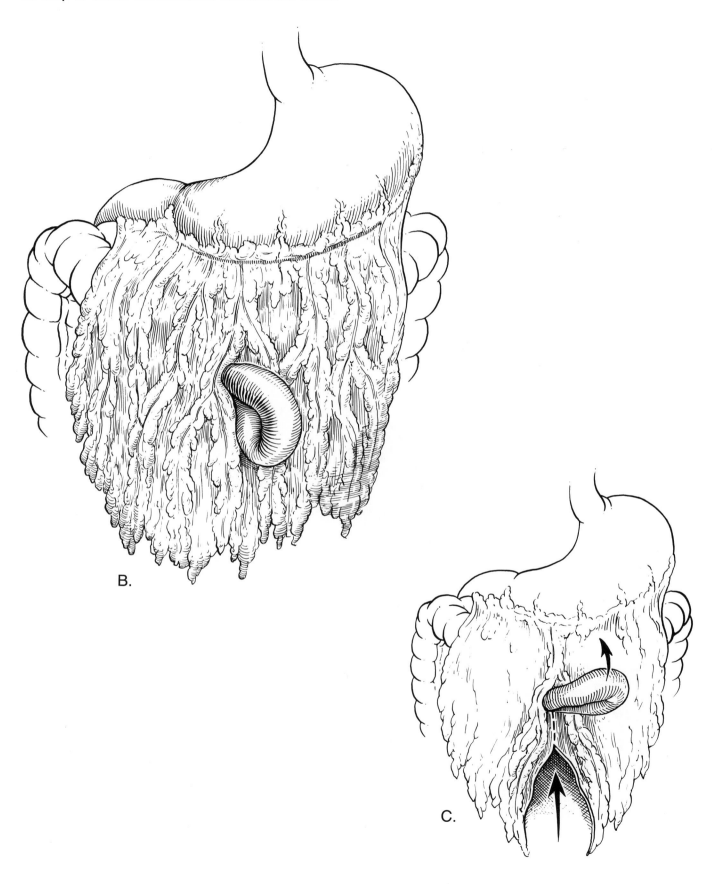

B.

C.

PLATE 86 (*Continued*)

Repair of Omental and Mesenteric Hernia

D. Alternatively, enlarge the ring by clamping it with Kelly clamps. Incise the omental tissue between clamps.

E. *Step 2.* Reduce the hernia. Ligate the clamped tissue with 00 silk.

F. *Step 3.* Close the omental defect with continuous or interrupted 00 catgut sutures.

Decompression of the proximal intestine without incising the ring will often permit reduction of the herniated loop and closure of the omental defect.

Mesenteric Hernia (Mesenteric, small bowel, sigmoid mesocolon, transverse mesocolon)

The repair procedure is similar to that for repair of hernia through the sigmoid mesocolon. Avoid vascular injury by not incising the neck. Decompress the dilated loop to permit reduction, and close the defect.

With a nonfatty mesentery, the vascular tree can be visualized and an incision of the neck is possible.

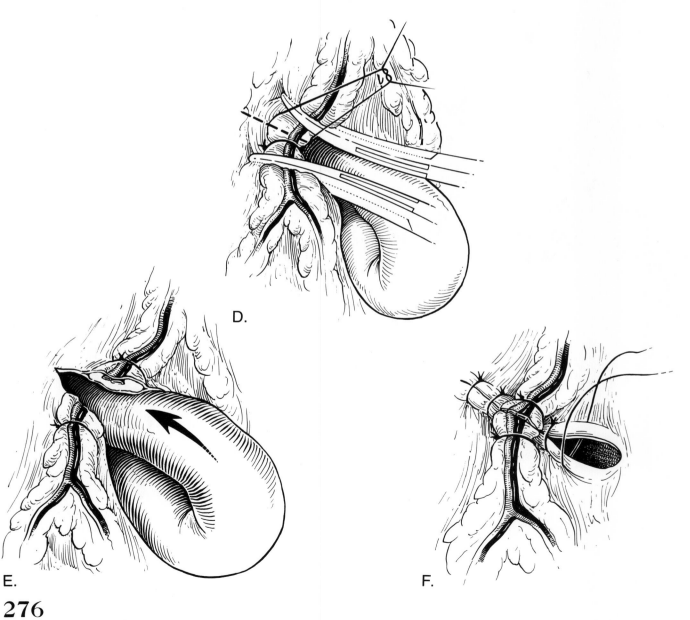

D.

E.

F.

PLATE 87

Repair of Hernia through the Sigmoid Mesocolon

The mesenteric defect may be located in (1) the mesentery of the small intestine, (2) the transverse mesocolon, or (3) the sigmoid mesocolon. At least one free edge of the ring is usually formed by a branch of the superior mesenteric or inferior mesenteric artery. Since there is no sac and the obstructed loop is visible, decompress the dilated loop only and do not incise the neck. Vascular injury ad portas must be avoided. The sigmoid artery is above and to the right of the fossa.

An ileal loop has passed through a defect in the sigmoid mesocolon beneath the sigmoid colon. At least one free edge of the ring is usually formed by a branch of the superior or inferior mesenteric artery.

Step 1. Decompress the dilated proximal loop to permit reduction without incision of the ring.

Step 2. Close the ring after reduction. If the sigmoid arteries are obvious, enlarge the ring by incision of an avascular area; the strangulated loop may be reduced without aspiration, thereby avoiding possible contamination.

Step 3. Close the defect with continuous or interrupted 00 chromic catgut sutures, avoiding incorporation of the sigmoid arteries.

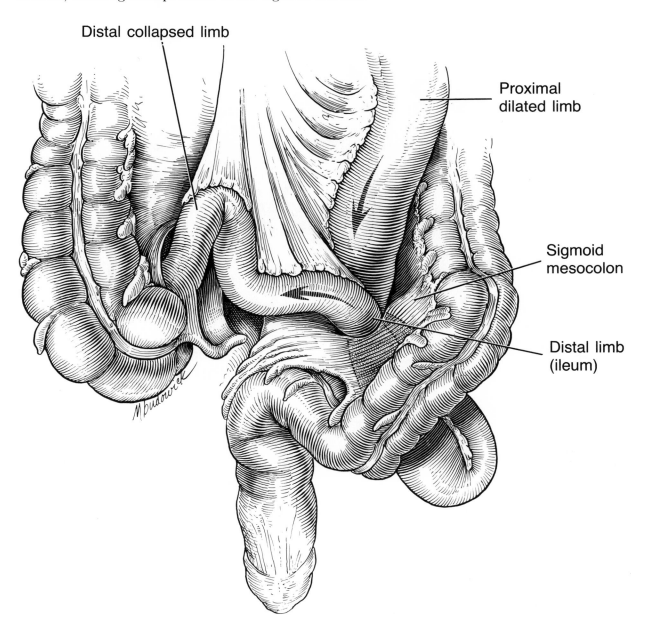

Distal collapsed limb

Proximal dilated limb

Sigmoid mesocolon

Distal limb (ileum)

277

PLATE 88

Repair of Hernia through the Broad Ligament

This is a rare hernia passing through a defect in the broad ligament of the uterus. Like other mesenteric defects, the cause is unknown.

     Incise the ring carefully in an avascular area; reduce the loop and close the defect.

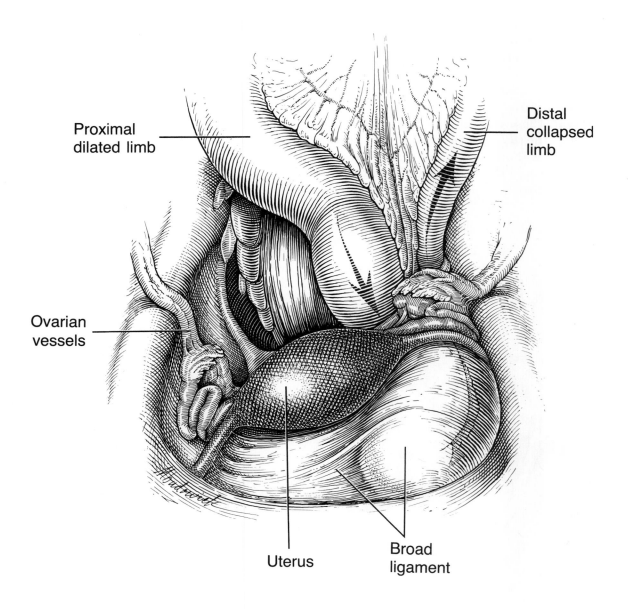

Proximal dilated limb

Distal collapsed limb

Ovarian vessels

Uterus

Broad ligament

PLATE 89
Repair of Hernia through the Falciform Ligament

A. This extremely rare hernia illustrates the possibility for hernia in an unlikely location.

B. After proximal and distal ligation, incise the falciform and round ligaments and reduce the hernia.

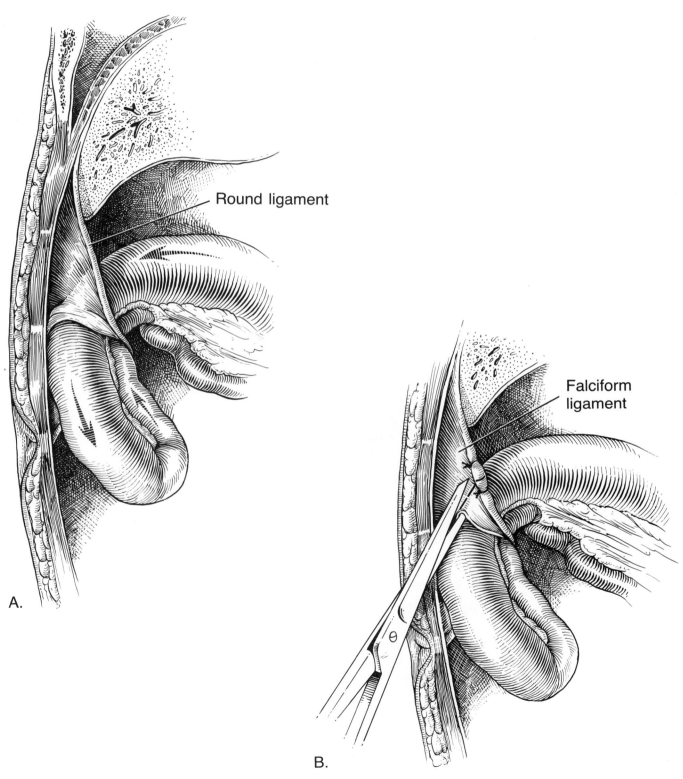

Round ligament

Falciform ligament

A.

B.

Hernias Beneath a Mesenteric or Peritoneal Fold

Surgical Anatomy

In this second group of internal hernias, there is no break in the peritoneum; the herniated viscus enters and enlarges a naturally occurring fold or pocket of peritoneum. A sac is always present. There are a number of possible sites of such hernias. Following is a discussion of some of them.

Hernia through the Epiploic Foramen of Winslow

Definition

This is a rare hernia in which an intestinal loop enters the epiploic foramen and passes into the lesser peritoneal sac. The hernia may be intermittent (chronic) or strangulated (acute).

It is not clear why this hernia should be so rare. If it can occur, one would expect it to do so frequently because the epiploic foramen is normally open.

Anatomy

The boundaries of the epiploic foramen are

Superior: The caudate process of the liver and the inferior layer of the coronary ligament.

Anterior: The hepatoduodenal ligament containing the portal vein, the hepatic artery, and the common bile duct. The cystic duct is also present in the free edge of the lesser omentum.

Posterior: The inferior vena cava.

Inferior: The first part of the duodenum and the transverse part of the hepatic artery.

Repair

Following reduction of the hernia, the epiploic foramen should be closed, taking care to protect the structures at the porta hepatis. Fixation of an abnormally mobile cecum or right colon may be helpful. Recurrence of the hernia in the absence of repair has not been reported. The hepatogastric ligament is opened and the strangulated proximal intestine is decompressed.

PLATE 90

Repair of Hernia through the Epiploic Foramen (of Winslow) ▶

A. A loop of small intestine has entered the epiploic foramen and is visible beneath the hepatogastric ligament containing the portal vein, hepatic artery, and common bile duct. The cystic duct forms the free edge of the hernial ring. Under no circumstance should the neck of the ring be incised.

B. *Step 1.* Open the hepatogastric ligament and decompress the strangulated intestine.

Inset: Close the aspiration site with a purse-string suture.

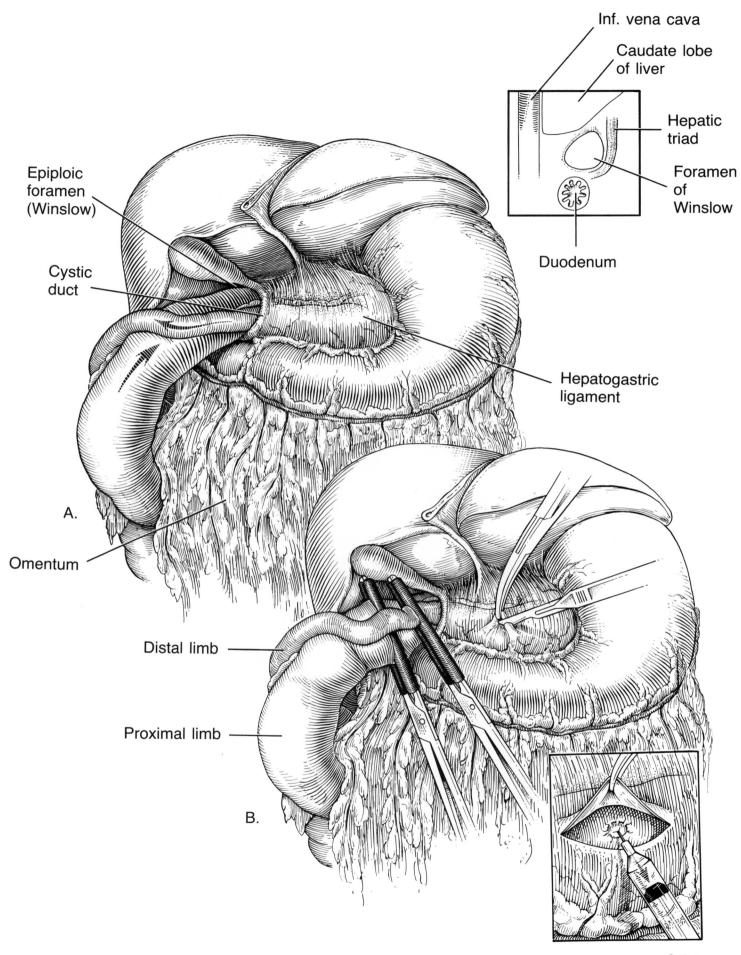

Inf. vena cava

Caudate lobe
of liver

Hepatic
triad

Foramen
of
Winslow

Duodenum

Epiploic
foramen
(Winslow)

Cystic
duct

Hepatogastric
ligament

A.

Omentum

Distal limb

Proximal limb

B.

281

PLATE 90 (*Continued*)

Repair of Hernia through the Epiploic Foramen (of Winslow)

C. *Step 2.* The herniated loop is released.

    Inset: Close the defect in the hepatogastric ligament with 00 silk.

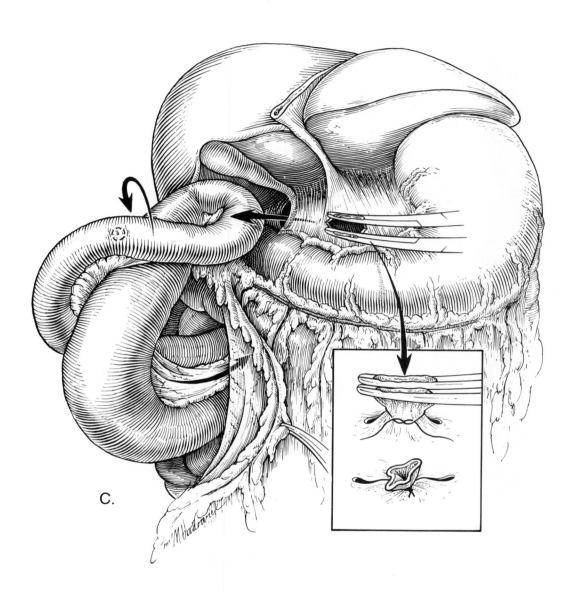

C.

The Paraduodenal Hernias

Surgical Anatomy

These hernias are formed in peritoneal pockets or "fossae" on the posterior abdominal wall. Moynihan[1] described no fewer than nine such fossae in which herniation might occur. These fossae are inconstant; any, all, or none may be present in a given individual. Precise identification of a specific fossa in the presence of a hernia is often impossible because of distortion of the orifice. We consider only five of these fossae to be constant enough to be of clinical importance. These are listed together with their relative frequency in Table 9.

More important than the location of the fossa is the direction of the herniated loop of intestine. If the loop passes to the right, it is a *right paraduodenal hernia;* if the loop passes to the left, it is a *left paraduodenal hernia,* without reference to the midline of the body or to the specific fossa concerned.

Paraduodenal sacs usually contain small intestine. Only rarely are cecum, ascending colon, or sigmoid colon reported.

Early writers believed that the paraduodenal fossae were congenital and that a hernia was acquired by gradual enlargement of the existing fossa. It is now believed that the hernias as well as the fossae are of congenital origin. A paraduodenal fossa is not the site of a potential hernia in later life; instead it marks the location in which a congenital hernia might have formed but failed to do so.

Both the ascending and descending limbs of the colon have mesenteries when the intestines return from the umbilical cord to the abdomen during the tenth embryonic week. These mesenteries come in contact with the posterior peritoneal wall and fuse with it by the fifth fetal month. Paraduodenal hernias are formed during this period of fixation of the colon.

A right paraduodenal hernia is produced by an intestinal loop entering a pocket in the yet unfused ascending mesocolon between its attachment and the superior mesenteric vein. When the mesocolon fuses with the peritoneum of the body wall, the pocket containing the intestinal loop becomes the hernial sac. The mouth of the sac may lie at the site of the mesentericoparietal fossa of Waldeyer, at the superior or inferior horn of the fossa of Treitz, or at the intermesocolic fossa of Broesike. The hernial sac is directed to the right.

A left paraduodenal hernia forms by a similar pocket in the unfused descending mesocolon, the mouth of which is the fossa of Landzert. The hernial sac is directed to the left.

TABLE 9
The Five Paraduodenal Fossae

Name	Direction of Hernia if Present	Relative Incidence, %
1. Superior duodenal fossa of Treitz	Right	30–50
2. Paraduodenal fossa of Landzert	Left	2
3. Inferior duodenal fossa of Treitz	Right	50–75
4. Intermesocolic fossa of Broesike	Right	Rare
5. Mesentericoparietal fossa of Waldeyer	Right	1

[1]Moynihan BGA: *Retro-peritoneal Hernia.* Balliere, London, 1889.

Repair

Surgical treatment of strangulated paraduodenal hernia is reduction of the hernia and eradication of the fossa. This may be by closure at the neck or by enlargement of the orifice. Injury to major blood vessels must be avoided. Enterostomy may be required for decompression. The herniated loop must be evaluated for viability and resected where necessary.

PLATE 91
Repair of Paraduodenal Hernia

A. The five major paraduodenal fossae. The transverse colon has been reflected upward and the duodenum has been reflected to the right to reveal the paraduodenal fossae.

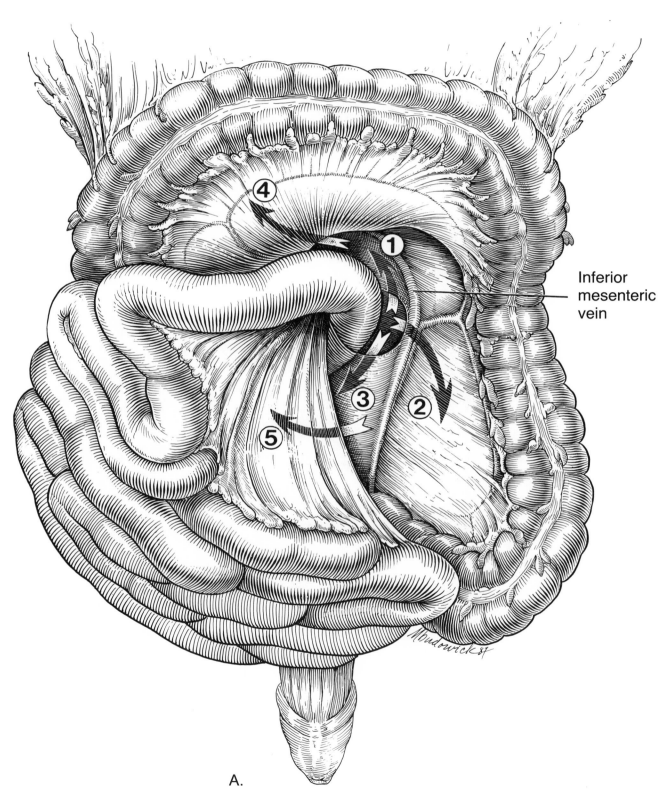

Inferior
mesenteric
vein

A.

PLATE 91 (*Continued*)

Repair of Paraduodenal Hernia

B. Right paraduodenal hernia. The mouth of the sac lies behind the superior mesenteric artery or the ileocecal artery at the base of the mesentery of the small intestine (mesentericoparietal fossa of Waldeyer). The mouth opens to the left. The sac is directed to the right and usually lies in the retroperitoneal space behind the right mesocolon or transverse mesocolon. The boundaries are

Superior: The duodenum
Anterior: The superior mesenteric artery or ileocolic artery
Posterior: The lumbar vertebrae

Repair
Incise the lower part of the mouth to avoid vascular injury. If vascular damage appears inevitable, the surgeon should open the mesentery and decompress the proximal intestinal loop before attempting reduction.

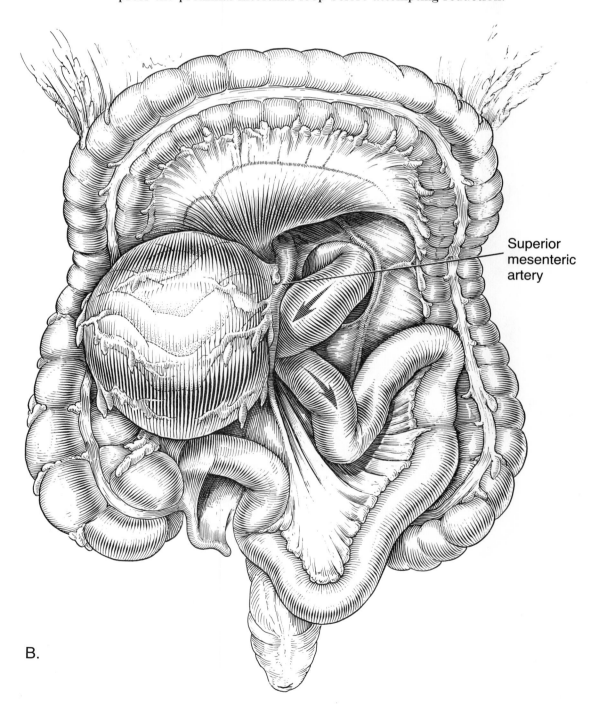

Superior
mesenteric
artery

B.

C. Left paraduodenal hernia. The mouth of the sac lies behind the inferior mesenteric vein and the left colic artery, at the left of the fourth part of the duodenum and the duodenojejunal flexure. The mouth opens to the right. The sac is directed to the left and usually lies in the retroperitoneal space behind the left mesocolon. The boundaries of the ring are

Superior: The duodenojejunal flexure or the beginning of the jejunum, pancreas, and renal vessels

Anterior: The inferior mesenteric vein and left colic artery

Right: The aorta

Left: The left kidney

Repair
Make the incision in the lower part of the mouth. A downward incision of the mouth will avoid sacrifice of the inferior mesenteric vein.

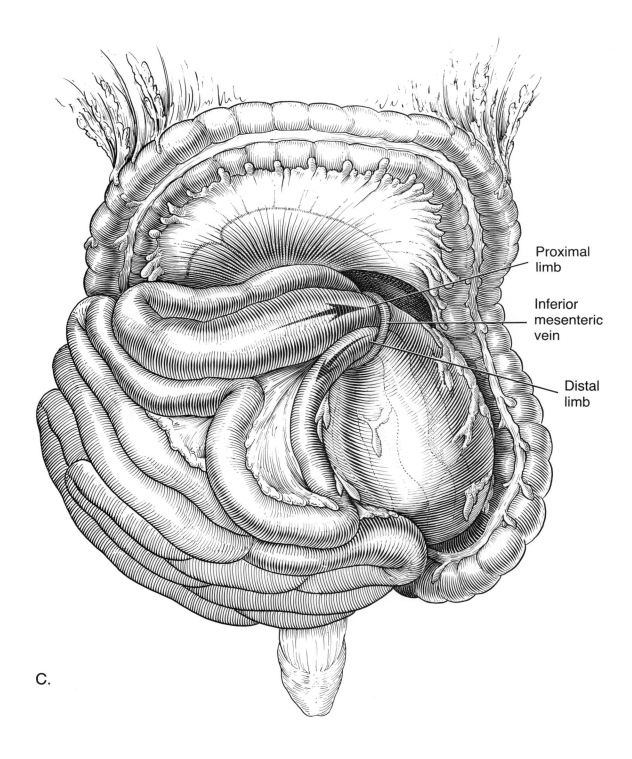

Proximal limb

Inferior mesenteric vein

Distal limb

C.

287

Hernia through the Ileocecal Fossae (Superior and Inferior)

These rare hernias are formed by the same developmental process as are paraduodenal hernias. Their repair is similar: reduction of the herniated loop and either closure or enlargement of the ring to prevent recurrence.

PLATE 92

Hernia into the Superior Ileocecal Fossa

A. Superior and inferior ileocecal folds forming fossae.

B. The intestinal loop has been trapped by the right mesocolon during the fusion with the peritoneum of the body wall.

Source: Skandalakis JE, Gray SW, Rowe JS: *Anatomical Complications in General Surgery.* McGraw-Hill, New York, 1983, p. 225, Fig. 12-7.

Repair
Avoid the right ileocolic and right colic arteries when incising the ring. Aspiration of the proximal loop should be considered.

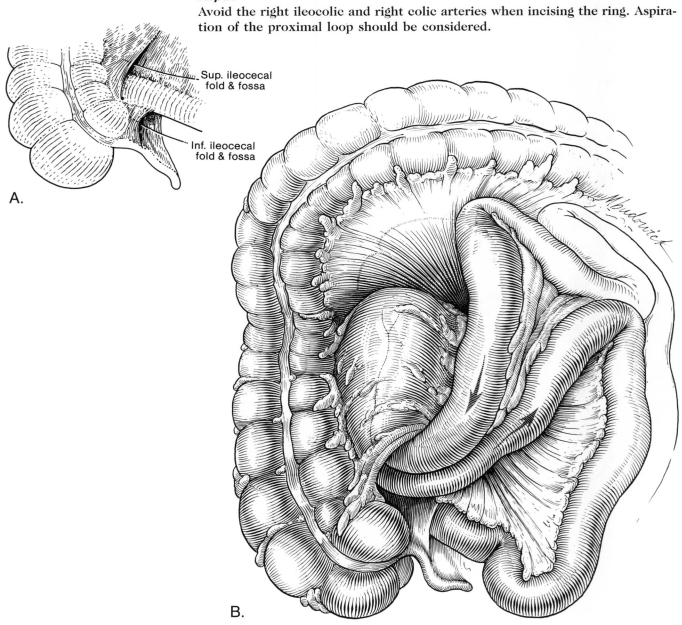

Sup. ileocecal fold & fossa

Inf. ileocecal fold & fossa

A.

B.

Retroanastomotic Hernia

A gastrojejunostomy automatically forms an internal hernial ring which may sooner or later admit an intestinal loop.

Surgical Anatomy

If the gastrojejunostomy is behind the transverse colon (retrocolic), the boundaries of the hernial ring are

Anterior: The gastrojejunostomy and the efferent or afferent jejunal loop, depending on whether the afferent loop is attached to the lesser or the greater curvature of the stomach

Posterior: The posterior parietal peritoneum

Superior: The transverse mesocolon and posterior wall of the gastric remnant

Inferior The ligament of Treitz and the duodenojejunal peritoneal fold

If the gastrojejunostomy is in front of the transverse colon (antecolic) with the afferent loop attached to the greater curvature of the stomach, the boundaries of the ring are

Anterior: The gastrojejunostomy and the afferent jejunal loop

Posterior: The omentum and mesocolon

Superior: The transverse colon and mesocolon

Inferior: The ligament of Treitz and the duodenojejunal peritoneal fold

With the afferent loop attached to the lesser curvature of the stomach, the boundaries of the ring are

Anterior: The afferent jejunal loop with its mesentery

Posterior: The omentum, transverse colon, and mesocolon

Superior: The gastrojejunostomy, ligament of Treitz, and the duodenojejunal peritoneal fold

Inferior: The jejunum with its mesentery

Repair

Do not incise the ring. An enterostomy may be required to facilitate reduction of the loop. Recurrence is prevented by closure of the ring.

PLATE 93
Repair of Retroanastomotic Hernia

A. The gastrojejunostomy has been constructed behind the transverse colon (retrocolic). An ileal loop has passed from right to left behind the anastomosis.

Step 1. Aspirate the incarcerated loop with a trocar or 18-gauge needle to facilitate reduction of the loop.

Step 2. Close the aspiration site with a purse-string suture and reduce the herniated loop.

Step 3. Close the ring with continuous or interrupted 00 catgut sutures, avoiding incorporation of the middle colic artery.

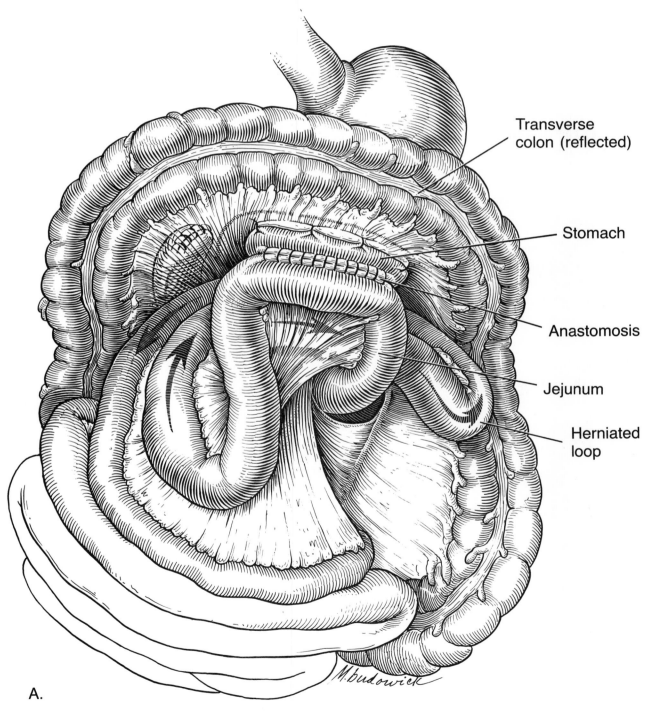

Transverse colon (reflected)

Stomach

Anastomosis

Jejunum

Herniated loop

A.

B. The gastrojejunostomy has been constructed in front of the transverse colon (antecolic). The hernia passes beneath the anastomosis as in part A above. Remember to follow the procedure described above and to avoid incising the ring.

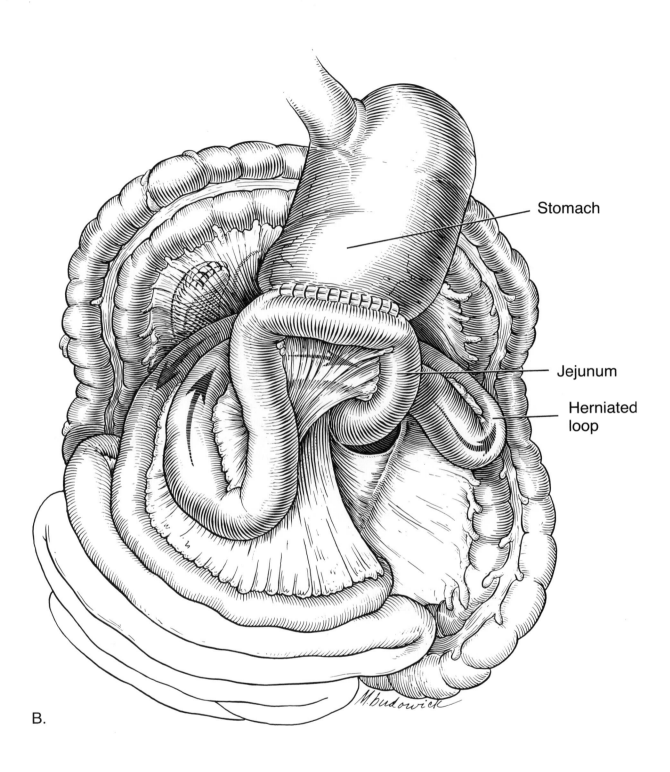

Stomach

Jejunum

Herniated loop

B.

Internal Supravesical Hernias

Definition
The hernial sac and its contents pass through the supravesical fossa of the anterior abdominal wall. They may then protrude through the abdominal wall as a direct inguinal hernia (external supravesical hernia), or they may remain within the abdomen, passing into spaces around the urinary bladder (internal supravesical hernia).

Surgical Anatomy of the Infraumbilical Anterior Abdominal Wall
The posterior surface of the anterior abdominal wall contains three shallow fossae on either side of the midline. The midline is marked by the median umbilical ligament, the adult remnant of the urachus of the fetus.

The lateral fossa is bounded medially by the inferior epigastric artery and is the site of the internal inguinal ring through which may pass *indirect inguinal hernias.*

The medial fossa lies between the inferior epigastric artery and the medial umbilical ligament (obliterated umbilical artery). It is the site of *direct inguinal hernias.*

The supravesical fossa lies between the medial umbilical ligament and the median umbilical ligaments. It partially overlies Hesselbach's triangle, as it is described today. It is the site of *supravesical hernias.* In practice, the lateral border of the rectus sheath may be a more constant landmark.

A *supravesical hernia,* anterior to the bladder, forms as a result of failure of the integrity of the transversus abdominis aponeurosis and the transversalis fascia, both of which insert on the pectineal ligament (of Cooper). The hernial sac may remain above the pelvis and form an external hernia (see page 97) or pass downward to become an internal supravesical hernia.

Although all internal supravesical hernias by definition start in the supravesical fossa, their subsequent course is variable. We have proposed a classification[1] based on whether this course is in front of, beside, or behind the bladder (Plate 94 A, B):

1. Anterior supravesical hernia
   a. Retropubic supravesical hernia
   b. Invaginating supravesical hernia
2. Right or left lateral supravesical hernia
3. Posterior supravesical hernia

The anterior retropubic and lateral hernias pass into the retropubic space (of Retzius) between the pubis and the bladder (Plate 94C). The invaginating type pushes in the anterior bladder wall and is very rare (Plate 94D). The posterior hernias enter the space between the bladder and rectum in the male (Plate 94E) and between the bladder and the uterus in the female (Plate 94F); they also are rare.

In the early stages of herniation, the anterior retropubic and lateral hernias are not easily distinguished from each other. Attempts at precise classification are in many cases futile.

These hernias result from the loss of integrity of the transversus abdominis muscle and the transversalis fascia. Most of these hernias pass downward as direct inguinal or femoral hernias. About half of direct inguinal hernias originate in the supravesical fossa between the middle umbilical ligament and the medial umbilical fold.

[1]Skandalakis JE, Gray SW, Burns WB, Sangmalee U, Sorg JL: Internal and external supravesical hernia. *Am Surg* 42:142–146, 1976.

The Retropubic Space of Retzius

The retropubic space is situated in front of, and to the sides of, the urinary bladder. Its boundaries are

Anterior: Symphysis pubis

Lateral: Pubic bone; fascia of obturator internus muscle; superior fascia of levator ani muscle; lateral puboprostatic ligament

Medial: Inferior lateral surface of bladder

Superior: Peritoneum bridging the upper surface of the bladder and the lateral pelvic wall

Posterior: Vascular stalk of the internal iliac artery and vein with their sheath, which will reach the posterolateral border of the bladder

Inferior: Puboprostatic or pubovesical ligaments; reflection of the superior fascia of levator ani muscle to the urinary bladder

Potentially, the space is larger. It extends upward and laterally to form a triangular space between the medial umbilical ligaments, with its apex at the umbilicus and its base the puboprostatic or pubovesical ligaments. The space is "an extensive bursa-like cleft in the areolar tissue at the front and sides of the bladder which allows the bladder to fill and empty without hinderance."[1]

The peritoneum of the bladder has a number of folds which attach it to the pelvic wall. These are called the ligaments of the bladder. The concept of "true" and "false" ligaments has been with us for over a century; it refers to the apparent strength ("true") or weakness ("false") as supports of the bladder. These terms are largely of mnemonic value. They are listed in Table 10. See also the discussion of peritoneal reflections in the chapter "Hernias of the Pelvic Wall."

TABLE 10
Ligaments of the Bladder

Ligament	Location
True Ligaments	
Median umbilical ligament (urachus) (unpaired)	Dome of bladder to umbilicus
Lateral true ligament	Lateral wall of bladder to tendinous arch of pelvic fascia
Medial umbilical ligament (obliterated umbilical aa)	Inguinal ligament
Medial puboprostatic ligament (male)	Pelvic wall to prostate gland
Lateral puboprostatic ligament	Pelvic wall to prostate gland
False Ligaments	
Superior false ligament (unpaired)	Covers the urachus
Lateral false ligament	Bladder to wall of pelvis
Lateral superior ligament	Covers the medial umbilical ligament
Posterior ligament (sacrogenital fold)	Side of bladder, around rectum to anterior aspect of sacrum

[1]Basmajian JV: *Grant's Method of Anatomy,* 8th ed. Williams & Wilkins, Baltimore, 1971, p. 287.

293

The Retrovesical Space

The boundaries of the retrovesical space in the male are

Anterior: Posterior surface of the bladder with vesical fascia; the lateral true ligament of the bladder

Superior: Peritoneum and transverse fold of bladder

Posterior: Anterior surface of the rectum with rectal fascia

Inferior: Rectourethralis ligament; pelvic diaphragm

Both the vesical and rectal fasciae are loose connective tissue. Between them lies a stronger fascia (Denonvilliers'), the anterior layer of the prostatoperitoneal membrane. Thus the true retrovesical space lies between the vesical fascia and the anterior layer of the prostatoperitoneal membrane in the male (Plate 94E).

Starting at the bottom of the transverse fold of the bladder, the hernia sac will pass between the vesical fascia and the peritoneum. It may then take either of two paths:

1. If the sac follows the bladder wall downward toward the seminal vesicles, its posterior boundary will be the prostatoperitoneal membrane as illustrated by path 1 in Plate 94E. This membrane, attenuated close to the peritoneum, becomes stronger as it descends toward the prostate.
2. If the sac travels more posteriorly through the upper, more attenuated, part of this membrane, then the posterior boundary becomes the rectal wall since the rectal fascia is too loose to form a barrier. The prostatoperitoneal membrane forms the anterior boundary in this case, as seen in path 2 of Plate 94E.

If the sac originates in the rectovesical pouch instead of the transverse fold, it will pass into the same space, between the prostatoperitoneal membrane and the wall of the rectum (path 3, Plate 94E). Thus, a hernia sac in the retrovesical space may have its mouth (1) at the bottom of the transverse fold of the bladder, or (2) at the bottom of the rectovesical pouch.

In either case, the end of the sac lies on the intact pelvic floor. Should there be a defect in this floor through which the sac may pass, it will become a perineal hernia.

PLATE 94

Surgical Anatomy of Internal Supravesical Hernia

A. The anterior portion of the abdominal wall viewed from the posterior surface. Internal supravesical hernias result from the loss of integrity of the transversus abdominis muscle and the transversalis fascia. Most of these hernias pass downward as direct inguinal or femoral hernias. About half of direct inguinal hernias originate in the supravesical fossa between the middle umbilical ligament and the medial umbilical fold.

Source: From Gray SW, Skandalakis JE: *Atlas of Surgical Anatomy for General Surgeons.* Williams & Wilkins, Baltimore, 1985, p. 317, Plate 14-10.

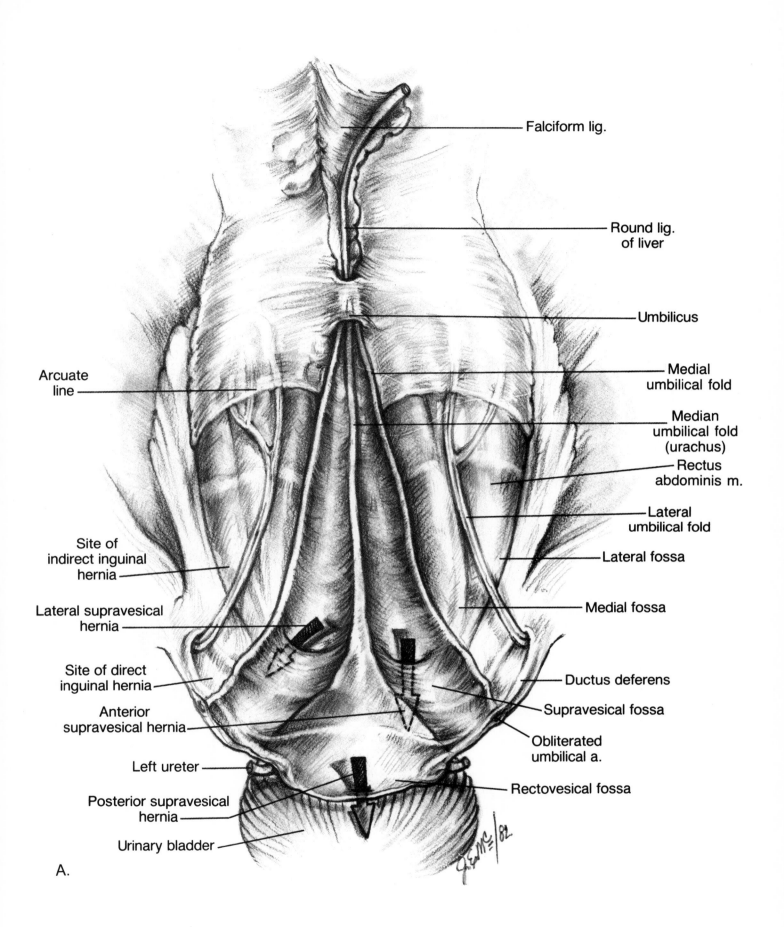

Falciform lig.

Round lig.
of liver

Umbilicus

Medial
umbilical fold

Median
umbilical fold
(urachus)

Rectus
abdominis m.

Lateral
umbilical fold

Lateral fossa

Medial fossa

Ductus deferens

Supravesical fossa

Obliterated
umbilical a.

Rectovesical fossa

Arcuate
line

Site of
indirect inguinal
hernia

Lateral supravesical
hernia

Site of direct
inguinal hernia

Anterior
supravesical hernia

Left ureter

Posterior supravesical
hernia

Urinary bladder

A.

295

PLATE 94 (*Continued*)

Surgical Anatomy of Internal Supravesical Hernia

B. Highly diagrammatic section of the body at the level of the acetabulum showing some of the landmarks of the spaces around the bladder.

Inset

1. Location of sac in anterior internal supravesical hernia.
2. Location of sac in lateral internal supravesical hernia.
3. Location of sac in posterior internal supravesical hernia.

C. Comparison of anterior and posterior internal supravesical hernias. The majority are of the anterior type. The diagram of the posterior hernia illustrates a case in a patient who had previously undergone hysterectomy.

D. Invaginating type of anterior internal supravesical hernia.

Source: Plate 94B from Skandalakis JE, Gray SW: Supravesical hernia, in *Hernia,* 2d ed, Nyhus LM, Condon RE (eds). Lippincott, Philadelphia, 1978, p. 399, Fig. 23-4; Plate 94C from Skandalakis JE et al: Internal and external supravesical hernia. *Am Surg* 42:142–146, 1976, Fig. 2.

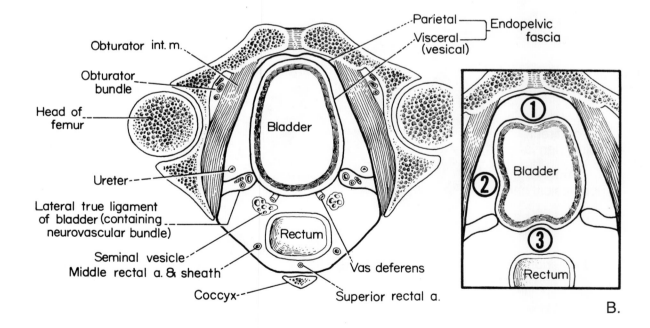

B.

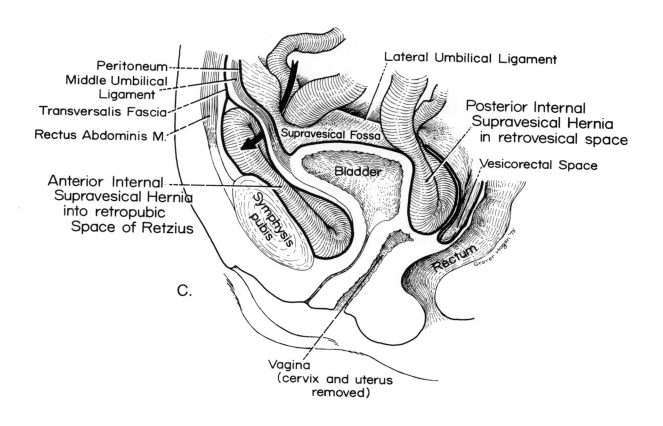

Peritoneum
Middle Umbilical Ligament
Transversalis Fascia
Rectus Abdominis M.

Lateral Umbilical Ligament

Posterior Internal Supravesical Hernia in retrovesical space

Supravesical Fossa

Bladder

Vesicorectal Space

Anterior Internal Supravesical Hernia into retropubic Space of Retzius

Symphysis pubis

Rectum

C.

Vagina (cervix and uterus removed)

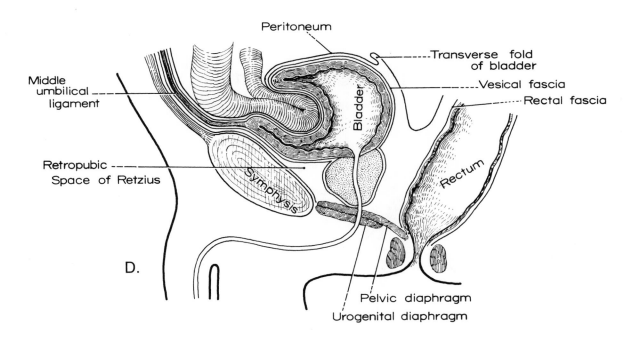

Peritoneum

Transverse fold of bladder

Middle umbilical ligament

Bladder

Vesical fascia

Rectal fascia

Retropubic Space of Retzius

Symphysis

Rectum

D.

Pelvic diaphragm

Urogenital diaphragm

297

PLATE 94 (*Continued*)

Surgical Anatomy of Internal Supravesical Hernia

E. Three possible pathways of posterior internal supravesical hernias in the male:

1. Path of true retrovesical hernia.
2. Path of rectovesical hernia.
3. Path of hernia through rectovesical pouch.

F. Two possible pathways of a posterior internal supravesical hernia in the female:

1. Path of true retrovesical hernia.
2. Path of hernia through the vesicovaginal pouch.

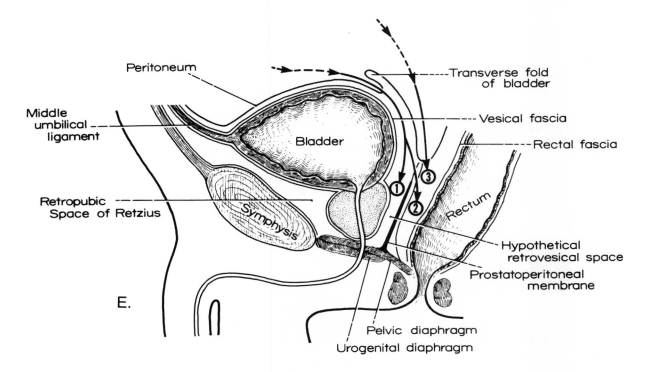

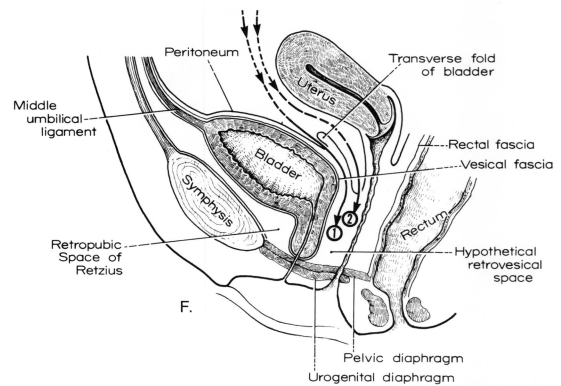

G. Posterior superior view of the right abdominal wall from inside.

Source: Plate 94D, E, F from Skandalakis JE, Gray SW: Supravesical hernia, in *Hernia,* 2d ed, Nyhus LM, Condon RE (eds). Lippincott, Philadelphia, 1978, pp. 401–3, Figs. 23-6, 23-7, 23-8.

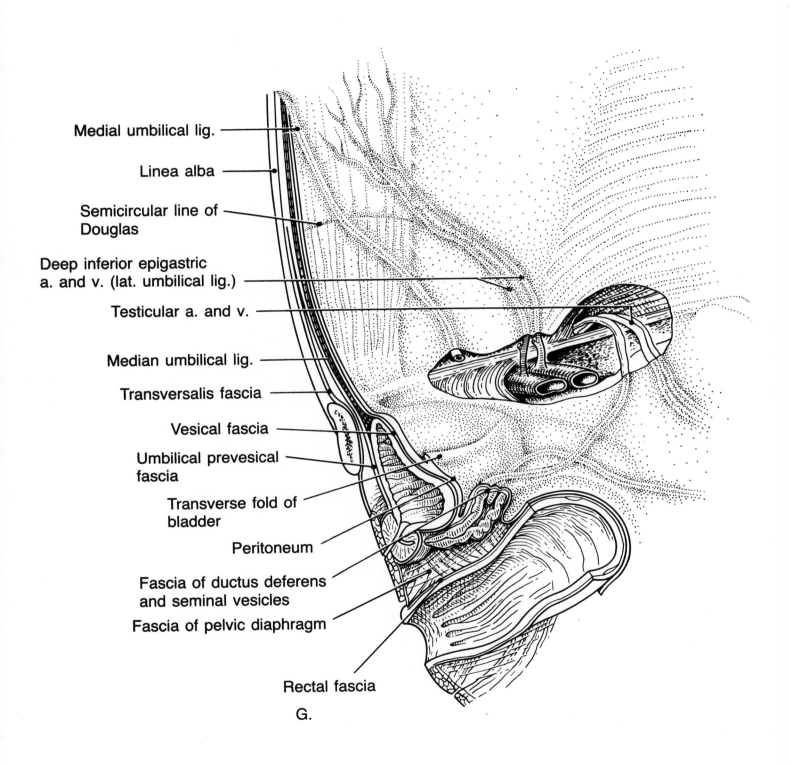

Medial umbilical lig.

Linea alba

Semicircular line of Douglas

Deep inferior epigastric a. and v. (lat. umbilical lig.)

Testicular a. and v.

Median umbilical lig.

Transversalis fascia

Vesical fascia

Umbilical prevesical fascia

Transverse fold of bladder

Peritoneum

Fascia of ductus deferens and seminal vesicles

Fascia of pelvic diaphragm

Rectal fascia

G.

299

PLATE 94 (*Continued*)
Surgical Anatomy of Internal Supravesical Hernia

H. Diagram of the bladder and some of its ligaments.

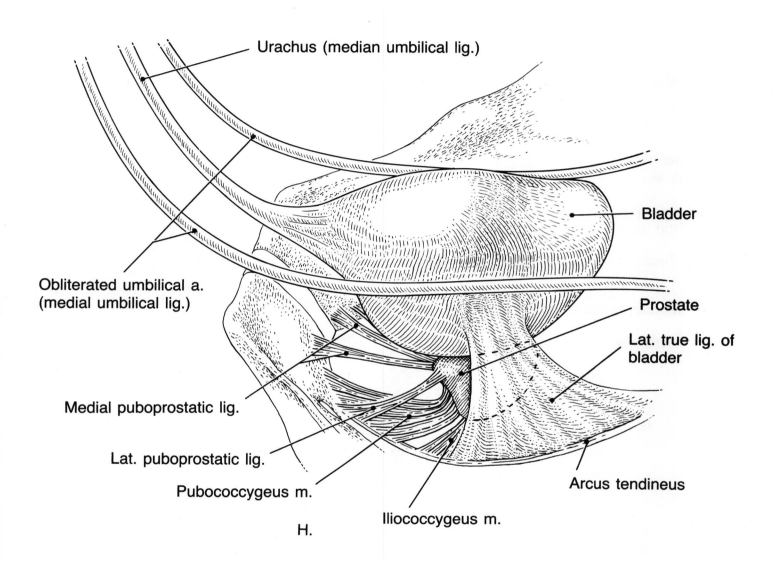

Urachus (median umbilical lig.)

Bladder

Obliterated umbilical a.
(medial umbilical lig.)

Prostate

Lat. true lig. of
bladder

Medial puboprostatic lig.

Lat. puboprostatic lig.

Pubococcygeus m.

Arcus tendineus

Iliococcygeus m.

H.

PLATE 95
Repair of Internal Supravesical Hernia

A. A loop of ileum is incarcerated in the retrovesical space forming a posterior supravesical hernia.

B. *Step 1.* Reduce the hernia and evert the hernial sac.

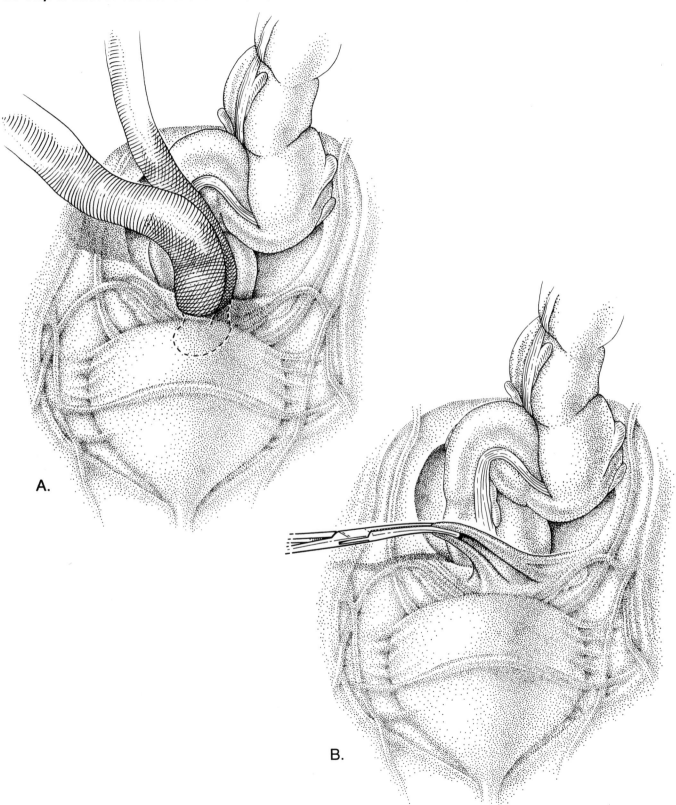

A.

B.

PLATE 95 (*Continued*)
Repair of Internal Supravesical Hernia

C. *Step 2.* Ligate and excise the sac.

D. *Step 3.* Close the peritoneal defect with Prolene mesh.

Complications
Viscus and ureteral injury

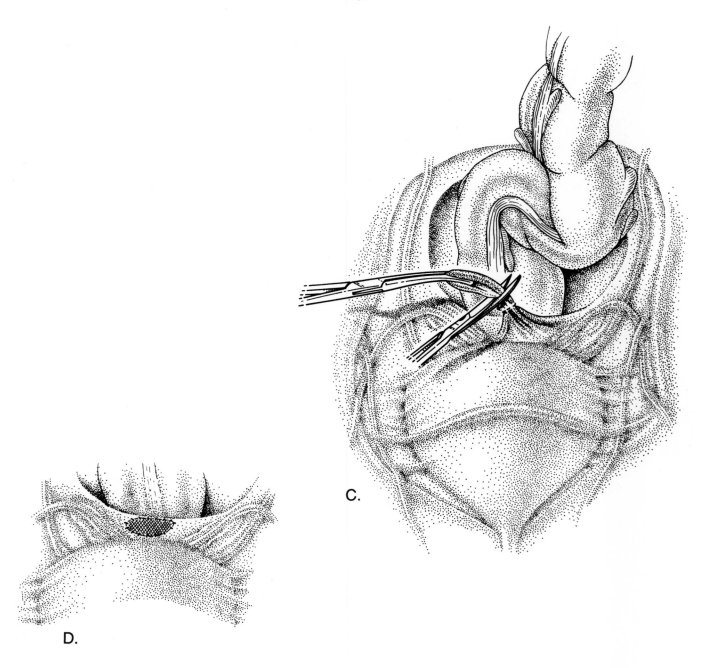

C.

D.

SECTION FOUR
HERNIAS OF THE DIAPHRAGM

The orifice of the stomach . . . was extremely large, as the gula which is continued therefrom was also, to the height of, at least, four inches above the stomach, in the hole of which tract it was more red, internally, than the other parts.

. . . the foramen, which is open'd in the septum transversum, in order to transmit the oesophagus, was much bigger than usual, particularly in its breadth, and that it terminated, at its upper extremity, by a right line transversely, instead of an angle.

MORGAGNI,
De Sedibus, Letter XXXVII, Article 30, 1769

EMBRYOLOGY AND ANATOMY OF THE DIAPHRAGM

And the Lord God caused a deep sleep
to fall upon Adam, and he slept:
and he took one of his ribs,
and closed up the flesh instead thereof.

GENESIS, 3;21

Definition

A diaphragmatic hernia, acquired or congenital, is a protrusion of abdominal viscera through a defect in the diaphragm into the low pressure of the mediastinal space or pleural cavity from the high pressure of the abdominal cavity.

Embryology of the Diaphragm

The diaphragm develops from four embryonic components.

Transverse Septum

The growing head fold of the embryo brings a wall of mesoderm to a position cranial to the open midgut and caudal to the heart during the third embryonic week. This mesoderm forms the ventral component of the future diaphragm.

The cranial surface of the transverse septum also contributes to the connective tissue of the pericardium, and the caudal surface contributes to the capsule and stroma of the liver.

Mediastinum

The mediastinum is the thick dorsal mesentery of the foregut, containing the future esophagus and the inferior vena cava. It is continuous anteriorly with the transverse septum and posteriorly with the axial mesoderm. By posterior and caudal extension it splits to form the diaphragmatic crura.

Pleuroperitoneal Membranes

The pleuroperitoneal membranes close the right and left communication between the pleural and peritoneal cavities at about the eighth embryonic week. Originally they form a large part of the developing diaphragm, but relative growth of other elements reduces their contribution to a small area.

Muscles of the Body Wall

Myotomes of the seventh to twelfth segments contribute the lateral component of the diaphragm by caudal excavation of the thoracic wall to form the costodiaphragmatic recesses. This process produces the final domed shape of the diaphragm.

Phrenic nerve fibers are present in the diaphragm by the seventh week, and muscle fibers can be found a week later. Before birth there is a preponderance of white, fast-twitch, low oxidative fibers. An increase in red, slow-twitch, high oxidative fibers takes place until, by the eighth postnatal month, about 55 percent of the fibers are of the red, slow-twitch type. These fibers are less easily fatigued than are white fibers.

It is not certain whether all muscle fibers originate from the thoracic wall and migrate centrally or originate in the transverse septum and migrate peripherally. With the data presently available, it is not possible to delineate in the adult diaphragm the exact boundaries of the four embryonic components.

Descent of the Diaphragm

In the third week, the transverse septum lies at the level of the third cervical vertebra, and the developing diaphragm descends to its final position at the level of the first lumbar vertebra by the eighth week. The phrenic nerve, which originates from the third to fifth cervical levels, is carried caudad with the descending diaphragm.

During the first 2 months of fetal life, there is no pressure on the developing diaphragm from above or below. Above, the lungs are not inflated; below, the growth of the gut is taking place extraabdominally into the umbilical cord. The first mechanical pressure on the diaphragm comes during the tenth week when the intestines return from the umbilical cord to the abdomen. By that time all of the diaphragmatic components are normally in place and have sufficient strength to contain the abdominal viscera. This may not be the case if the normal development timetable is disturbed.

A number of areas of the diaphragm may give way under pressure from the abdominal viscera. Most diaphragmatic hernias start in these small areas of weakness and enlarge with age. The specific hernias are described in this section and summarized in Tables 11 and 12.

Anatomy of the Diaphragm

Note: The subphrenic spaces and the lymphatics are not presented in this text. The reader is referred to JE Skandalakis, SW Gray, JS Rowe Jr.: *Surgical anatomy of the diaphragm,* vol 1, in *Mastery of Surgery,* Nyhus LM, Baker RJ (eds), Little, Brown, Boston, 1984.

Origins and Insertions of the Diaphragmatic Musculature

The diaphragm is composed of a central tendinous area from which muscle fibers radiate in all directions toward their peripheral attachments.

Sternal Portion (Anterior)

Paired slips of muscle originate from the xiphoid process and the aponeurosis of the transversus abdominis muscle. Small triangular spaces (foramina of Morgagni) separate those slips from the costal fibers and from each other.

Costal Portion (Anterolateral)

Muscle fibers arise from the cartilages of the seventh and eighth ribs, the cartilage and bony portions of the ninth rib, and the distal bony portions of the tenth to twelfth ribs. Anteriorly, these origins are related to those of the transversus abdominis; on the twelfth rib, they are related to the attachment of the thoracolumbar fascia.

Lumbar Portion (Posterior)

Posteriorly the diaphragmatic muscle arises from the crura and the medial and lateral arcuate ligaments (lumbocostal arches).

The Crura

The crura arise from the anterior surface of the first to fourth lumbar vertebrae on the right, and the first two or three lumbar vertebrae on the left, as well as from the intervertebral disks and the anterior longitudinal ligament. The crural fibers pass superiorly and anteriorly, forming the muscular arms that surround the openings for the aorta and the esophagus; they insert on the central tendon. At their origin on the vertebrae, the crura are tendinous, becoming increasingly muscular as they ascend into the diaphragm proper. In our studies of cadavers, we found the crura to be tendinous, posteriorly and medially from their vertebral origins to the level of the tenth thoracic vertebra, in 90 percent of cadavers. Sutures to approximate the crura should always be placed through the tendinous portions.

The pattern of the crural arms at the esophageal hiatus is variable. In one-half or more of persons, both right and left arms arise from the right crus. In another one-third or more, the left arm arises from the right crus, and the right arm arises from both crura. The remainder of subjects present a variety of uncommon patterns. Hiatal hernia is not associated with any specific hiatal pattern.

The Arcuate Ligaments

The lateral arcuate ligaments (lumbocostal arches) are thickened bands in the fascia covering the anterior surface of the superior ends of the quadratus lumborum muscles, which attach to the twelfth ribs laterally and to the transverse processes of the first lumbar vertebra medially. The medial arcuate ligaments (medial arches) are tendinous bands or similarly thickened fascia of the superior ends of the psoas muscles, which attach to the transverse processes of the first lumbar vertebra laterally and to the body of the first or second lumbar vertebra medially. The medial arcuate ligaments are separated from each other by the crura and the median arcuate ligament, to be described later. From these two pairs of arcuate ligaments on either side arise the muscle fibers of the posterior portion of the diaphragm.

The Central Tendon

All the musculature described above inserts on the fibrous central tendon of the diaphragm. The thickened portion anterior to the esophageal hiatus and to the left of the caval aperture is sometimes called the *cruciform* (transverse) *ligament*. Fibers on the superior surface of the central tendon blend with those of the fibrous pericardium. Patches of muscle are often present among the fibers of the central tendon.

The Openings of the Diaphragm

The Hiatus of the Inferior Vena Cava

The hiatus of the inferior vena cava lies in the right dome of the central tendon about 2 cm to the right of the midline and at the level of the eighth thoracic vertebra. The margins of the hiatus are fixed to the vena cava, which is accompanied by branches of the right phrenic nerve.

The collagen fiber bundles forming the right margin of the caval hiatus cross inferiorly to the bundles forming the medial and posterior margins to form a fibrous limb that may be traced to the edge of the central tendon. The tendinous fibers forming the medial margin of the hiatus are attached to the muscle fibers of the right crus. Whether this arrangement of fibers constricts or enlarges the caval hiatus during inspiration has been a source of controversy for many years. Constriction of the vena cava during inspiration is known to occur in diving mammals such as the seal. In these animals, a muscular sphincter takes the place of the fibrous bundles found in the human diaphragm. No parallel can be drawn between seal and human.

The Esophageal Hiatus

The elliptical esophageal hiatus is in the muscular portion of the diaphragm 2 cm or less to the left of the midline at the level of the tenth thoracic vertebra. The anterior and lateral margins of the hiatus are formed by the muscular arms of the crura, and the posterior margin is formed by the median arcuate ligament. The anterior and posterior vagal trunks and the esophageal arteries and veins from the left gastric vessels pass through the hiatus with the esophagus. This is a region in which the portal circulation (left gastric vein) communicates with the systemic circulation (esophageal branches of the azygos veins).

The Aortic Opening

The oblique course of the aorta takes it behind the diaphragm rather than through it. At the level of the twelfth thoracic vertebra, the anterior border of the opening is the median arcuate ligament; laterally the diaphragmatic crura form its margins. The thoracic duct and sometimes the azygos vein accompany the aorta.

The Median Arcuate Ligament

The esophageal hiatus is separated from the aortic hiatus by fusion of the arms of the left and right crura. If the tendinous portions of the crura are fused, the median arcuate ligament is present as a fibrous arch passing over the aorta, connecting the right and left crura. If the fusion is muscular only, the ligament is ill-defined or absent.

The median arcuate ligament passes in front of the aorta at the level of the first lumbar vertebra just above the origin of the celiac trunk. The celiac ganglia lie just below and anterior to the celiac trunk. In 16 percent of patients, a low median arcuate ligament covers the celiac artery and may compress it. At angiography such compression may simulate atherosclerotic plaques. Adequate collateral circulation exists, since such patients usually do not have symptoms.

If there is no true ligament, and the muscular arms of the crura are thinned by posterior extension of the esophageal hiatus, the aortic and esophageal openings may become practically confluent, although there is always some connective tissue between them.

In about half of the cadavers with hiatal hernia that we examined, the ligament was sufficiently well developed to use in surgical repair of the esophageal hiatus. In the remainder, there was enough preaortic fascia lateral to the celiac trunk to perform a posterior fixation of the gastroesophageal junction. The celiac ganglion, just below the arcuate ligament, must be avoided.

Other Openings in the Diaphragm

Anteriorly the superior epigastric vessels pass through the parasternal spaces (foramina of Morgagni). In the dome of the diaphragm, the phrenic nerves pierce the upper surface to become distributed over the lower surface between the muscle and the peritoneum.

The azygos vein may pass behind the diaphragm with the aorta, to the right of the right crus, or it may pierce the right crus. Also passing through the crura are the greater, lesser, and least splanchnic nerves.

Diaphragmatic-Mediastinal Relations

Over much of the anterosuperior surface of the diaphragm the fibrous tissue of the central tendon is continuous with the fibrous pericardium.

In addition to the pericardium, the mediastinum on the right contains the inferior vena cava, the right phrenic nerve, the right pulmonary ligament, the esophagus with the right vagal trunk, the azygos vein, the vertebral bodies, and the right sympathetic trunk.

In the left mediastinum are the pericardium, the left phrenic nerve, the esophagus, the left vagal trunk, the descending aorta, the vertebral bodies, and the left sympathetic trunk. The triangle (of Truesdale) formed by the pericardium, the aorta, and the diaphragm contains the left pulmonary ligament and the distal esophagus. In sliding hiatal hernia, the stomach is in this triangle.

The remainder of the superior surface of the diaphragm is covered with the parietal pleura. The approximation of the right and left pleurae between the esophagus and the aorta forms the so-called mesoesophagus. The right pleura is in contact with the lower third of the esophagus almost down to the esophageal hiatus. This creates the risk of accidental entrance into the pleural cavity during abdominal operations on the esophageal hiatus. In spite of this proximity of the right pleura, the surgeon, working on the right side of the operating table, is more likely to produce a pneumothorax or hemopneumothorax on the left.

Peritoneal Reflections of the Inferior Surface of the Diaphragm and the Gastroesophageal Junction

The primitive dorsal and ventral mesenteries of the abdomen form a number of ligaments related to the diaphragm and the gastroesophageal junction.

Falciform, Coronary, and Triangular Ligaments

The falciform ligament, a remnant of the primitive ventral mesentery, arises from the anterior abdominal wall and extends to the anterior surface of the liver and the diaphragm. In its free edge runs the round ligament, the obliterated left umbilical vein.

The leaves of the falciform ligament separate over the liver to form the anterior and posterior layers of the coronary ligament. Enclosing the bare area on the right, these leaves unite laterally to form the right triangular ligament. On the left, the leaves are in apposition to each other, forming the left triangular ligament. One approach to the gastroesophageal junction is to section the left triangular and left portion of the posterior layer of the coronary ligament.

Gastrohepatic (Hepatogastric) Ligament

The abdominal esophagus lies between the two layers of the gastrohepatic ligament. This area is the superior part of the lesser omentum, derived from the primitive ventral mesentery. The inferior portion is the hepatoduodenal ligament. The gastrohepatic ligament extends from the porta hepatis to the lesser curvature of the stomach and the abdominal esophagus; it separates the lesser sac from the rest of the abdominal cavity. The gastrohepatic ligament is formed by the anterior leaf; the posterior leaf does not reach the gastroesophageal junction. Thus, a small bare area is left on the posterior wall of the stomach that lies over the left crus of the diaphragm and is easily separated from it by the surgeon's finger.

The ligament contains the left gastric artery and vein, the hepatic division of the left vagus nerve, and the lymph nodes. It may also contain both vagal trunks, branches of the right gastric artery and vein, and the left hepatic artery if it arises from the left gastric artery.

Gastrosplenic (Gastrolienal) Ligament

On the right, the gastrohepatic ligament divides to enclose the abdominal esophagus; its leaves rejoin on the left to form the gastrosplenic ligament, which is part of the primitive dorsal mesentery. The upper portion of the gastrosplenic ligament contains the short gastric vessels and the pancreaticosplenic lymph nodes; the lower portion contains the left gastroepiploic vessels, lymph nodes, and the terminal branches of the splenic artery.

Gastrophrenic Ligament

The gastrophrenic ligament, the superior portion of the dorsal mesentery, arises from the greater curvature of the fundus and extends upward to the diaphragm. The upper part is transparent and avascular, continuous with the posterior layer of the coronary ligament on the left. The lower part is continuous with the gastrosplenic ligament and contains some short gastric vessels and lymph nodes.

The upper avascular area may be perforated by the surgeon's finger in order to insert a Penrose drain around the cardia. The surgeon can thus apply gentle traction on the esophagus, a useful maneuver in vagotomy.

310

Vascularization of the Diaphragm

Arteries
The arterial supply to the superior surface of the diaphragm consists of two branches from the internal thoracic arteries—the pericardiophrenic and musculophrenic arteries—and two branches from the thoracic aorta—the superior phrenic arteries. All these branches are small.

The major blood supply to the diaphragm is to the inferior surface and comes from the inferior phrenic arteries, which arise from the aorta or the celiac axis just below the median arcuate ligament of the diaphragm. In a small percentage of individuals, the right inferior phrenic artery arises from the right renal artery. The inferior phrenic arteries also supply branches to the suprarenal glands.

Veins
On the superior surface of the diaphragm, small tributaries form the pericardiophrenic and musculophrenic veins, which run with the corresponding arteries and empty into the internal thoracic veins. Posteriorly there is some local drainage into the azygos and hemiazygos veins.

On the inferior surface, the right inferior phrenic vein runs with the arteries and empties into the inferior vena cava, but it may have a posterior branch that descends posteriorly to enter the left suprarenal vein.

Nerve Supply to the Diaphragm

The right phrenic nerve enters the diaphragm through the central tendon just lateral to the opening for the inferior vena cava. Occasionally it passes through that opening with the vena cava. The left phrenic nerve pierces the superior surface of the muscular portion of the diaphragm just lateral to the left border of the heart.

Both nerves divide at or just above the diaphragm, and the branches travel together into the musculature. Small sensory branches are given off to the pleura and to the peritoneum over the central part of the diaphragm. The larger motor branches separate within the diaphragm into three or four major nerve trunks: sternal, anterolateral, posterolateral, and crural. The last two usually have a common trunk. These nerve trunks travel partly within the diaphragmatic musculature and partly on the inferior surface covered only by the peritoneum. The sternal branches of the two sides may anastomose behind the sternum.

The peripheral portions of the pleura and peritoneum have an independent sensory innervation that arises from the seventh to the twelfth intercostal nerves.

In addition to the phrenic and intercostal nerves, fibers to the inferior surfaces of the right posterior portion of the diaphragm arise from the celiac ganglion, often forming a phrenic ganglion before their distribution. A connection has been claimed between these fibers and a posterior branch of the right phrenic nerve.

The Distal Esophagus and the Diaphragm

The Gastroesophageal Junction
The external gastroesophageal junction may be described as the point at which the esophageal tube becomes the gastric pouch. From 0.5 to 2.5 cm of

the tube lies in the abdomen. The external junction lies at the level of the eleventh or twelfth thoracic vertebra.

Internally, the junction is marked by an irregular boundary between stratified squamous esophageal epithelium and columnar gastric epithelium. This boundary may lie as far as 1 cm above the external junction. A biopsy specimen of esophageal mucosa should be taken at least 2 cm above the external junction.

The columnar epithelium below the internal junction contains mucus-secreting glands, the cardiac glands of the body of the stomach. The term *junctional epithelium* has been proposed by Hayward.[1]

The external and internal junctions do not coincide; in addition, the loose submucosal connective tissue permits considerable movement between the mucosa and the muscularis externa, changing the relation between them as the stomach fills with food. Plate 101A shows the gastroesophageal junction from several points of view.

The Lower Esophageal Sphincter

A sphincter at the distal end of the esophagus normally permits swallowing but not reflux. No specialized muscular ring guards this opening, such as is found in the pylorus, although several investigators have reported a thickening of the circular muscle in most individuals.

A number of mechanisms for closing the distal esophagus have been suggested: the angle (of His) at which the esophagus enters the stomach; the pinchcock action of the diaphragm; a plug of redundant mucosa (mucosal rosette); the sling of oblique fibers of the gastric musculature; and factors relating to wall tension of the stomach as a force contributing to sphincter opening. Regardless of the mechanism, the lower esophageal sphincter at rest withstands a pressure of about 15 cm of water. This permits one to stand on one's head without losing one's lunch. Incompetence of this closing mechanism with esophageal reflux may or may not be associated with sliding hiatal hernia.

The Phrenoesophageal Ligament (Membrane)

A strong, flexible, airtight seal is necessary at the esophageal hiatus of the diaphragm. The seal is provided by the pleura above and the peritoneum below; strength and flexibility are provided by the phrenoesophageal ligament.

The major component of the ligament is formed by collagenous and elastic fibers that arise as a continuation of the endoabdominal (transversalis) fascia beneath the diaphragm. One leaf of this fascia passes upward through the hiatus forming a truncated cone that inserts in the adventitia and intermuscular connective tissue of the esophagus 1 or 2 cm above the diaphragm. A second leaf of the fascia turns downward and inserts into the adventitia of the abdominal esophagus and the stomach. A weaker and less constant component may arise from the endothoracic fascia, passing upward to join the fibers of the endoabdominal fascia. The relations of these components of the phrenoesophageal ligament are shown in Plate 101B.

Much of the variation in descriptions of the ligament is due to changes with age. In the fetus, the esophagus and diaphragm are tightly joined at the hiatus by connective tissue. With the onset of respiratory movements and swallowing in postnatal life, the two structures become less firmly attached and the space between them fills with loose connective tissue and fat.

---

[1]Hayward J: Sliding esophageal hiatus hernia, in *Hernia,* Nyhus LM, Harkins HN (eds). Lippincott, Philadelphia, 1964, p. 401.

The development of the phrenoesophageal ligament may be summarized as follows:

1. In newborn infants, the phrenoesophageal ligament is present.
2. In adults, the ligament is attenuated and subperitoneal fat accumulates at the hiatus.
3. In adults with hiatal hernia, the ligament for all practical purposes does not exist.

Structures at or near the Esophageal Hiatus

A number of structures lie close to the esophageal hiatus of the diaphragm and hence may be injured in surgical procedures on the hiatus.

Left Inferior Phrenic Artery and Left Gastric Artery

The abdominal esophagus and the proximal stomach are supplied by esophageal branches of the left gastric artery. These branches usually, but not always, anastomose above the diaphragm with esophageal arteries from the aorta. In some persons, the lower esophagus also receives twigs from the left inferior phrenic artery. In still others, branches of the inferior phrenic artery supply the lower esophagus, whereas branches of the left gastric artery are confined to the cardia and fundus of the stomach. The margin of the hiatus is always supplied by a branch of the left inferior phrenic artery.

Left Inferior Phrenic Vein

The left inferior vein may drain into the left suprarenal vein or the inferior vena cava, or both. The branch draining into the vena cava passes in front of the esophagus closely enough to be injured.

Left Gastric (Coronary) Vein

The left gastric vein passes upward along the lesser curvature to a point 2 to 3 cm from the esophageal hiatus, where it receives one to three esophageal tributaries. From this point it turns downward and obliquely to the right to join the portal vein or backward to enter the splenic vein.

In our own dissections of 22 cadavers, we found the left gastric vein entering the portal vein in 16 and entering the splenic vein in 6 instances. It is important to remember that the severed distal tributaries of the left gastric vein bleed from anastomoses with esophageal and hemiazygos veins in the thorax.

Aberrant Left Hepatic Artery

An aberrant left hepatic artery arising from the left gastric artery lies in the gastrohepatic ligament in about 11 percent of persons. The possibility of such an artery must be considered before dividing the ligament to reach the gastro-esophageal junction.

Other Vessels

The celiac trunk, the aorta, and the inferior vena cava are all close enough to the esophageal hiatus to be at risk during operations on the hiatus.

Vagal Trunks

Among 100 cadavers dissected by our group, the anterior and posterior vagal trunks passed through the hiatus with the esophagus in 88. In three others, the esophageal plexus was present at the hiatus and the trunks lay entirely within the abdomen. In another nine, the trunks had divided above the hiatus and their major divisions passed through the hiatus.

TABLE 11
Congenital Hernias of the Diaphragm

Congenital Hernias	Anatomy	Sac and Herniated Organs	Remarks
Eventration of the diaphragm.	Congenital hernia. Diaphragm is thin with sparsely distributed, but normal muscle fibers. Either or both sides may be affected. Phrenic nerve appears normal.	"Sac" is formed by the attenuated diaphragm. Contents: Normal abdominal organs under elevated dome of hemidiaphragm.	Heart and mediastinum shifted to contralateral side. Ipsilateral lung collapsed, but normal. Malrotation and inversion of abdominal viscera are common.
Hernia through the foramen of Bochdalek. Posterolateral hernia of the diaphragm.	Congenital hernia through the lumbocostal trigone. May expand to include almost whole hemidiaphragm. More common on left.	Sac present in 10 to 15%. Contents: Small intestine, usual; stomach, colon, spleen, frequent. Pancreas and liver, rare. Liver only in right-sided hernia.	Heart and mediastinum shifted to contralateral side. Ipsilateral lung collapsed but usually not hypoplastic. Secondary malrotation is common. Craniorrhachischisis, tracheoesophageal fistula and heart defects are common.
Hernia through the foramen of Morgagni. Retrosternal hernia. Parasternal hernia. Anterior diaphagramatic hernia.	Congenital potential hernia through muscular hiatus on either side of the xiphoid process. Usually on the right; bilateral cases are known. Actual herniation usually the result of postnatal trauma.	Sac present at first. May rupture later, leaving no trace. Contents: Infants: Liver. Adults: Omentum. May be followed by colon and stomach later.	Rare in infants and children.
Peritoneopericardial hernia. Defect of the central tendon. Defect of the transverse septum.	Congenital hernia through central tendon and pericardium.	Sac rarely present. Contents: Stomach, colon.	Has been seen in newborns and in adults. Perhaps traumatic in adults. Very rare.

Source: Gray SW, Skandalakis JE: *Atlas of Surgical Anatomy for General Surgeons*, 1985, p. 62, Plate 3-4, p. 63, Plate 3-4,

Celiac Ganglia
The celiac ganglia lie on the crura at or below the level of origin of the celiac trunk. Sutures to approximate the crura must be placed above the ganglia and behind the celiac division of the posterior vagal trunk.

Thoracic Duct
The cisterna chyli, when present, lies on the bodies of the first and second lumbar vertebrae between the right crus of the diaphragm and the aorta. Division of the thoracic duct or other large lymph vessels in this area can result in chylous ascites. Ligation of the thoracic duct produces no ill effects.

Esophagus
Extensive mobilization or skeletonization of the esophagus may result in perforation during surgery, or afterward, from subsequent local ischemia.

TABLE 12
Acquired Hernias of the Diaphragm

Acquired Hernias	Anatomy	Sac and Herniated Organs	Remarks
Hiatal hernia. Sliding hiatal hernia. Fixed hiatal hernia.	Congenital potential hernia. The enlarged esophageal hiatus of the diaphragm permits the cardia of the stomach to enter the mediastinum above the diaphragm. The phrenoesophageal ligament is attenuated and stretched. The gastroesophageal junction may be freely movable or fixed in the thorax.	Sac lies anterior and lateral to the herniated stomach. Contents: Cardiac stomach.	A large hiatus (admitting three fingers) may be a predisposing factor; actual herniation usually occurs in late adult life. It has been seen in newborn infants.
Paraesophageal hernia.	Congenital potential hernia. The cardia is in the normal position. The fundus has herniated through the hiatus into the thorax.	Sac lies anterior to the esophagus and posterior to the pericardium. Contents: Fundus of stomach. Body of stomach, transverse colon, omentum and spleen may enter the sac later.	An esophageal hiatus larger than normal may be the predisposing factor. Actual herniation occurs in later adult life.
Acquired eventration.	Paralysis of normal muscle resulting from phrenic nerve injury.	Diaphragm elevated. No true hernial sac.	Heart and mediastinum shifted to contralateral side. Ipsilateral lung collapsed but normal. No malrotation.
Traumatic hernia.	Acquired hernia. Tear, usually from esophageal hiatus across dome to left costal attachment of diaphragm.	There is no sac. Herniated organs: None at first. Spleen, splenic flexure of colon, stomach, left lobe of liver later.	

Source: Gray SW, Skandalakis JE: *Atlas of Surgical Anatomy for General Surgeons* 1985, p. 62, Plate 3-4.

Most perforations are in the posterior wall, the result of a blind search for the posterior vagal trunk. It should be kept in mind that the posterior trunk lies closer to the aorta than to the esophagus and is slightly to the right of the midline.

Periesophageal Space

The periesophageal space involving the abdominal esophagus and the cardia of the stomach was first described by Philip E. Donahue and Lloyd M. Nyhus in 1981.[1] The space is bounded anteriorly by the peritoneal reflection, posteriorly by the aorta, on the right by the hepatogastric ligament which encloses the esophagus, and on the left by the beginning of the gastrosplenic ligament. We would like to call this space the Donahue-Nyhus space (Plate 102).

[1]Donahue PE, Nyhus LM: Exposure of the periesophageal space. *Surg Gynecol Obstet* 152:218–220, 1981.

PLATE 96
Embryology of the Diaphragm

A. The four embryonic components of the diaphragm.

B. The adult diaphragm. The sites of the closed pleuroperitoneal canals occupy a relatively small area in the adult diaphragm.

Source: Plate 96A,B,C from Skandalakis JE, Gray SW, Rowe JS Jr.: Surgical anatomy of the diaphragm, vol. 1, in *Mastery of Surgery,* Nyhus LM, Baker RJ (eds). Little, Brown, Boston, 1984, p. 303, Figs 38-2A,B, Fig. 38-3.

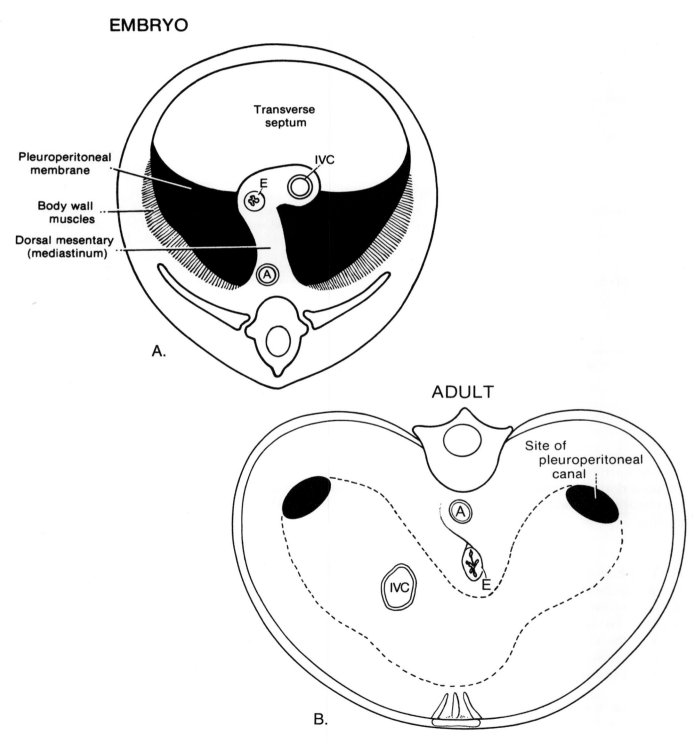

C. The descent of the diaphragm during development. The phrenic nerve arises from the third to the fifth cervical segments and follows the diaphragm down to its final position.

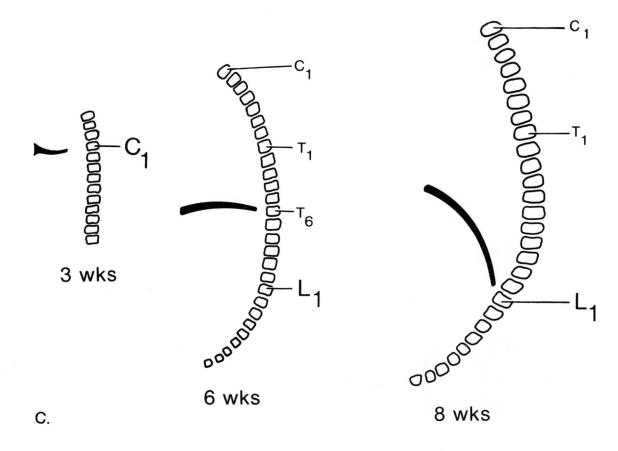

3 wks

6 wks

8 wks

C.

PLATE 97
Origins and Insertions of the Diaphragmatic Musculature

A. The diaphragm from below, showing the foramen of Bochdalek and the foramen of Morgagni. Both are weak areas of potential herniation. Arrows indicate the direction of enlargement after herniation has begun.

Source: From Skandalakis JE, Gray SW, Rowe JS Jr.: Surgical anatomy of the
diaphragm, vol. 1, in *Mastery of Surgery,* Nyhus LM, Baker RJ (eds).
Little, Brown, Boston, 1984, p. 306, Fig. 38-5.

B. The crura consist of both tendinous and muscular tissue; only the tendinous
portion holds sutures. In 9 out of 10 persons, the medial edge of the crura is
tendinous.

Source: From Gray SW, Rowe JS Jr., Skandalakis JE: Surgical anatomy of the
gastroesophageal junction. *Am Surg* 45:575, 1979, Fig. 2.

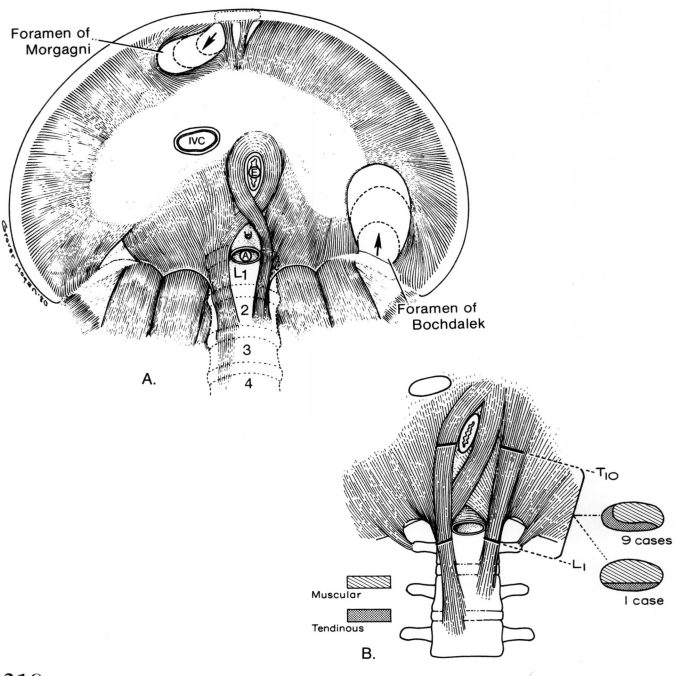

C. The most common patterns of the diaphragmatic crura. A-1 and B-1 seen from below. A-2, A-3, and B-2, B-3 seen from above.

Source: Data from Pataro VA, Piombo HS, Suarez DZ, Acrich MW: Anatomic aspects of the esophageal hiatus: Distribution of the crura in its formation. A study of sixty fresh human specimens. *J Int Coll Surg* 35:154, 1961.

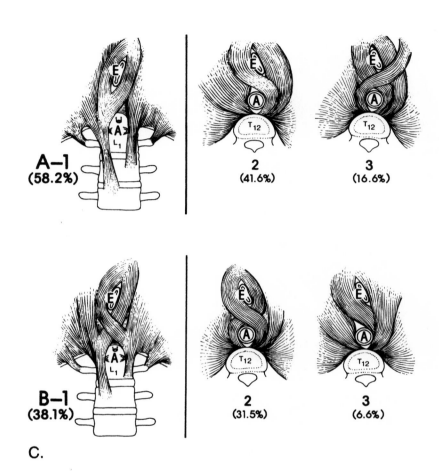

C.

PLATE 98
Openings of the Diaphragm

A. The diaphragm viewed from above. The area in contact with the pericardium is indicated. The pericardial fibrous tissue is continuous with that of the diaphragm.

B. The apertures of the diaphragm seen from below and the structures traversing them.

Source: Plate 98A, B from Skandalakis, JE, Gray SE, Rowe JS Jr.: Surgical anatomy of the diaphragm, in *Mastery of Surgery,* Nyhus LM, Baker RJ (eds). Little, Brown, Boston, 1984, p. 309, Figs. 38-11, 38-12.

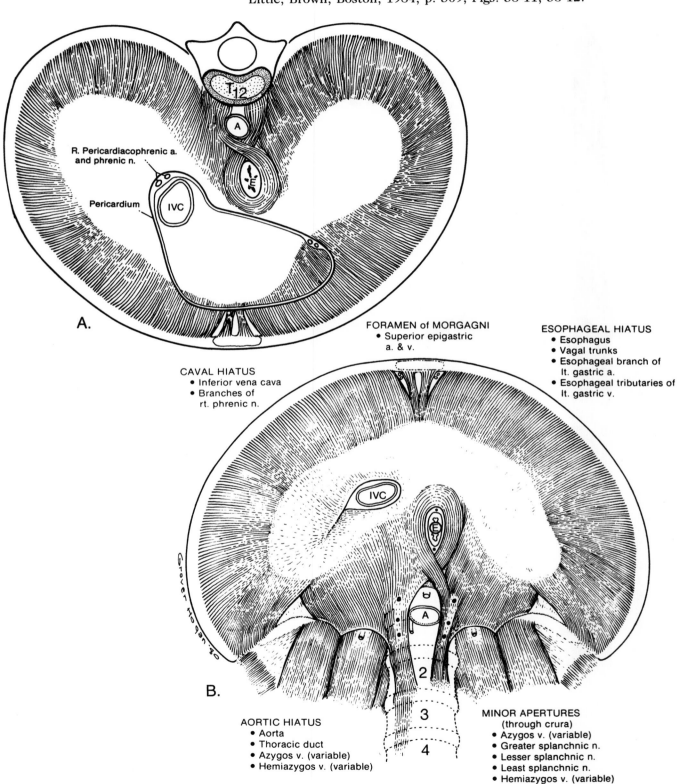

R. Pericardiacophrenic a. and phrenic n.

Pericardium

IVC

A.

CAVAL HIATUS
- Inferior vena cava
- Branches of rt. phrenic n.

FORAMEN of MORGAGNI
- Superior epigastric a. & v.

ESOPHAGEAL HIATUS
- Esophagus
- Vagal trunks
- Esophageal branch of lt. gastric a.
- Esophageal tributaries of lt. gastric v.

AORTIC HIATUS
- Aorta
- Thoracic duct
- Azygos v. (variable)
- Hemiazygos v. (variable)

MINOR APERTURES
(through crura)
- Azygos v. (variable)
- Greater splanchnic n.
- Lesser splanchnic n.
- Least splanchnic n.
- Hemiazygos v. (variable)

B.

PLATE 99

Peritoneal Reflections of the Inferior Surface of the Diaphragm and Gastroesophageal Junction

Peritoneal reflections of the stomach, gastroesophageal junction, and bare area of the diaphragm.

Source: From Skandalakis JE, Gray SW, Rowe JS Jr.: Surgical anatomy of the diaphragm, in *Mastery of Surgery,* Nyhus LM, Baker RJ (eds). Little, Brown, Boston, 1984, p. 312, Fig. 38-17.

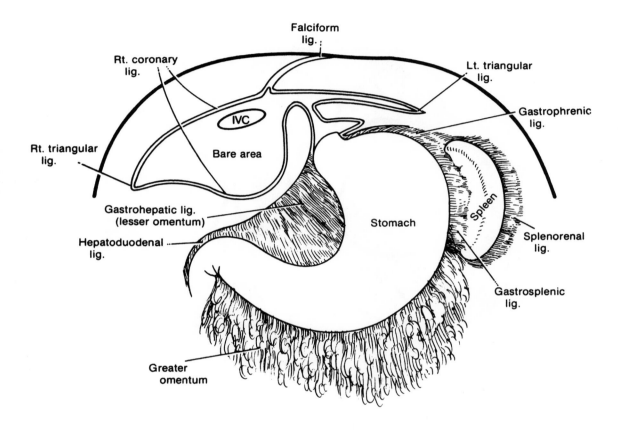

PLATE 100

Nerve Supply to the Diaphragm

The major branches of the phrenic nerves from below. Each phrenic nerve divides just before entering the diaphragm from above.

Source: From Skandalakis JE, Gray SW, Rowe JS Jr.: Surgical anatomy of the diaphragm, in *Mastery of Surgery,* Nyhus LM, Baker RJ (eds). Little, Brown, Boston, 1984, p. 314, Fig. 38-21.

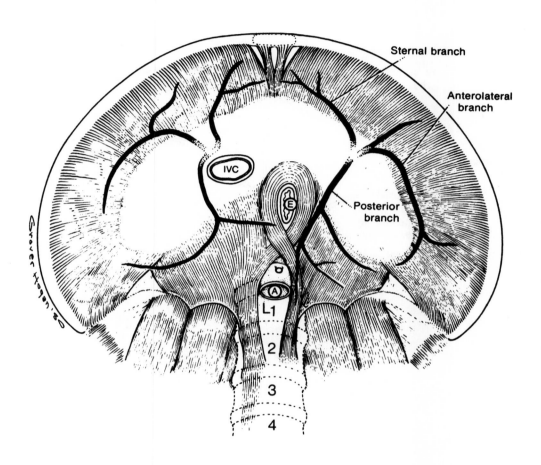

322

PLATE 101

The Distal Esophagus and the Diaphragm

A. The gastroesophageal junction from the point of view of (1) the anatomist, (2) the surgeon, (3) the radiologist, and (4) the endoscopist.

Source: From Skandalakis JE, Gray SW, Rowe JS Jr.: Surgical anatomy of the diaphragm, in *Mastery of Surgery,* Nyhus LM, Baker RJ (eds). Little, Brown, Boston 1984, p. 315, Fig. 38-22.

B. Structures at the gastroesophageal junction and the diaphragmatic hiatus.

Source: From Skandalakis JE, Gray SW, Rowe JS Jr.: Surgical anatomy of the diaphragm, in *Mastery of Surgery,* Nyhus LM, Baker RJ (eds). Little, Brown, Boston 1984, p. 315, Fig. 38-23.

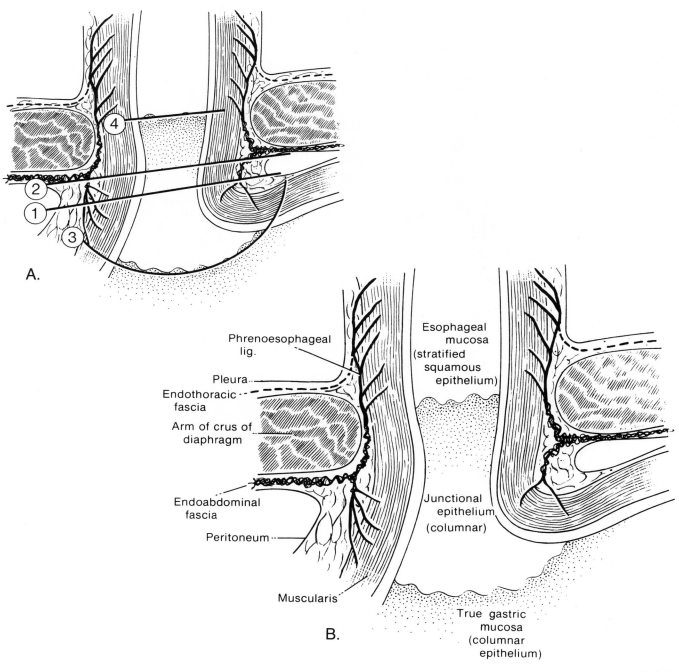

PLATE 101 (*Continued*)

The Distal Esophagus and the Diaphragm

Variations in the blood supply to the distal esophagus and the esophageal hiatus.

C. The inferior phrenic artery supplies the margin of the hiatus. An esophageal branch of the left gastric artery supplies the esophagus and anastomoses with thoracic esophageal arteries. This is the most frequent pattern.

D. The esophagus is supplied by esophageal branches of the left gastric and the inferior phrenic arteries without cranial anastomoses.

E. The esophagus is supplied entirely by a branch of the inferior phrenic artery, which anastomoses with thoracic esophageal arteries. This pattern is rare.

Source: From Skandalakis JE, Gray SW, Rowe JS Jr.: Surgical anatomy of the diaphragm, in *Mastery of Surgery,* Nyhus LM, Baker RJ (eds). Little, Brown, Boston 1984, p. 316, Fig. 38-24.

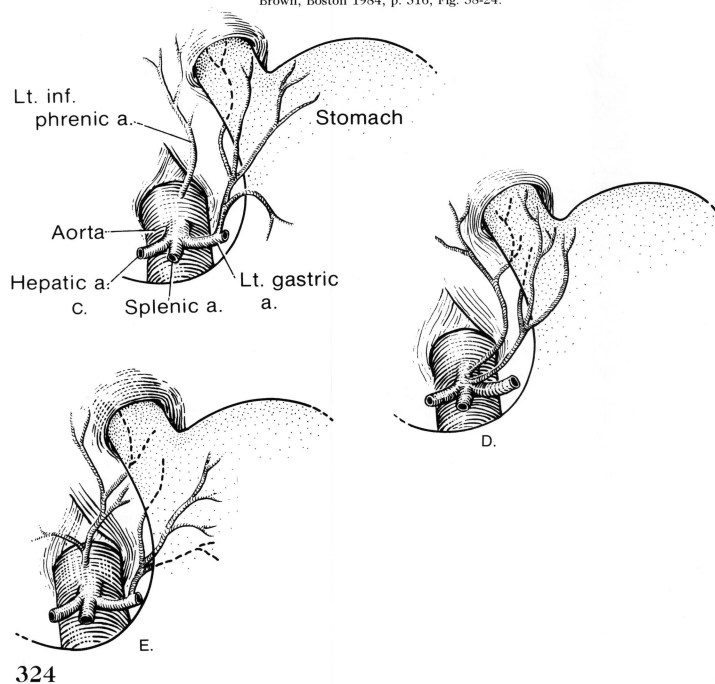

PLATE 102

Exposure of the Periesophageal Space

A. *Step 1.* Incise from the peritoneal reflection over the gastroesophageal junction on the right to the angle of His on the left.

B. *Step 2.* Clean up the fat between the peritoneal reflection and the periesophageal plane, dividing the adventitial and adipose tissue between clamps.

C. *Step 3.* Use finger to identify the abdominal esophagus. Insert the index finger slowly from left to right around the posterior area of the space between the aorta and the posterior esophageal wall.

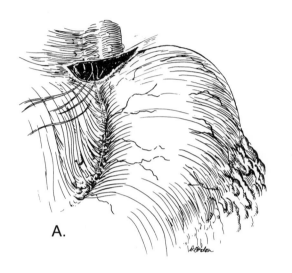

A.

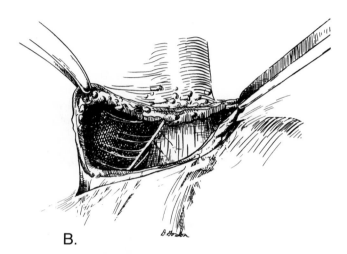

B.

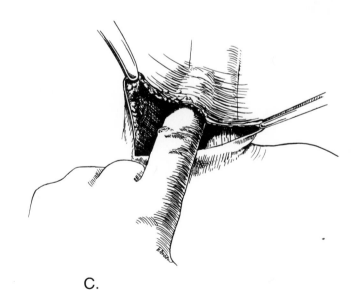

C.

PLATE 102 (*Continued*)

Exposure of the Periesophageal Space

D. *Step 4.* The "stout" or dorsal mesoesophagus is disrupted by digital pressure and final perforation. If the mesoesophagus is "very stout," divide between clamps with direct vision, avoiding the posterior right esophageal wall.

E. *Step 5.* The esophagus is retracted. Mobilize at least 5 cm of the distal esophagus. The surgeon should now be able to see and feel (a) the longitudinal musculature; (b) the left anterior vagus trunk at the right anterior esophageal wall; (c) the right posterior vagus trunk, a cordlike formation at the extensor surface of the second phalanx of the finger.

Source: Plate A through E from Donahue PE, Nyhus LM. Exposure of the periesophageal space. *Surg Gynecol Obstet* 152: 218–220, 1981, Fig. 1-5.

Remember

The anterior vagus trunk is fixed to the esophageal wall.
The posterior vagus trunk is close to the aorta.
A Penrose drain should be inserted around the esophagus. Be sure to mobilize at least 5 cm of distal esophagus.

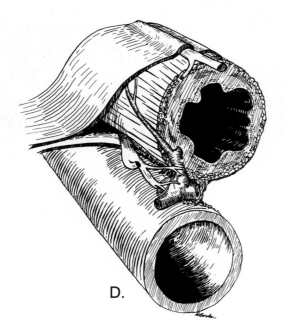

D.

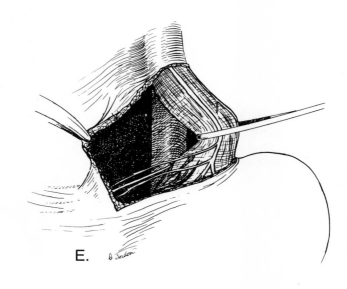

E.

THE SURGICAL TREATMENT OF HIATAL HERNIA

*No good physician quavers incantations when the malady
he is treating needs the knife.*

SOPHOCLES

Sliding Hiatal Hernia

Definition

Enlargement of the esophageal hiatus of the diaphragm allows the abdominal
esophagus and the cardia of the stomach to enter the thoracic cavity. Pressure from below further enlarges the hiatus and attenuates and weakens the
phrenoesophageal ligament, which normally attaches the distal esophagus to
the margins of the hiatus. When herniation actually occurs, there is an empty
peritoneal hernial sac on the left side of the stomach and a small bare area
without peritoneal covering on the right side of the stomach. The gastroesophageal junction is displaced upward.

Repair of Sliding Hiatal Hernia

Treatment of hiatal hernia is directed mainly to the prevention of gastroesophageal reflux which may or may not accompany hiatus hernia. Hiatal hernia repair is the surgical approach to the prevention of reflux. Hiatal hernia
without significant reflux is not an indication for repair. Surgical repair is
advised for those patients who do not respond to conservative management.

    We present seven effective surgical procedures for repair of hiatal hernia.

Abdominal Approach

An upper midline transverse or oblique incision is made. If necessary, the
xiphoid process may be removed. An exposure of approximately 4 cm of
esophagus may be obtained. The incision of the peritoneum should be made
slightly to the left of the midline to avoid the round ligament at the free edge
of the falciform ligament. If the falciform ligament is in the way or is bleeding,
do not hesitate to ligate both round and falciform ligaments. Should a thoracic
extension of the upper midline incision become necessary, it can be made
through the left eighth intercostal space.

327

An exploratory laparotomy must be performed. Special attention should be paid to the gastroduodenal area to determine the presence or absence of a duodenal ulcer or a stenosis secondary to scarring and fibrosis.

Expose the gastroesophageal junction by careful mobilization of the left lobe of the liver; reduce the hernial sac.

Push down the left lobe of the liver and divide the left triangular and left coronary ligaments. These ligaments are practically a single unit because of the close apposition of the anterior and posterior layers of the coronary ligament which form the left triangular ligament. Long scissors are advisable. The blood supply of the abdominal esophagus and the inferior surface of the diaphragm is very variable. Proceed very carefully when cutting in the area to the right of the falciform ligament. At this point there is danger of injury to the left hepatic vein or the "common" left hepatic vein with a long tear to the inferior vena cava.

Now the left lobe of the liver may be displaced downward, inward, and to the right. Wet laparotomy pads can keep the lobe in this position.

The index finger of the surgeon will penetrate the avascular peritoneal reflection which forms several ligaments such as gastrohepatic, gastrosplenic, and, of course, the peculiar phrenoesophageal ligament. A Penrose drain is inserted for traction of the esophagus.

Remember:

Avoid injury to the vagus nerves.

Avoid injury to the mediastinal pleura.

Avoid injury to the left hepatic vein.

Avoid perforation of the esophagus.

Watch for an aberrant blood supply to the left triangular ligament.

Watch for accessory bile ducts.

The hernia should be reduced after careful dissection of some of the ligaments mentioned above and by dissecting the proximal lesser curvature (approximately 5 cm). If it is necessary, the fundus of the stomach at the greater curvature should be dissected (5 to 10 cm). Some short gastric vessels may be ligated. By gentle downward pulling of the stomach or of the gastroesophageal junction, the stomach is reduced. The mediastinal sac should be excised.

At this point, the surgeon should evaluate the hiatus and decide about

1. Insertion of a mercury bougie
2. Simple periesophageal closure
3. Gastropexy or gastrostomy
4. Antireflux procedure

Anterior closure of the hiatus is accomplished with deep bites of 0 silk or 0 Surgilon if the gastroesophageal junction is quite mobile and not fixed posteriorly. Posterior closure is also acceptable, depending upon the local topographical anatomy.

PLATE 103
Repair of Sliding Hiatal Hernia

A. *Step 1.* A transverse, oblique, or vertical midline incision may be used.

B. *Step 2.* Incise the triangular ligament.

C. *Step 3.* Retract the left lobe of the liver.

   Step 4. Incise the peritoneal coverings of the esophagus.

   Step 5. Pass a Penrose drain beneath the esophagus for traction.

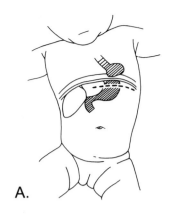

A.

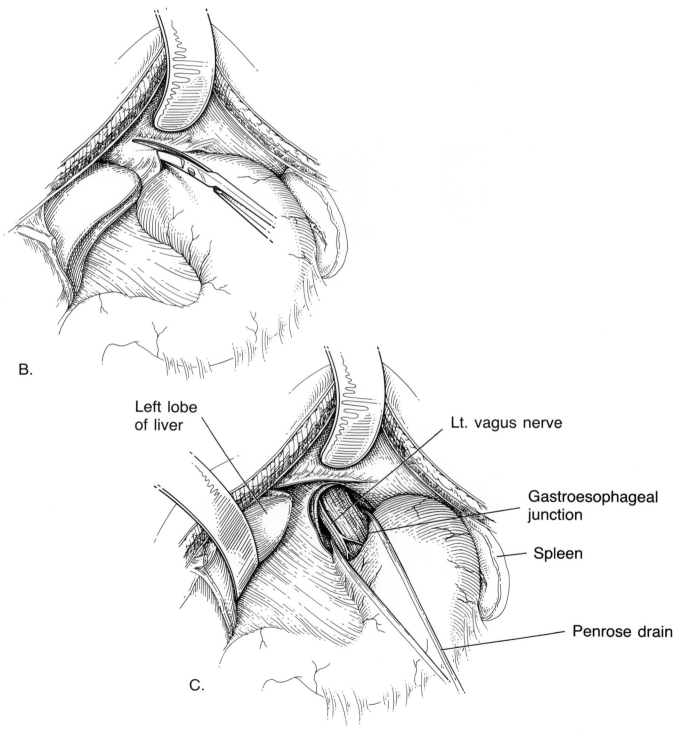

B.

Left lobe
of liver

Lt. vagus nerve

Gastroesophageal
junction

Spleen

Penrose drain

C.

329

PLATE 103 (*Continued*)

Repair of Sliding Hiatal Hernia

D. *Step 6.* Dissect the greater curvature of the stomach beginning at the cardia and continuing toward the gastrosplenic ligament and the vasa breva. One or two vasa breva may be divided, but damage to the spleen must be avoided.

E. *Step 7.* Dissect the diaphragm and the tissue beneath the esophagus.

Step 8. At this stage, a widened hiatus can be repaired with 00 silk sutures, carefully avoiding the underlying aorta, celiac axis, and pleura. Tie these loosely and do not constrict the esophagus.

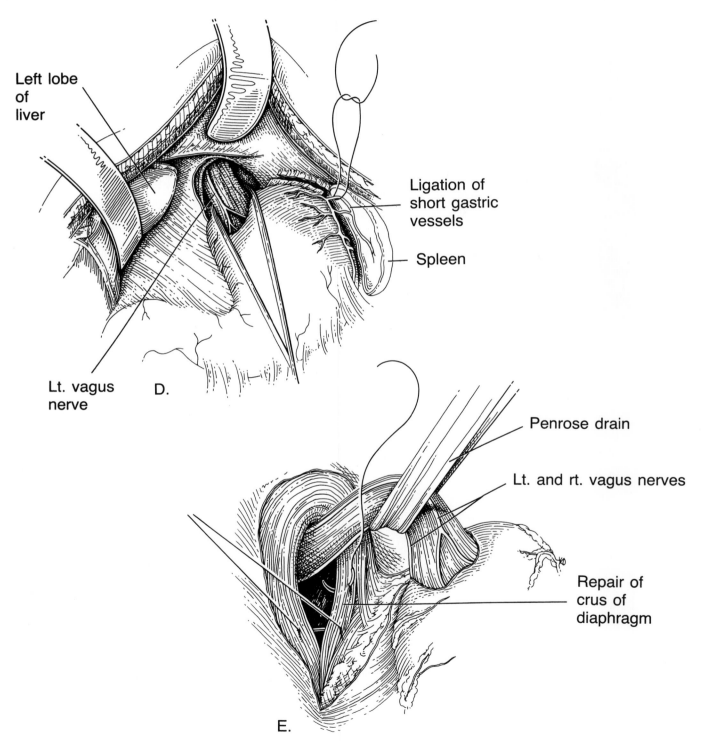

THE NISSEN FUNDOPLICATION

This procedure will allow the patient to belch and vomit at infrequent and appropriate occasions while controlling pathological reflux, thus simulating the normal condition of the gastroesophageal junction and achieving a more desirable clinical result after operation.

A no. 50 French dilator is passed into the esophagus by the anesthesiologist to limit constriction. Prior to fundoplication, a nasogastric tube (18F Levin tube) is passed through the dilator. The mobilized fundus is pushed behind and around the lower esophageal segment, producing a right and left fold. The folds are approximated by nonabsorbable 00 silk, with generous bites of the seromuscular layers. All the sutures of the fundoplication incorporate the anterior esophageal wall superficially, securing the wrapping in place and preventing falling down of the fundus. The dilator may be removed.

At this point, a temporary Stamm gastrostomy will serve as a gastropexy to avoid volvulus and will aid in the postoperative evacuation of gastrointestinal secretion. It will also ensure that the fundoplication remains within the abdomen.

Remember:
1. Avoid the gas-bloat syndrome by
    Protecting the vagus nerve
    Maintaining an adequate lumen in the distal esophagus.
2. If the vagus nerve is transected, pyloroplasty is the recommended procedure.
3. If the pylorus is stenotic, pyloroplasty is again recommended.
4. If chronic peptic ulcer disease (duodenal ulcer) is present, vagotomy and pyloroplasty should be performed.

PLATE 104
Nissen Fundoplication[1]

A. *Step 1.* A no. 50 French dilator is passed by the anesthesiologist into the esophagus to prevent constriction by an excessively tight fundic wrap.

B. *Step 2.* The fundus of the stomach is then wrapped around the lower esophagus 360°, and 00 silk sutures are inserted to include stomach, esophagus, and stomach.

C. *Step 3.* Place at least four sutures to complete the wrap.

[1]These steps follow the exposure of the abdominal esophagus described in the preceding section (see p. 329).

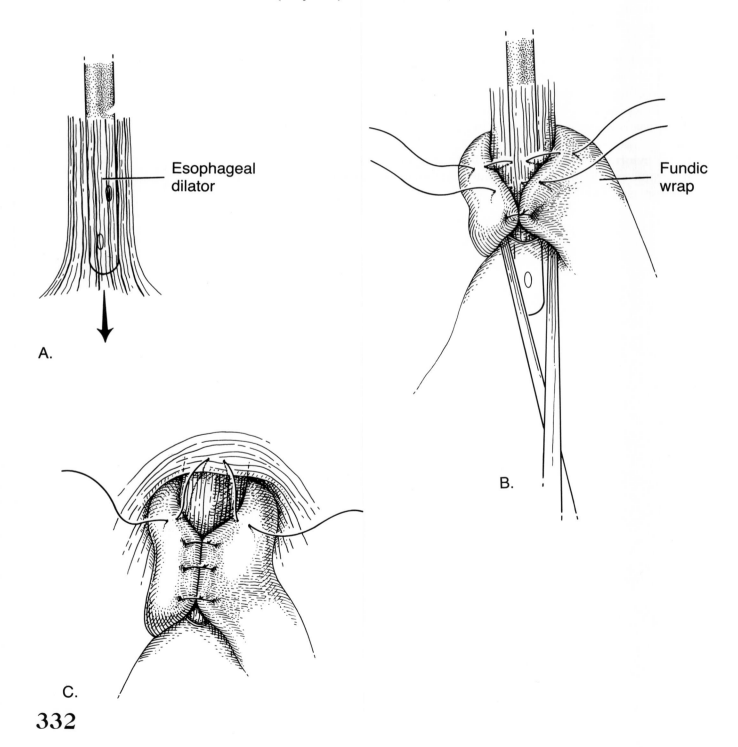

Esophageal dilator

Fundic wrap

A.

B.

C.

D. *Step 4.* Remove the dilator and the Penrose drain.

E. *Step 5.* Perform a Stamm gastrostomy.

F. *Step 6.* Close the incision.

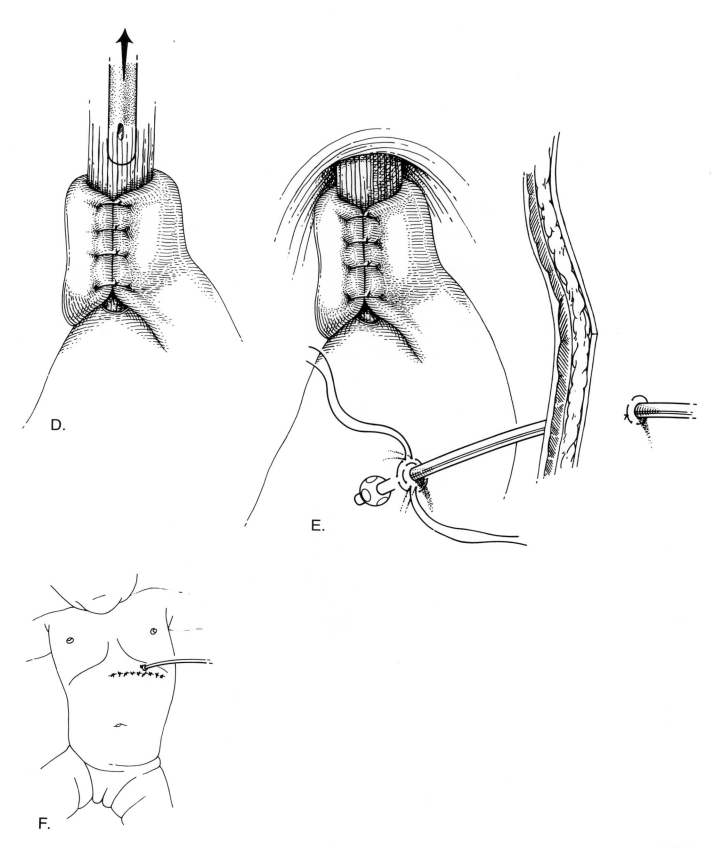

D.

E.

F.

DeMeester[1] has proposed three modifications of the Nissen procedure:

1. The size of the intraesophageal dilator is increased to no. 60 French. This reduces the initial temporary discomfort of swallowing.
2. The length of the gastric wrap is decreased from 4.0 to 1.0 cm. This decreases postoperative dysphagia.
3. The short gastric vessels are divided in order to mobilize the fundus and allow it to participate in the gastric wrap.

These modifications may be employed in both transabdominal and transthoracic procedures.

[1]DeMeester TR, Bonavina L, Albertucci M: Nissen fundoplication for gastroesophageal reflux disease. *Ann Surg* 204:9, 1986.

PLATE 105

Nissen Fundoplication—DeMeester Modification

A. *Step 1.* Isolate the distal esophagus by blunt dissection. The esophagus is retracted to the left. The right (posterior) vagus nerve is excluded from the retraction.

Step 2. Mobilize the fundus by ligating and dividing the short gastric vessels. Care must be taken to divide such vessels that pass retroperitoneally and fix the fundus to the posterior abdominal wall.

Step 3. Close the esophageal hiatus by approximation of the crura with interrupted 0 silk sutures. Six such sutures are usually needed. The crural closure should be too loose rather than too tight.

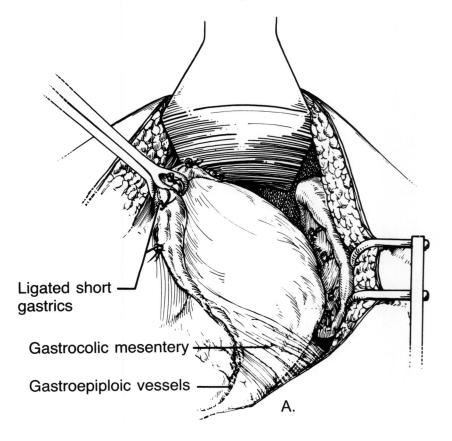

Ligated short gastrics

Gastrocolic mesentery

Gastroepiploic vessels

A.

B. *Step 4.* Construct the fundic wrap. Pass a no. 60 French dilator into the stomach to identify the gastroesophageal junction. The wrap should be large enough to include the surgeon's index finger besides the esophagus as well as the no. 60 French dilator within it.

C. Schematic cross section of Nissen fundoplication showing the use of Teflon felt pledgets in forming the wrap. Arrows illustrate (1) intragastric pressure, (2) intraabdominal pressure, and (3) gastric muscle tone.

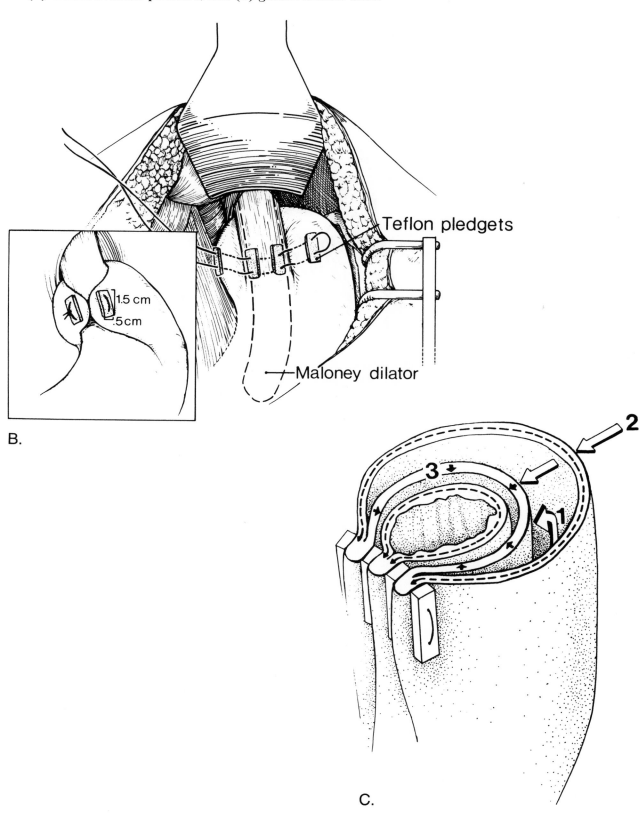

Teflon pledgets

1.5 cm

.5 cm

Maloney dilator

B.

C.

PLATE 105 (*Continued*)

Nissen Fundoplication—DeMeester Modification

D. Transthoracic repair. The gastric fundus has been brought up through the hiatus and rotated to the right for an easier placement of the holding U stitch. The complete fundoplication consists of an anterior fundic wrap secured posteriorly by a U stitch reinforced with Teflon felt pledgets.

Source: DeMeester TR, Bonavina L, Albertucci M: Nissen fundoplication for gastroesophageal reflux disease. *Ann Surg* 204:9–20, 1986, Figs. 5–8.

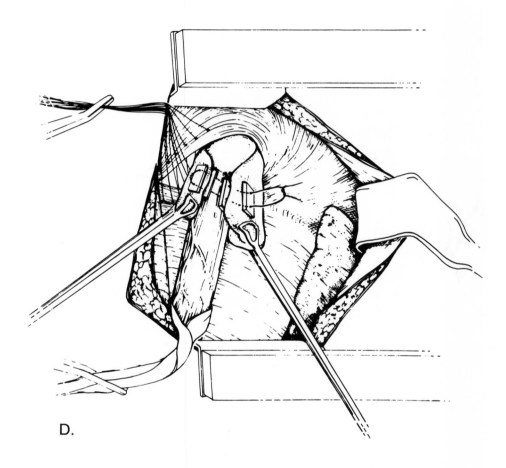

D.

THE FLOPPY NISSEN FUNDOPLICATION

This adaptation of the Nissen procedure, described by Donahue et al.,[1] has as its purpose the construction of the fundic wrap in a manner that will allow normal reflux at appropriate occasions while preventing pathological reflux.

A typical Nissen fundoplication is performed with a no. 50 French dilator and a no. 20 French nasogastric tube in the esophageal lumen. The fundic wrap is loose enough to allow a 15 Hegar dilator or an index finger to pass freely beneath it.

"Collar" fundoesophageal interrupted sutures are inserted to keep the fundoplication in situ, and the dilator is removed.

A gastrostomy is recommended.

THE HILL PROCEDURE OR POSTERIOR GASTROPEXY WITH SOME APPLICATIONS BY OTTINGER

For practical purposes, the Hill procedure is a combination of a Nissenlike fundoplication and posterior gastropexy. The significant characteristics are

1. The use of the median arcuate ligament.
2. Intraoperative monitoring of pressure in the high-pressure zone of the lower esophageal sphincter by manometry.

Hill stated that if the pressure exceeds 40 mmHg, the sutures are too tight and must be loosened to avoid dysphagia. Pressure is recorded by insertion of a nasogastric tube to which is attached a special polyethylene tube with a side opening to be located at the gastroesophageal junction. Pressure is measured by attaching the tube to a strain gauge and a recording device (Physiocontrol Corporation). The initial reading should be 0 to 5 mmHg.

The abdomen should be explored through an upper midline or a right or left paramedian incision.

The esophageal hiatus is exposed by division of the left triangular ligament and other peritoneal reflections and ligaments. The abdominal esophagus and the gastroesophageal junction are mobilized. Avoid injury to the vagus nerve and the spleen. Some short gastric vessels may be sacrificed.

The stomach is retracted to the left and the aorta, the celiac axis, and the celiac ganglion are identified. This will permit identification of the preaortic fascia and its thickened edge, the median arcuate ligament, which covers the aorta and the origin of the celiac axis. In about 50 percent of individuals, the ligament is absent. To avoid injury to the celiac axis or the aorta, careful use of the preaortic fascia is necessary if the ligament is absent.

The diaphragmatic crura can now be seen and the state of the hiatus fully evaluated. The hiatus is narrowed by through and through deep, wide 0 silk sutures. The sutures must be deep to include the tendinous part of the crura, and wide to avoid muscle cutting. A finger should pass easily between the crural suture line and the abdominal esophagus and the gastroesophageal junction. The sutures should be placed above the ganglion and behind the celiac division of the posterior vagal trunk. Remember to identify and preserve both vagal trunks.

Babcock clamps are placed on the anterior and posterior gastric wall. A malleable retractor is placed beneath the median arcuate ligament to protect the aorta. The peritoneal edges on each side of the gastroesophageal junction are picked up with clamps. Sufficient tissue is grasped to give a solid hold to the sutures; stomach wall may be included. By traction on the clamps, the gastroesophageal junction is rotated to expose its posterior aspect. Inter-

[1]Donahue PE, Larson GM, Stewardson RH, Bombeck CT: Floppy Nissen fundoplication. *Rev Surg* 34:223, 1977.

rupted 0 silk sutures are placed to include tissue on both sides of the junction and the median arcuate ligament. When tied, these will partially wrap the proximal part of the stomach around the junction. Additional imbricating sutures are passed through the anterior and posterior gastric wall beneath the median arcuate ligament.

One by one, the sutures are tied and the esophageal pressure is measured. If the mean pressure is greater than 40 mmHg, the sutures should be loosened to avoid the gas-bloat syndrome and dysphagia.

The tightness of the repair should be checked with the finger also.

Ottinger sutures the fundus of the stomach to the diaphragm using 000 silk.

PLATE 106

The Hill Procedure—Posterior Gastropexy

A. Diagram of a sagittal section through the gastroesophageal junction showing normal pressure and pH. HPZ = high pressure zone.

Source: From Hill LD: Surgical management of hiatal hernia, in *Hernia,* 2d ed, Nyhus LM, Condon RE (eds). Lippincott, Philadelphia, 1978, p. 697, Fig. 42-2.

B. *Step 1.* Divide the anterior and posterior leaves of the left triangular ligament. Carry the dissection very carefully to approach the area of the left hepatic vein. Fold and retract the left lateral segment of the liver.

C. *Step 2.* Retract the esophagus preserving the vagal trunks. Divide the posterior part of the phrenogastric ligament if present. The superior pole of the spleen is visible; a superior short gastric artery may be ligated between ligatures. If a left accessory hepatic artery is present, it should be ligated.

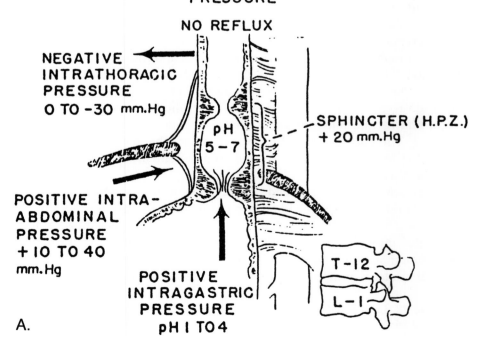

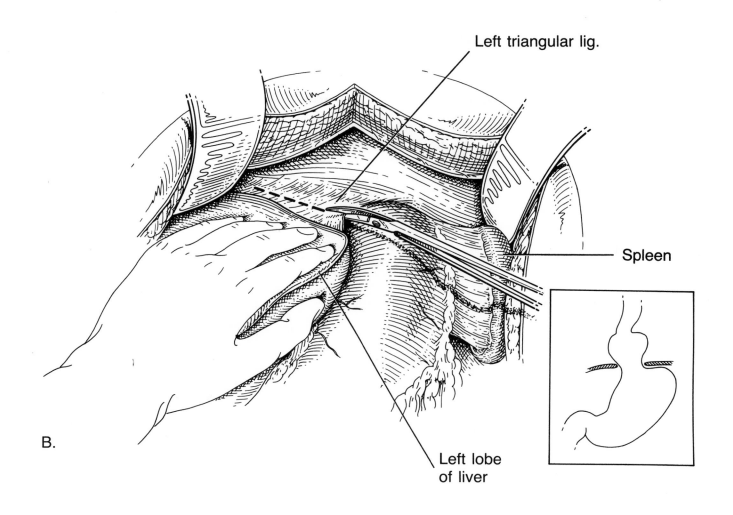

Left triangular lig.

Spleen

B.

Left lobe
of liver

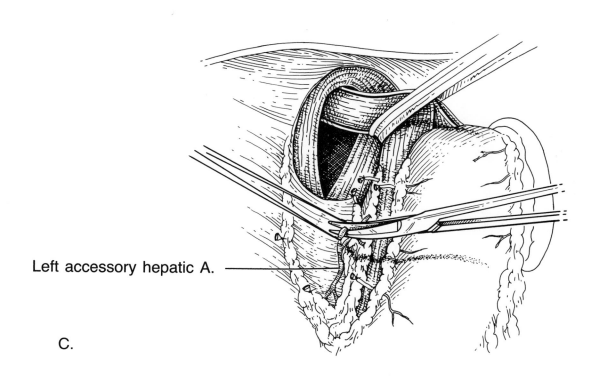

Left accessory hepatic A.

C.

339

PLATE 106 (*Continued*)

The Hill Procedure—Posterior Gastropexy

D. *Step 3.* Retract the stomach to the patient's left to expose the preaortic fascia. Aorta, celiac axis, and median arcuate ligament may be palpated. It may be necessary to ligate a phrenic artery as well as some short gastric vessels.

E. *Step 4.* The hiatus is narrowed by interrupted 0 silk sutures through the crura.

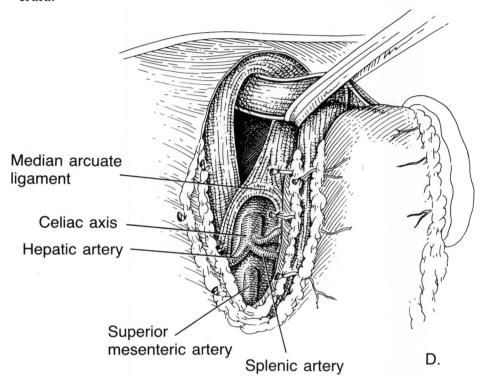

Median arcuate ligament

Celiac axis

Hepatic artery

Superior mesenteric artery

Splenic artery

D.

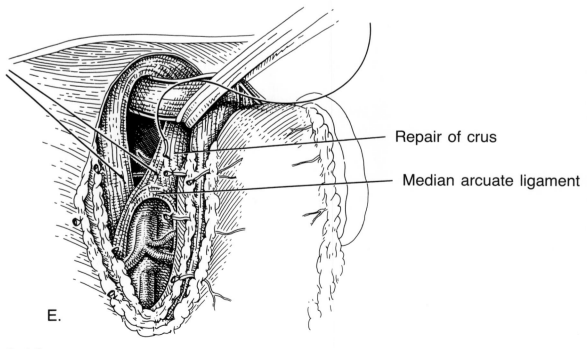

Repair of crus

Median arcuate ligament

E.

340

F. *Step 5.* This is a Nissen fundoplication and posterior gastropexy. Place sutures through the posterior and anterior gastric wall, including the median arcuate ligament. Tie the sutures and the partial wrapping of the gastroesophageal junction will be completed.

G. *Step 6.* Test the size of the opening before cutting the fixation sutures. Palpate the esophageal opening into the stomach with the tip of the finger. Some adjustment of the fixation sutures may be necessary if the tip of the finger is not admitted after the invagination of the gastric wall into the esophagus.

H. *Step 7.* Complete the repair by further fixation of the gastric fundus to the diaphragmatic crura with 000 silk sutures.

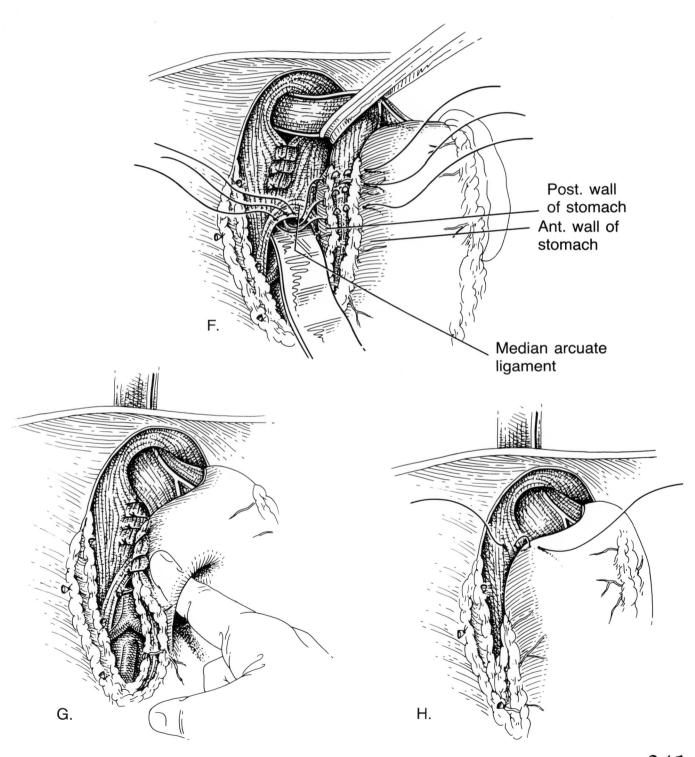

Post. wall of stomach

Ant. wall of stomach

Median arcuate ligament

F.

G.

H.

The purpose of this procedure is to create a longer intraabdominal esophagus using the lesser curvature of the stomach to form the "neoesophagus" of Chassin.

PLATE 107

The Collis Gastroplasty

A. *Step 1.* Completely mobilize the distal esophagus, the gastroesophageal junction, and the fundus of the stomach, and place a no. 56–60 French Maloney dilator into the stomach along the lesser curvature. The greater curvature is pulled to the left by a Babcock clamp, and a GIA staple is applied at the angle of His.

B. *Step 2.* Transect between the two lines of staples for 4 to 6 cm parallel to the lesser curvature. The staple lines should be inverted with 000 or 0000 interrupted silk sutures. The "neoesophagus" may be further elongated if necessary.

C. *Step 3.* Form a Nissen type of fundoplication 280 or 360° counterclockwise.

D. *Step 4.* Suture the wrapped portion of fundus to itself around the neoesophagus with 000 silk sutures. The sutures may incorporate seromuscular bites into the neoesophagus. Remove the dilator and insert a nasogastric tube.

E. *Step 5.* Close the hiatus with heavy 0 silk interrupted sutures, making sure that a finger can be inserted in the hiatus.

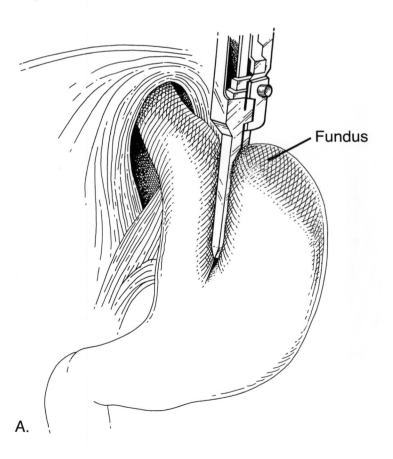

Fundus

A.

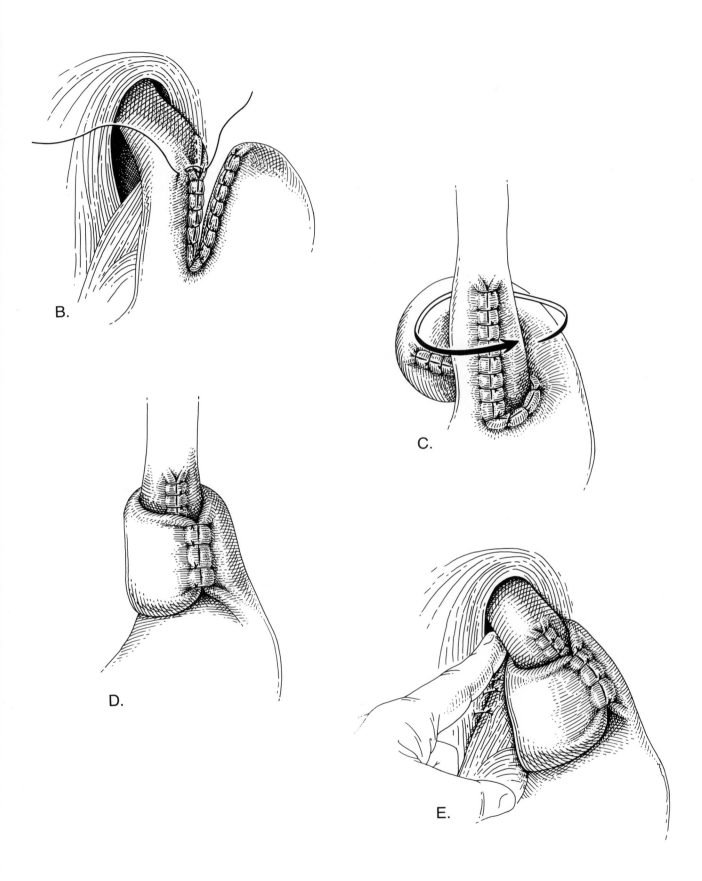

B.

C.

D.

E.

343

The purpose of this procedure is to maintain the abdominal position of the distal esophagus without complicated surgery and without recurrence of the hernia.

PLATE 108

The Angelchik Prosthetic Repair

A. *Step 1.* Mobilize, but do not skeletonize, the distal esophagus and the gastro-esophageal junction.

B. *Step 2.* Insert a horseshoe-shaped prosthesis behind the distal esophagus. The strings are tied anteriorly. Gastropexy is optional; approximation of the crura is not necessary.

C. *Step 3.* The strings are adjusted to permit the insertion of the surgeon's finger under the prosthesis.

Source: Plate 108 from Angelchik JP: In *Surgery of the Oesophagus.* Jamieson GG (ed). Churchill Livingstone, Edinburgh, in press.

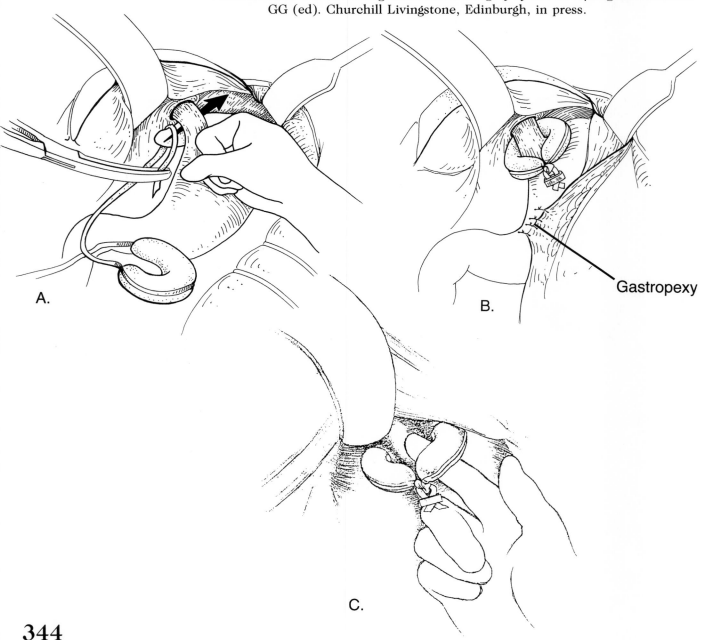

A.

B.

Gastropexy

C.

WOODWARD PROCEDURE

The patient is placed in the right lateral position with the left side of the thorax up. A no. 50–60 French Maloney dilator is passed into the stomach. The skin is incised from the tip of the scapula through the sixth or seventh intercostal space to the costal margin.

The latissimus dorsi muscle and the underlying serratus anterior muscle are divided with electric cautery close to the incision. This will preserve muscle function and avoid postoperative winged scapula. Working with fingers under the muscles will help to control the cutting. Divide the intercostal muscles at the upper border of the rib to avoid injury to the neurovascular unit.

It is up to the surgeon whether or not to resect the sixth to seventh ribs. A segmented resection, usually 1 to 2 cm posteriorly under the spinal muscles, will facilitate the operation. The periosteum should be separated from the rib, and intercostal vessels and nerves should be ligated with heavy silk at the inferior border of the rib.

The pleura is opened along the superior border of the rib, and a rib spreader is inserted. The pulmonary ligament is divided by cautery or between ligatures. Identify and preserve the inferior pulmonary vein. Upward retraction of the left lower lobe of the lung will reveal the mediastinal pleura, which may be incised from the diaphragm to the aortic arch. The herniated stomach, the displaced gastroesophageal junction, and the distal esophagus may be seen.

PLATE 109
Transthoracic Hiatal Hernia Repair

A. *Step 1.* Place the patient in the right lateral position with the left hemithorax up. Pass a no. 56–60 French Maloney dilator into the stomach. Incise the skin from the tip of the scapula to the costal margin over the area of the sixth or seventh left intercostal space.

B. *Step 2.* Divide the latissimus dorsi and the underlying serratus anterior muscles with an electric cautery close to their costal origin and caudal to the skin incision.

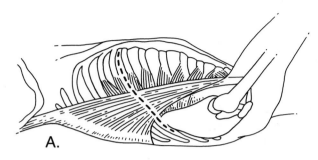

A.

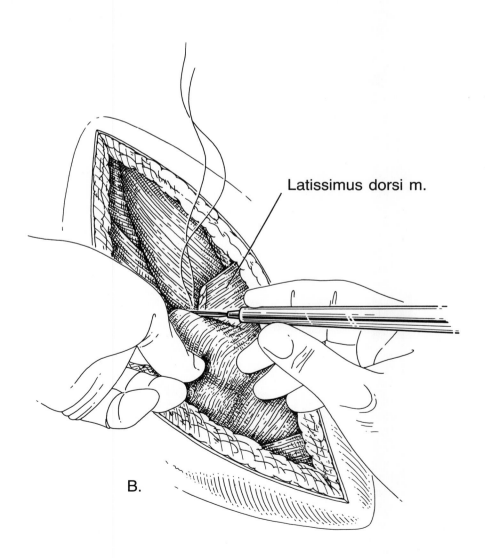

Latissimus dorsi m.

B.

C. *Step 3.* Divide the intercostal muscles at the upper border of the rib to avoid injury to the neurovascular unit.

D. *Step 4.* Separate the periosteum, divide vessels and nerve, and ligate with heavy silk sutures at the inferior border of the rib. Open the pleura along the upper margin of the rib.

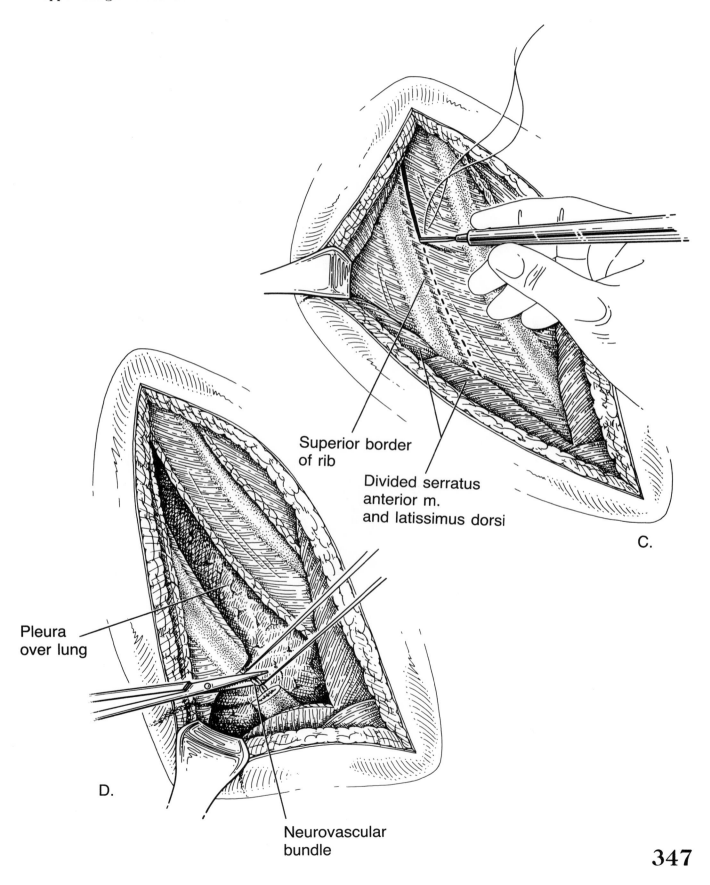

Superior border
of rib

Divided serratus
anterior m.
and latissimus dorsi

C.

Pleura
over lung

D.

Neurovascular
bundle

347

PLATE 109 (*Continued*)

Transthoracic Hiatal Hernia Repair

E. *Step 5.* Insert a rib spreader and open the thoracic cavity slowly and carefully to avoid rib fracture. Divide the pulmonary ligament with cautery or between ligatures. The mediastinal pleura may be seen and opened after upward retraction of the left lower lobe of the lung.

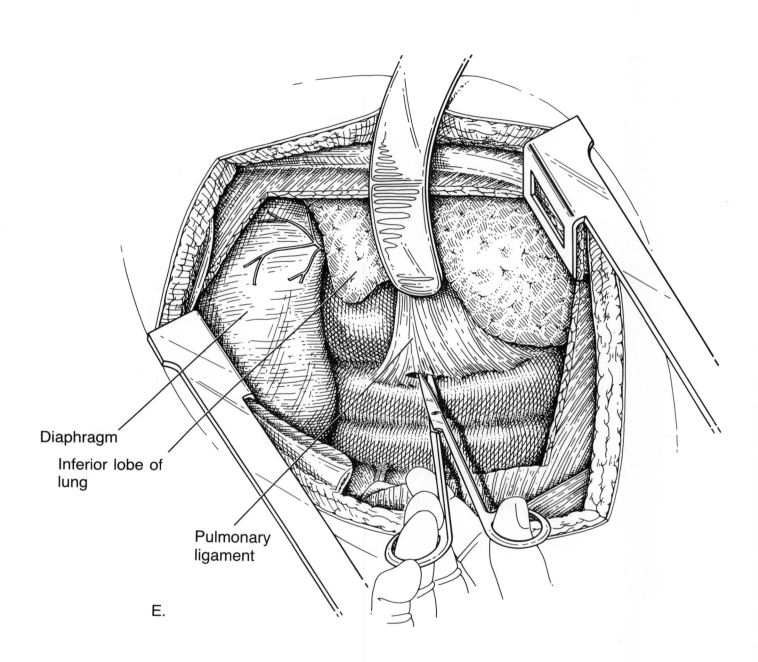

Diaphragm

Inferior lobe of lung

Pulmonary ligament

E.

F. *Step 6.* Incise the mediastinal pleura medial to the aorta from the diaphragm to the aortic arch. The herniated stomach, the gastroesophageal junction, and the distal esophagus are now visible.

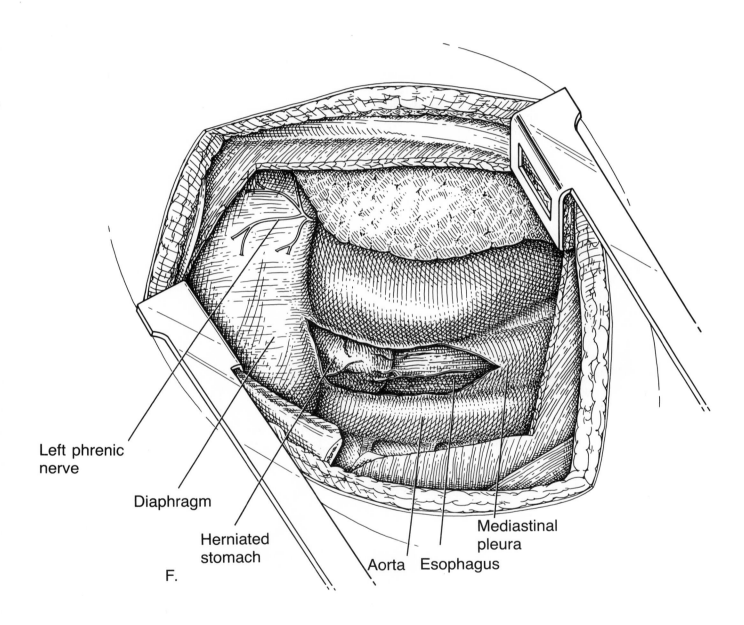

Left phrenic
nerve

Diaphragm

Herniated
stomach

F.

Aorta   Esophagus

Mediastinal
pleura

349

PLATE 109 (*Continued*)

Transthoracic Hiatal Hernia Repair

G. *Step 7.* Inspect the esophagus. If there is no fixation (evidence of esophagitis), esophageal mobilization by finger dissection is easy. The Maloney dilator is easily felt.

　　If the esophagus is fixed, careful mobilization with downward sharp dissection will be necessary. Locate and preserve both vagal trunks.

　　After mobilizing the esophagus from the diaphragm to the aortic arch or to the left pulmonary vein, insert a Penrose drain or umbilical tape around the esophagus.

H. *Step 8.* If a sac is present, incise all adhesions and the attenuated phrenoesophageal ligament. Elevate the sac; incise it inferiorly and laterally. Carefully continue the peritoneal incision medially, putting the index finger within the sac. The finger can now travel all the way into the lesser sac.

　　Incise the diaphragm from the hiatus to the central tendon to visualize the gastric fundus, the spleen, the proximal gastrohepatic ligament, and the short gastric vessels.

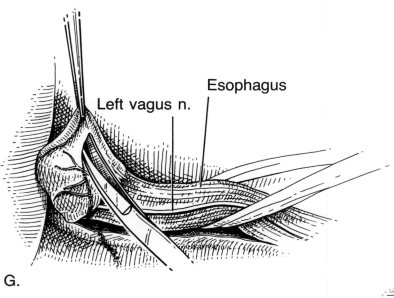

Left vagus n.　Esophagus

G.

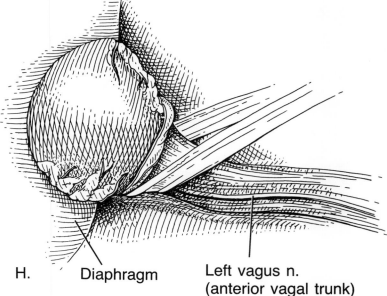

H.　Diaphragm　Left vagus n. (anterior vagal trunk)

I. *Step 9.* Ligate the short gastric vessels and branches of the right gastric artery at the greater curvature. Ligate a left hepatic accessory artery if it is present. Also ligate Belsey's artery, which is a communicating branch between the ascending branch of the left gastric and inferior phrenic arteries. The proximal stomach may be brought into the thorax.

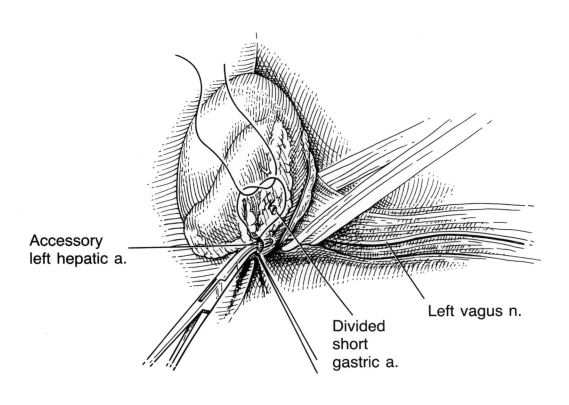

Accessory left hepatic a.

Divided short gastric a.

Left vagus n.

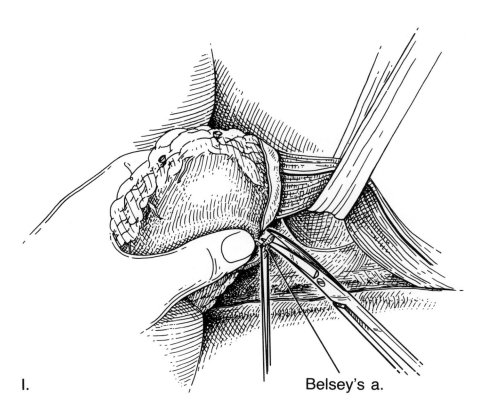

I.

Belsey's a.

PLATE 109 (*Continued*)

Transthoracic Hiatal Hernia Repair

J. *Step 10.* Fundoplication. Perform a fundoplication by wrapping the fundus of the stomach around the distal esophagus using 00 silk interrupted sutures. Suture the fundus to the esophageal musculature using 000 silk interrupted sutures.

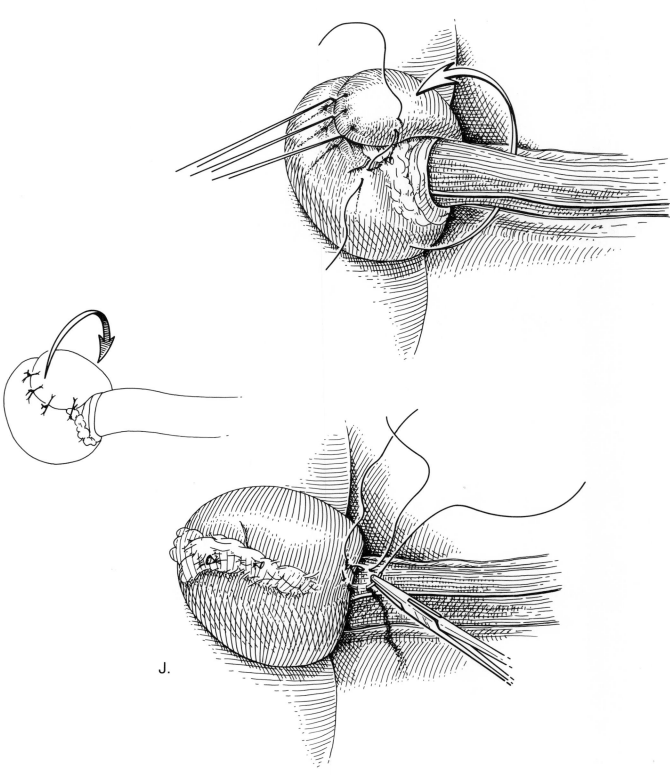

J.

K. *Step 11.* Suture the radial diaphragmatic incision to the thoracic portion of the fundus using 00 silk interrupted sutures.

L. *Step 12.* The suturing of the fundus of the stomach is complete. Place a posterior chest tube next to the descending aorta, fixed with a suture of 000 chromic catgut.

M. *Step 13.* Bring the chest tube externally through a separate stab wound. Anchor the tube to the skin and connect to closed chest drainage. Close the wound in layers.

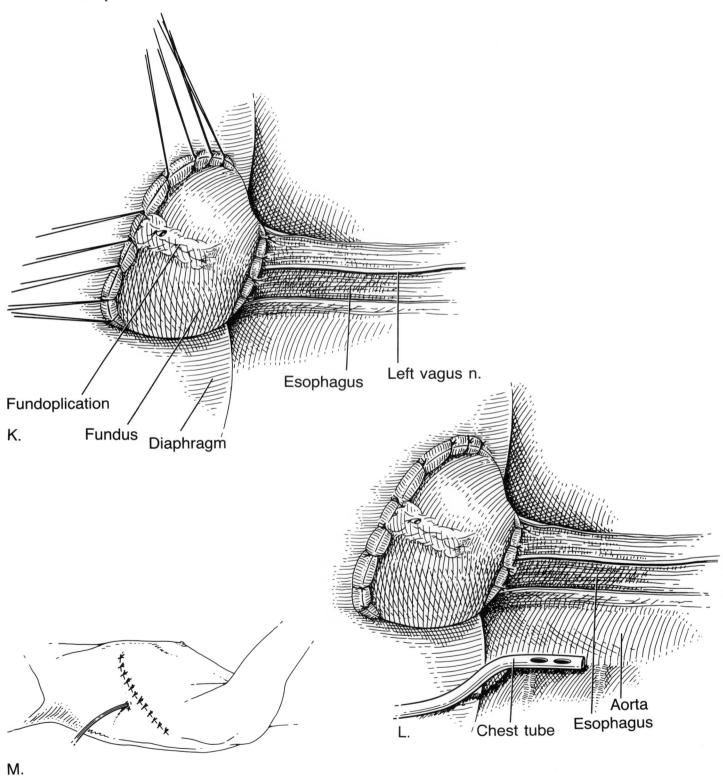

Fundoplication

K.

Fundus   Diaphragm

Esophagus   Left vagus n.

L.   Chest tube   Aorta
Esophagus

M.

The purpose of this procedure is the creation of a subdiaphragmatic esophagus which is anchored by three layers of sutures which plicate the distal two-thirds of the abdominal esophagus with the fundus of the stomach. The procedure begins with complete mobilization of the distal esophagus, the gastroesophageal junction, and the fundus of the stomach, as described in the Woodward procedure.

PLATE 110

Belsey Mark IV Transthoracic Cardioplasty

A. *Step 1.* Completely mobilize the distal esophagus, the gastroesophageal junction, and the gastric fundus through a left thoracotomy.

B. *Step 2.* Place mattress sutures of 000 silk between the muscular layer of the esophagus and that of the gastric cardia 1 to 2 cm above and below the gastroesophageal junction. Tie the sutures gently.

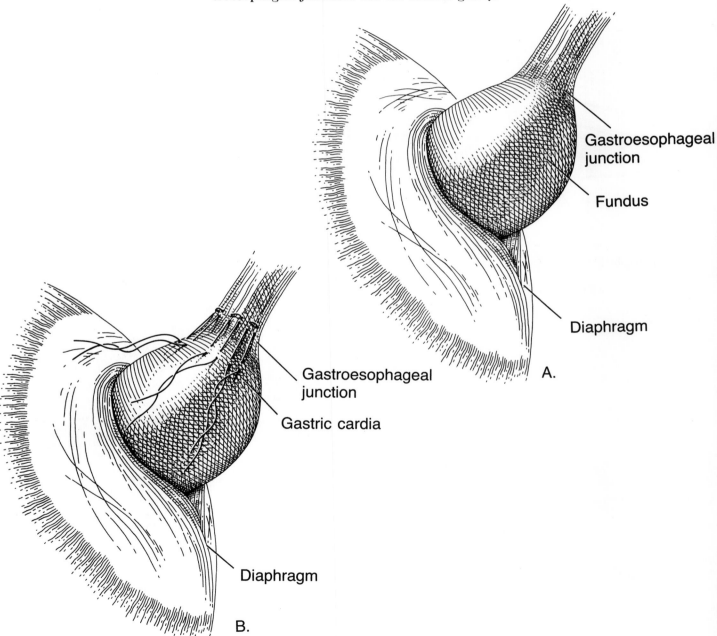

354

C. *Step 3.* Place a second line of mattress sutures between the muscular layer of the esophagus, that of the gastric fundus, and the tendinous portion of the diaphragm. Do not tie these sutures.

D. *Step 4.* Close the hiatus with 0 silk deep interrupted sutures. Two to three sutures are enough to approximate the diaphragmatic crura.

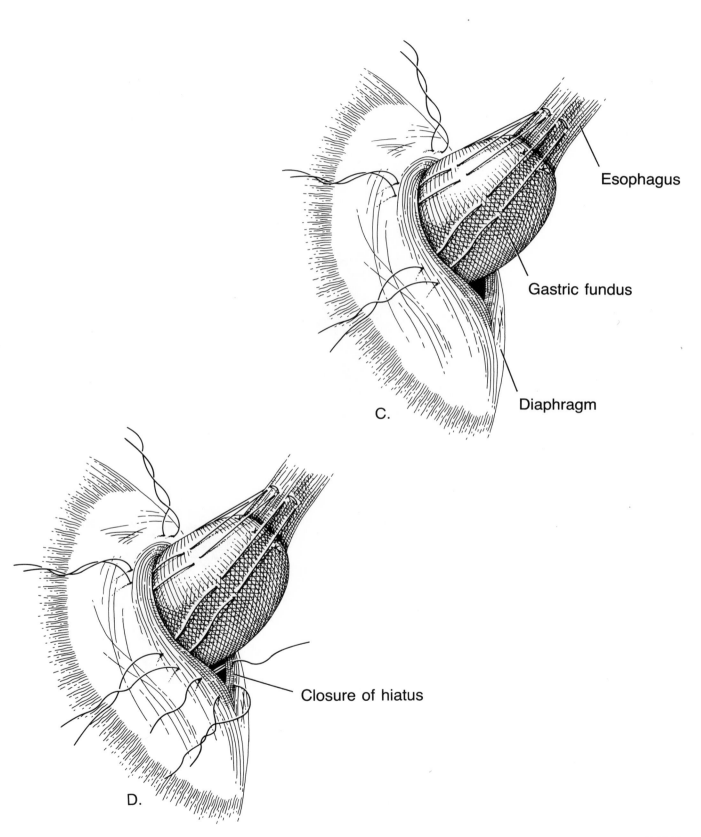

Esophagus

Gastric fundus

Diaphragm

C.

Closure of hiatus

D.

355

PLATE 110 (*Continued*)

Belsey Mark IV Transthoracic Cardioplasty

E. *Step 5.* Tie all sutures.

F. Sagittal section through the gastroesophageal junction showing the result of the completed Belsey Mark IV cardioplasty.

Source: Drawings modified from Payne WS, Ellis FH, Jr: Esophagus and diaphragmatic hernias, in *Principles of Surgery,* 4th ed, Schwartz SE (ed). McGraw-Hill, New York, 1984, p. 1080.

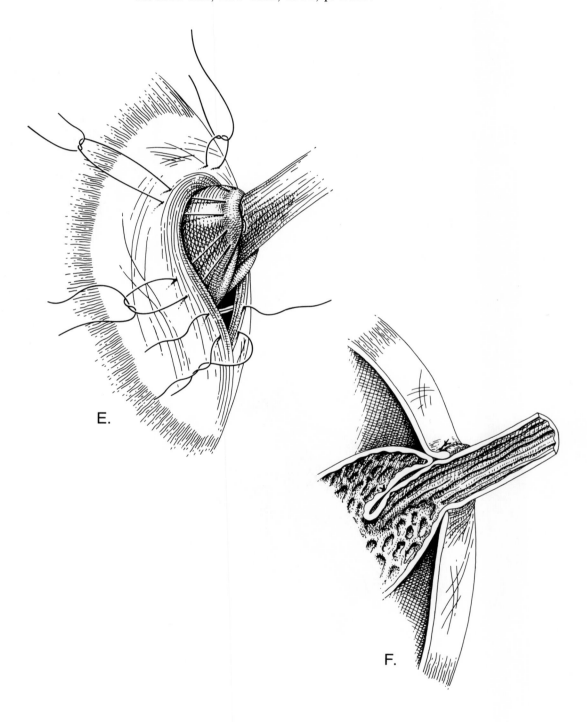

E.

F.

Paraesophageal Hiatal Hernia

Definition

In paraesophageal hiatal hernia, the gastroesophageal junction is in its normal position below the diaphragm, but the fundus of the stomach and part of the greater curvature have passed through the hiatus into the mediastinum anterior to the esophagus and behind the pericardium. Occasionally the entire stomach may be rolled into the thorax.

As the name paraesophageal hernia implies, the herniating stomach passes through the hiatus beside the normally situated esophagus. This is a "pure" paraesophageal hernia. In some patients, the gastroesophageal junction may be displaced upward; this conformation is a "mixed" paraesophageal hernia.

PLATE 111
Repair of Paraesophageal Hernia

A. *Step 1.* Open the abdomen as for sliding hiatal hernia (a midline supraumbilical incision from the xiphoid process to just above the umbilicus with downward extension if necessary).

B. *Step 2.* Incise the left triangular ligament of the liver.

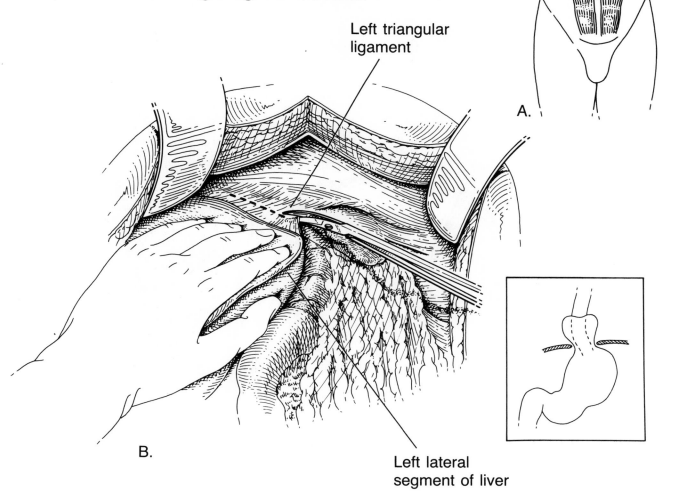

Left triangular ligament

A.

B.

Left lateral segment of liver

PLATE 111 (*Continued*)
Repair of Paraesophageal Hernia

C-1,C-2. *Step 3.* Reduce the stomach and esophagus into the abdomen.

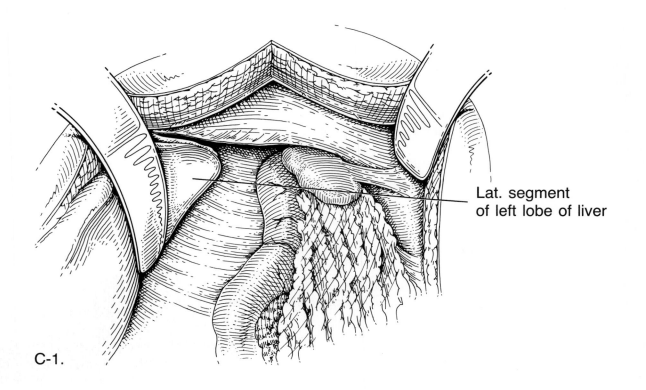

Lat. segment
of left lobe of liver

C-1.

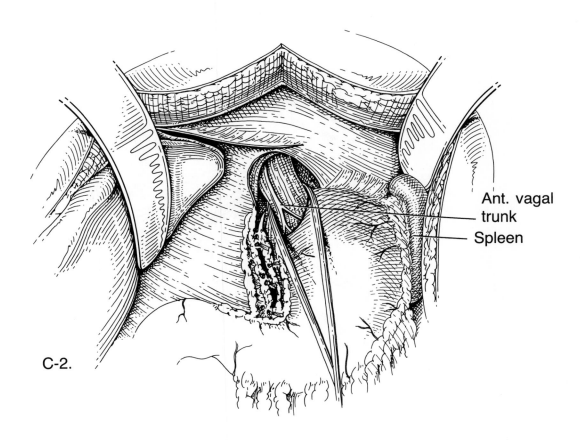

Ant. vagal
trunk

Spleen

C-2.

D. *Step 4.* Open the hernia sac and expose the esophagus. Protect the anterior vagal trunk. Excise the sac.

E. Anterior approximation of the crura (interrupted 00 silk sutures).

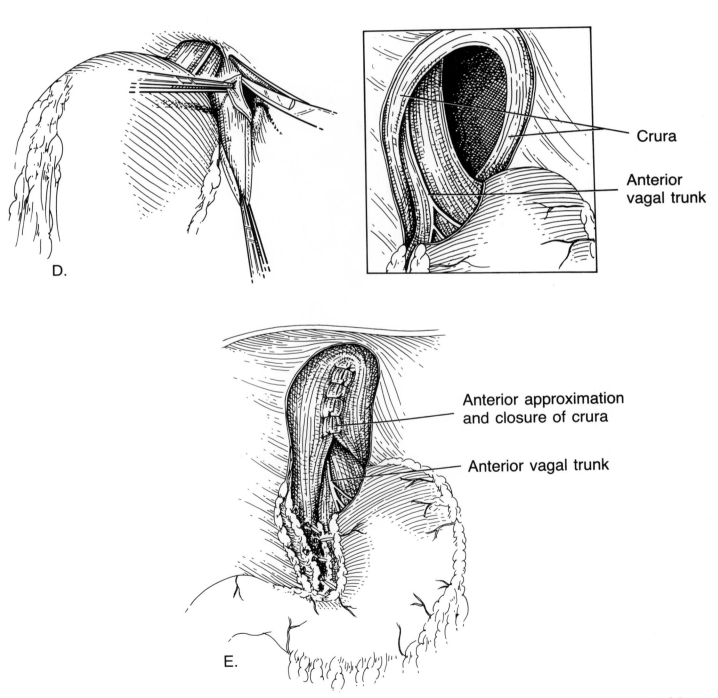

Crura

Anterior vagal trunk

Anterior approximation and closure of crura

Anterior vagal trunk

D.

E.

PLATE 111 (*Continued*)

Repair of Paraesophageal Hernia

F. Posterior approximation of the crura. Occasionally the lesser curvature of the stomach is sutured to the left crus posteriorly with interrupted 00 silk sutures. The diaphragm should admit one finger between it and the esophagus.

G. The fundus of the stomach may be sutured to the undersurface of the diaphragm with 000 silk to add stability to the anatomical repair.

H. A fundic wrap (see "Nissen Fundoplication") may be added to the repair in those unusual instances when a mixed paraesophageal hernia with reflux is present.

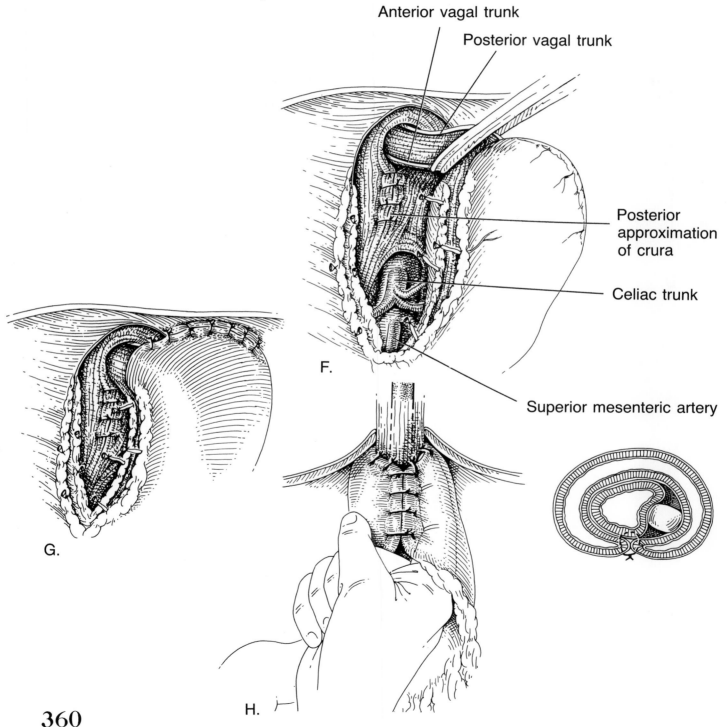

Anterior vagal trunk

Posterior vagal trunk

Posterior approximation of crura

Celiac trunk

F.

Superior mesenteric artery

G.

H.

Traumatic Diaphragmatic Hernia

Definition

Traumatic hernia of the diaphragm usually results from violent injury to the lower chest, often in an automobile accident. The left side is injured more often than the right. This may cause acute respiratory distress or may be accompanied by other serious injuries. The rupture may be an emergency problem requiring immediate repair.

The diagnosis is not uncommonly missed on initial evaluation. The examining surgeon must maintain a high index of suspicion to avoid delayed diagnosis.

PLATE 112

Repair of Traumatic Diaphragmatic Hernia

A. *Step 1.* A combined thoracoabdominal incision may be necessary, depending on the intraabdominal trauma accompanying the diaphragmatic rupture. Open the chest through the bed of the seventh rib on the affected side.

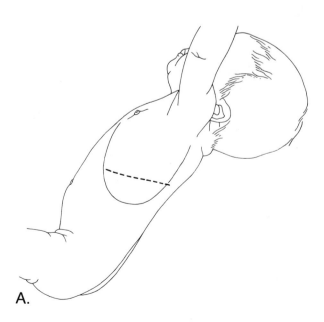

PLATE 112 (*Continued*)
Repair of Traumatic Diaphragmatic Hernia

B. *Step 2.* Identify the defect and determine its extent. Inspect the intestines, as well as any other organs in the chest cavity for injury.

C. *Step 3.* Debride the edges of the diaphragm of devitalized tissue. Note the position of the phrenic nerve when beginning repair.

D. *Step 4.* Approximate the edges of the diaphragm with interrupted 00 silk mattress sutures and pledgets of Dacron for reinforcement.

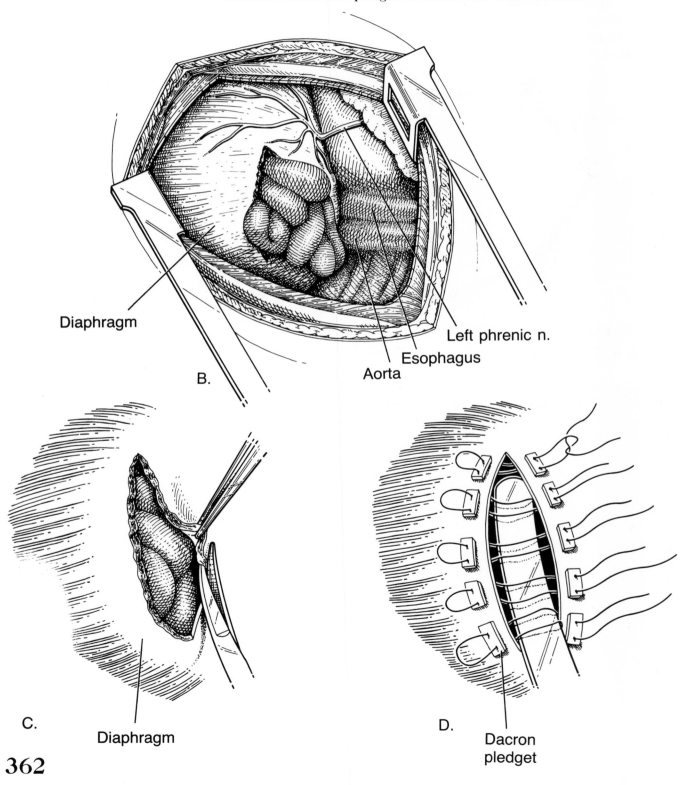

Diaphragm

Left phrenic n.

Esophagus

Aorta

B.

C.

Diaphragm

D.

Dacron pledget

E. *Step 5.* Insert a chest tube into the chest cavity and suture it to the skin of the chest wall with a purse-string suture of 00 silk.

F. *Step 6.* Close the chest with 00 chromic catgut pericostal sutures and the latissimus muscle with a 00 chromic suture. Close the skin. The chest tube is connected to a water seal and continuous negative suction of 10 to 15 cm of water.

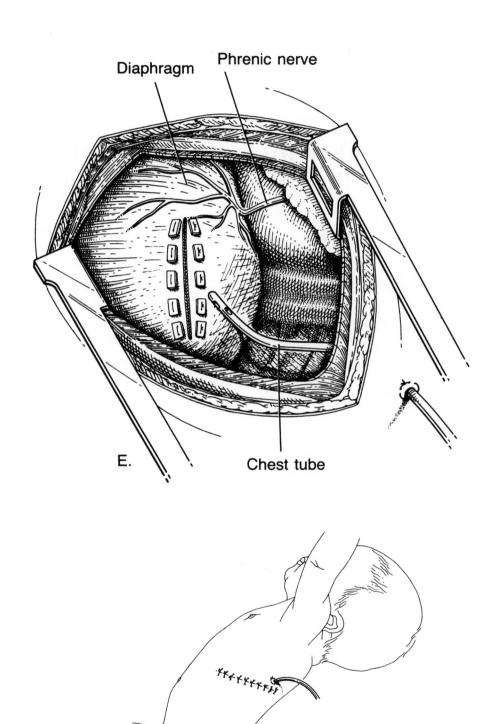

Diaphragm

Phrenic nerve

E.

Chest tube

F.

CONGENITAL DIAPHRAGMATIC HERNIAS

Congenital Diaphragmatic Hernia (through the Foramen of Bochdalek)

Definition

Posterolateral diaphragmatic hernia, or hernia through the foramen of Bochdalek, is a herniation of the intestines and occasionally the spleen and liver through a defect in the posterolateral aspect of the diaphragm. The defect in the diaphragm may vary from a small opening to the absence of the entire diaphragm. A sac of pleuroperitoneum is present in 10 percent of cases. The left side is affected in 80 to 90 percent of patients.

Embryology

The diaphragm is formed from septum transversum and pleuroperitoneal membrane. A pleuroperitoneal canal is progressively closed, and ingrowth of mesenchyme between pleuroperitoneal membranes completes the muscular sheet of the diaphragm. This occurs by the ninth week, with the left posterolateral aspect the last to close. The intestines return to the abdomen from an extracelomic position by the tenth week. A failure of closure of the diaphragm results in herniation into the pleural cavity (Plate 113). This herniation takes place during the period of lung development and may prevent maturation of lung tissue. Additionally, there is reduced growth of the abdomen and failure of normal rotation.

Pathophysiology

After birth, increasing air volume in the intestines progressively compresses lung tissue. Hypoplasia of pulmonary parenchyma further diminishes diffusion, resulting in hypercarbia, hypoxemia, and respiratory acidosis. As a consequence, pulmonary hypertension and persistent fetal circulation occur. A patent ductus may shunt unoxygenated blood into the systemic circulation. These events, if uncorrected, lead to myocardial failure and death.

364

Preoperative Treatment

Congenital posterolateral diaphragmatic hernia is a true surgical emergency. As soon as possible, the following steps should be taken:

1. Turn the baby to the side of the hernia, thereby decreasing contralateral pressure on the lung.
2. Maintain body temperature.
3. Insert an endotracheal tube with assisted ventilation of oxygen.
4. Insert an orogastric or nasogastric tube with suction.
5. The infant should be transported to a pediatric center with tertiary facilities for emergency surgical correction and intensive neonatal care as expeditiously as possible.
6. Avoid sodium bicarbonate.

PLATE 113

Hernia through the Foramen of Bochdalek

A. The diaphragm from below, showing the foramen of Bochdalek and the foramen of Morgagni. Both are weak areas of potential herniation. Arrows indicate the direction of enlargement after herniation has begun.

Source: From Skandalakis JE, Gray SW, Rowe JS Jr.: Surgical anatomy of the diaphragm, in *Mastery of Surgery,* Nyhus LM, Baker RJ (eds). Little, Brown, Boston, 1984, p. 306, Fig. 38-5.

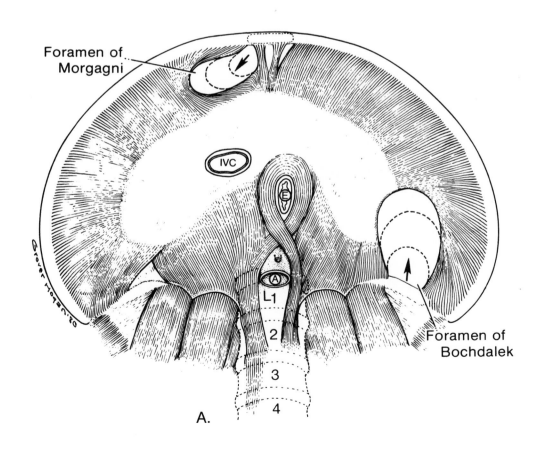

PLATE 113 (*Continued*)

Hernia through the Foramen of Bochdalek

B. Herniation of intestines through the foramen of Bochdalek compressing the left lung. The mediastinum is shifted to the right, reducing the volume of the right lung also.

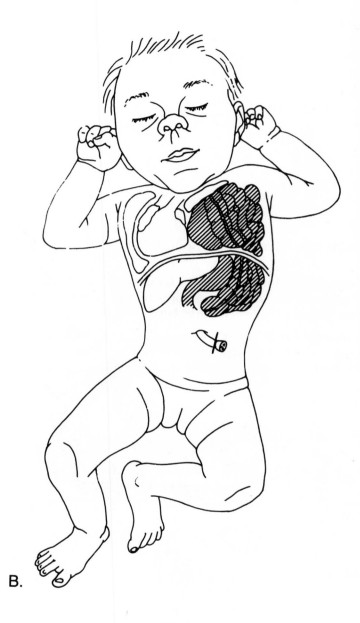

B.

PLATE 114
Repair of Hernia through the Foramen of Bochdalek

Inset:

A. *Step 1.* Make a transverse upper abdominal incision starting slightly to the right of the midline, across the abdomen to the left flank.

Step 2. Retract the intestines to expose the diaphragmatic defect through which the intestines have herniated into the chest cavity. Insert a soft red rubber catheter through the defect to allow air pressure in the chest to equalize as the intestines and other herniated organs are withdrawn.

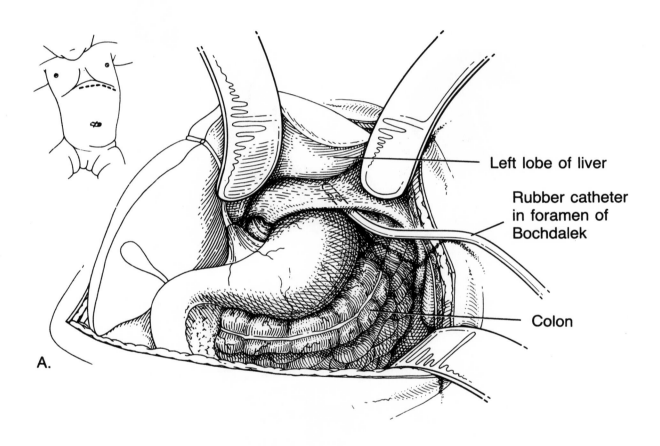

Left lobe of liver

Rubber catheter in foramen of Bochdalek

Colon

A.

PLATE 114 (*Continued*)

Repair of Hernia through the Foramen of Bochdalek

B. *Step 3.* In the unusual instance where a sac is present, a small opening in it will allow it to be pulled into the abdomen and excised.

C. *Step 4.* Do not disturb the hypoplastic lung within the chest. Avoid attempts to expand the hypoplastic lung with excess intrabronchial pressure which may cause aveolar rupture.

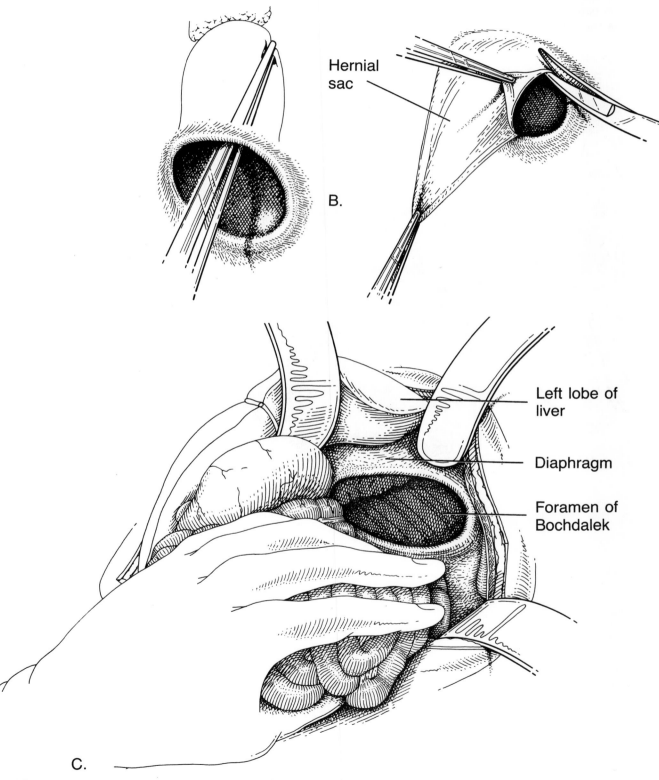

Hernial
sac

B.

Left lobe of
liver

Diaphragm

Foramen of
Bochdalek

C.

D. *Step 5.* Suture the diaphragm with interrupted 00 silk sutures passing through the anteromedial edge and the posterolateral margin of the diaphragm.

As the lateral margin is approached, pass the sutures through the chest wall or even the rib for anchoring purposes. (Rarely, a synthetic material is needed for closure; Prolene or Dacron-reinforced Silastic sheeting may be used.) Insert a chest tube prior to closure of the diaphragm.

E. *Step 6.* Evaluate the abdomen for closure. If closure appears to cause excessive intraabdominal pressure, the skin alone should be closed, leaving a ventral hernia to be repaired later.

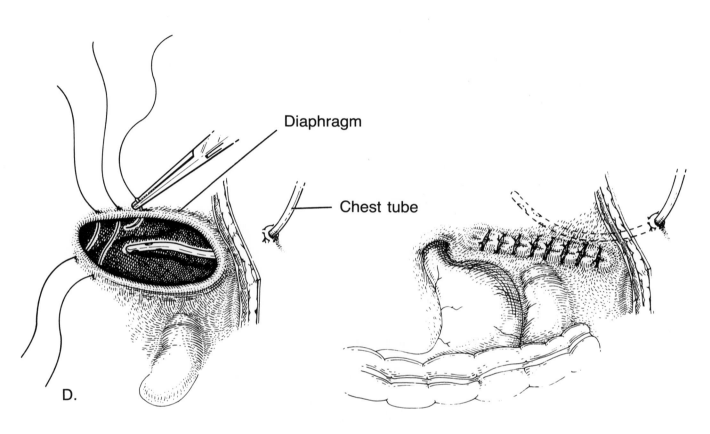

Diaphragm

Chest tube

D.

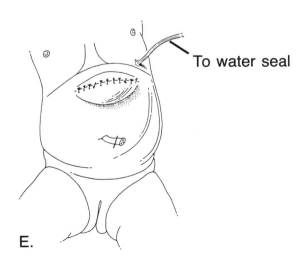

To water seal

E.

PLATE 114 (*Continued*)

Repair of Hernia through the Foramen of Bochdalek

F. *Step 7.* An alternative is to suture a Dacron-reinforced Silastic silo over the bowel. Suture the silo to the skin with 00 Prolene continuous sutures. This requires later closure. (See "Treatment and Repair" of omphalocele.)

G. *Step 8.* If the abdominal pressure is not too great, primary closure can be effected.

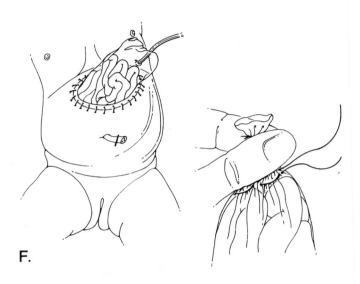

F.

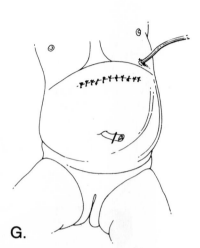

G.

Postoperative Treatment

This is a critical period requiring intensive neonatal care, as follows:

1. Delivery of humidified oxygen.
2. Ventilatory support with hyperventilation to reduce P_{CO_2} may be indicated.
3. Sedation and paralytic agents may be needed.
4. Monitoring arterial blood gases.
5. IV, pharmacologic agents (tolazoline, dopamine, etc.,) may be needed.
6. Chest tube care—water level in water seal drainage should be no more than 1 or 2 cm above lower end of line attached to intrathoracic catheter.
7. IV fluids, electrolytes, blood, antibiotics, etc.
8. Temperature control.

Retrosternal Hernia (through the Foramen of Morgagni)

Thus also, anteriorly, betwixt the fibres that come from the xiphoid cartilage and the neighbouring fibres, there generally is an interval through which something similar [herniation] may happen.

MORGAGNI
De Sedibus, Letter LIV, Article 11

Definition

A retrosternal hernia is a herniation of an intestinal loop through small triangular areas of the diaphragm on either side of the inferior end of the sternum. They are bounded medially by muscle fibers from the xiphoid process and laterally by fibers from the costal cartilages. These "foramina of Morgagni," "spaces of Larrey," or "parasternal spaces" permit the passage of the superior epigastric vessels and may be also the site of herniation of abdominal contents. Herniation is usually on the right, but bilateral defects are known. A sac is always formed but it may have ruptured, leaving no trace.

The spaces represent the junction of the embryonic septum transversum, the lateral component of the diaphragm, and the anterior thoracic wall. A dual herniation is often the result of trauma.

371

PLATE 115

Repair of Retrosternal Hernia (Foramen of Morgagni)

A. *Step 1.* An upper transverse abdominal incision will provide sufficient exposure of the hernia.

B. *Step 2.* Open the peritoneum and identify the defect in the anterior portion of the diaphragm.

C. *Step 3.* Withdraw any hernial contents. A sac is usually present and should be excised.

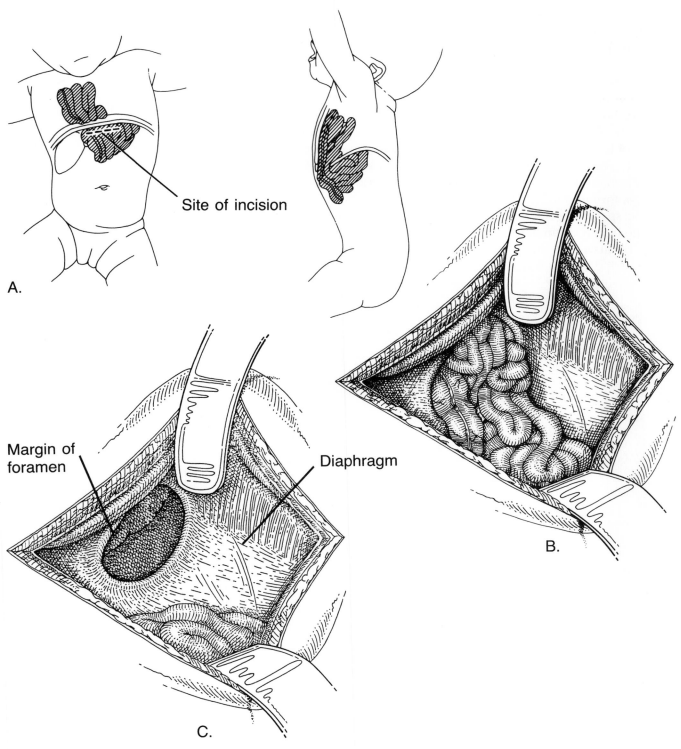

Site of incision

A.

Margin of foramen

Diaphragm

B.

C.

D. *Step 4.* Close the defect by suturing the inferior edge of the diaphragm to the posterior rectus fascia.

If the thorax is entered, insert a chest tube via the seventh or eighth intercostal space, anchoring it to the skin with 00 silk.

Close the defect by tying the anchoring sutures. Prosthetic materials are rarely needed.

E. *Step 5.* Close the abdomen.

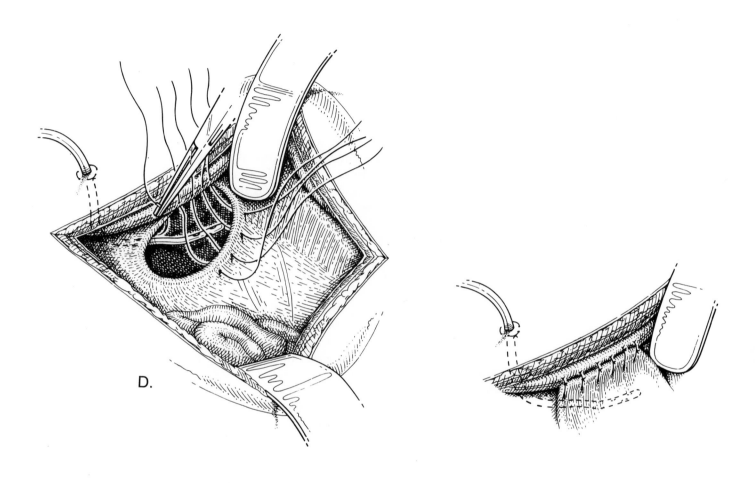

D.

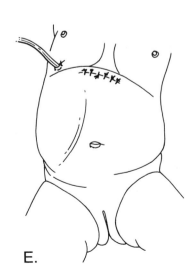

E.

Pericardial Hernia

Definition

This is a hernia through the central tendon of the diaphragm and the pericardium. A sac is rarely present. It may be associated with pentalogy of Cantrell, which includes a distal sternal defect, an omphalocele, the anterior diaphragmatic defect with pericardioperitoneal defect, a ventricular septal defect, and a left ventricular diverticulum. Fewer than 50 cases are known.

Embryology

The defect is in the transverse septum, the earliest of the diaphragmatic components to be formed. Since the septum is not paired, there is no fusion defect. We suggest that there is a secondary rupture of the embryonic septum during the fourth embryonic week. This is in contrast to other hernias of the diaphragm in which the defect is the congenital result of failure of fusion.

Surgical Repair of Pericardial Hernia

1. Make an upper midline incision for an abdominal approach.
2. Visualize the pericardial defect.
3. If a ventricular diverticulum is present, remove it by placing a noncrushing vascular clamp across its base and excising it. Repair the cardiac muscle with interrupted 00000 Prolene mattress sutures tied over pledgets of Dacron.
4. Close the edges of the pericardium with interrupted 000 silk sutures.
5. Close the abdomen with continuous absorbable Vicryl sutures.
6. Close the skin.

Diaphragmatic Eventration

Definition

This is a congenital lesion in which the muscular layer of one leaf of the diaphragm, usually the left, is absent or greatly reduced. The affected leaf is thin and membranous and is grossly elevated. The ipsilateral lung is partly collapsed but not hypoplastic; the mediastinum is shifted to the contralateral side, which further reduces ventilation. The phrenic nerve is normal.

Treatment is required only when decreased pulmonary function resulting from the deformity is sufficient to warrant surgical correction.

Embryology

The frequent disruption of the normal pattern of gut rotation and abnormal mesenteric attachments are the strongest arguments that the defect existed in fetal life. The presence of a normal phrenic nerve, shown by histologic section at autopsy in some cases and implied by a synchronous motion of the halves of the diaphragm in many other cases, is evidence that phrenic nerve injury is not responsible for most eventrations.

Congenital eventration is a failure of muscularization of the diaphragm, not a failure of fusion of its parts. Whether the defect is primarily muscular or is secondary to a distribution of phrenic nerve fibers is not known. It is more readily explained as failure of the migration of myoblasts along the phrenic nerve than by Bremer's theory of muscle formation from the thoracic wall.

PLATE 116

Diaphragmatic Eventration

Eventration of the (left) diaphragm. The herniated abdominal organs remain beneath the attenuated but intact leaf of the diaphragm. Both lungs are compressed and the mediastinum is shifted to the right.

Source: From Skandalakis JE, Gray SW, Rowe JS Jr.: Surgical anatomy of the diaphragm, in *Mastery of Surgery,* Nyhus LM, Baker BJ (eds.). Boston, Little, Brown, vol. 1, 1984, p. 306, Fig. 38-7.

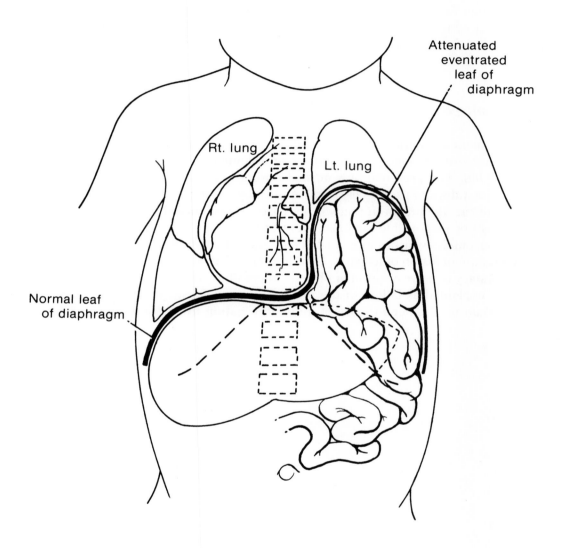

PLATE 117
Repair of Diaphragmatic Eventration

The surgical approach to eventration may be thoracic or abdominal. The thoracic approach has the advantage of direct vision of the diaphragm as well as avoiding injury to the intestines.

A. *Step 1.* Enter the chest through the bed of the seventh or eighth rib on the side of the lesion.

B. Site of the incision.

C. *Step 2.* Retract the lung to expose the eventrated diaphragm.

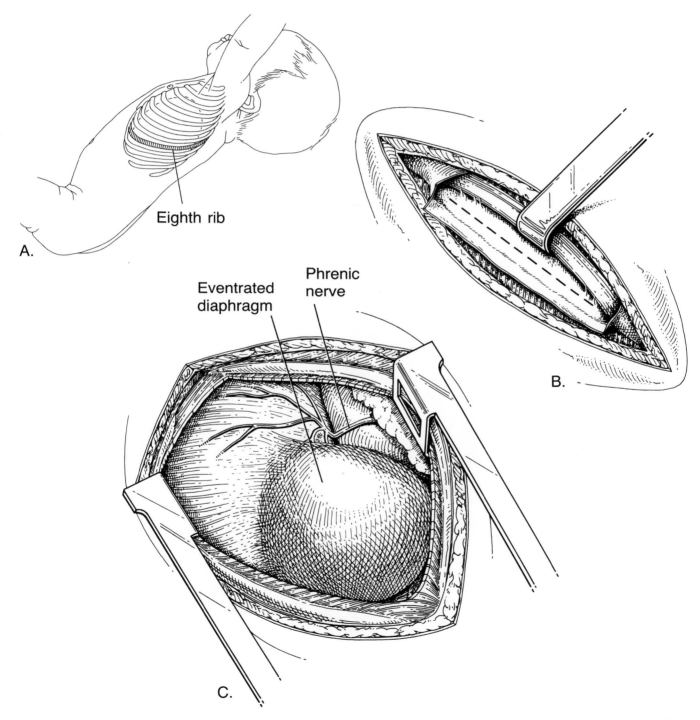

Eighth rib

A.

B.

Eventrated diaphragm

Phrenic nerve

C.

PLATE 117 (*Continued*)

Repair of Diaphragmatic Eventration

D. *Step 3.* Invert the diaphragm and suture its edges with 00 or 000 silk interrupted sutures or mattress sutures.

E. *Step 4.* Use pledgets of Dacron to reinforce the sutures if the tissue of the diaphragm is friable. Insert a chest tube into the thorax by tunneling under the skin. Secure the tube with a silk suture and a 00 purse-string suture to prevent pneumothorax and ensure retention.

F. *Step 5.* Close the chest with two pericostal sutures of 00 or 000 chromic catgut. Connect the chest tube with a water seal, and apply continuous negative suction of 10 to 15 cm of water.

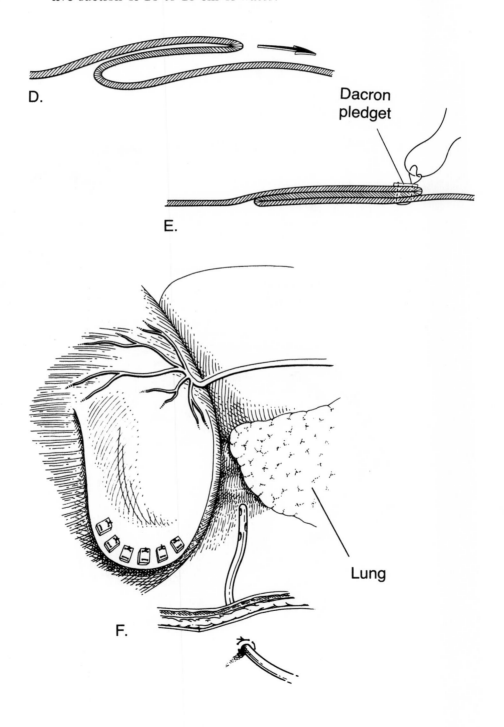

D.

Dacron
pledget

E.

Lung

F.

SECTION FIVE
EPONYMOUS HERNIAS

Good humor . . . helps enormously both in the study and practice of medicine.

SIR WILLIAM OSLER

A peculiar feature of much of the literature of the anatomy of hernia is its tendency to use proper names in place of structural designations.

METTLER
History of Medicine, 1947

Aren't there any structures named for Smith or Jones?

FIRST-YEAR MEDICAL STUDENT

Hernias have produced a long list of eponyms (Table 13). They have been applied to the hernias themselves, to structures through which the hernias pass, and to repair procedures. The list reads like a roster of great surgeons of the first half of the nineteenth century.

Most of the eponymous hernias are completely obscure, to be found only in the dictionary. A few have persisted to this day. Posterior hernia of the diaphragm is still called hernia through the foramen of Bochdalek. Is it the rhythm of the name, together with its improbability (to English-speaking people) that helps it survive?

Eponymous hernias are the result of (1) a good description of the lesions believed to be unlike any previously reported, (2) a reorganization of material from the literature, or (3) frequent use of the eponym by colleagues, students, or surgeons who popularized an old procedure. The last of these is the best way to transitory or even permanent fame.

A glance at Table 13 will show many repetitions. Professional jealousy and national pride are important factors in the presentation of eponyms. Hernia through the superior lumbar triangle of Grynfelt occurs in France, but in Germany the hernia passes through the triangle of Lesgaft!

In the anterior diaphragm, the name of Morgagni has survived even though there is an alternative eponym: the spaces of Larrey. Here the great pathologist appears to be taking precedence over the great military surgeon. Morgagni is more readily available in translation than is Larrey.

Spigelian hernia of the anterior abdominal wall has preserved its eponymy largely because more descriptive terms have proved to be too cumbersome.

Two other eponymous hernias have a curiously intermingled history. In 1778, Richter described a case in which a portion of the antimesenteric border of the ileum was incarcerated or strangulated in a firm and rigid ring, usually, but not always, in the femoral region. Early in its development, the intestinal lumen is only partially obstructed; later, obstruction becomes total. Three-quarters of a century earlier (1699) Littre described an inguinal hernia containing a Meckel's diverticulum. As the diverticulum itself was yet to be described by Meckel (1809), there was at first confusion between Richter's and Littre's hernias. In both lesions, the lumen of the ileum is only partially obstructed.

Littre's hernia can be described as "hernia of a persistent omphalomesenteric duct" or reduced to "hernia of Meckel's diverticulum," thereby substituting one eponym with another. "Littre's hernia" will probably persist with surgeons and in textbooks, especially since it is very uncommon.

Within the inguinal region, most of the major structures were at first eponymous (Table 14). By the end of the nineteenth century many of the eponyms were replaced by descriptive names. Only the pectineal ligament retains the name "Cooper's ligament," even by authors who grant no other eponyms. It is fitting that Sir Astley Cooper's name has survived, as his two-volume work (1804, 1807) on hernia was the greatest single contribution to the anatomy of the inguinal region. "Cooper's ligament" deserves this honor.

In the femoral triangle (of Scarpa) eponyms are legion because the pathway of the hernial sac may have varying relations to the femoral blood vessels. Seven such hernias are shown in Plate 118.

Two other names are a little less commonly used. The inguinal ligament is Poupart's and the lacunar ligament is Gimbernat's. While not descriptive, these eponyms are no harder to remember than are the "official" names. Whether they will survive remains to be seen.

TABLE 13
Eponymous Hernias

Eponym	Date	Description
Barth		H. of loops of intestine between the abdominal wall and the persistent vitelline duct
Beclard	1835	Eventration of the diaphragm
Berger		H. into pouch of Douglas
Berkett		H. into the vaginal process of the peritoneum
Blake		H. through levator ani muscle
Blandin		H. into the foramen of Winslow
Boccard		H. through the pelvic floor
Bochdalek	1848	H. through posterior foramen of diaphragm
Broesike	1891	H. into intermesocolic fossa
Bruggiser		Parainguinal H.
Chase		See Blake above
Callisen-Cloquet	1817	H. through aponeurosis of pectineus muscle (femoral)
Cooper	1807	Femoral H. with multilocular sac
Dobson		Mesocolic H.
Eppinger		H. in which the vascular arch (Treitz) is behind the posterior wall of the fossa
Fagge		H. into the broad ligament
Gerdy		Adumbilical H.
Gibbon		H. with hydrocele
Goyrand	1836	H. between layers of abdominal wall (interstitial)
Gruber	1859	Right paraduodenal H.
Grynfelt	1866	H. through superior lumbar triangle
Hensig		Retroperitoneal H.
Hesselbach	1806	External femoral H.
Hey		Bilocular femoral H.
Holthouse		H. extending along Poupart's ligament—inguinal-crural H.
Honnesco		Retroperitoneal H.
Huschke		Retroperitoneal H.
Klob		Right duodenal H.
Krönlein	1876	Properitoneal inguinal H.
Kuster	1887	Inguinal superficial H.
Lacoste		Ischiorectal H.
Landzert	1871	H. into paraduodenal fossa
Laugier	1833	H. through lacunar ligament of Gimbernat (femoral)
Lesgaft	1870	See Grynfelt above
Linhart		Retroperitoneal H.
Littre	1714	Groin H. containing Meckel's diverticulum only
Loebel		H. through transverse mesocolon
Macready		H. through the pelvic outlet
Malgaigne		Infantile H. intestines preceding descent of testes
Maydl		H. of two loops of intestine through same hernial ring, "W" H.
Mery		Perineal H.
Molin		Infracolic H.
Morgagni	1769	H. through anterior foramen of diaphragm
Partridge		Femoral H. external to the femoral blood vessels
Petersen	1900	Retroanastomotic H.
Petit	1783	H. through inferior lumbar triangle
Quain		H. into the broad ligament
Richter	1785	H. of antimesenteric part only of circumference of intestine
Rieux		Retrocecal H.
Rokitansky	1836	Transmesenteric H.
Sandifort		Retroperitoneal H.
Santorini		H. into the pericecal fossa
Schwalbe		H. through hiatus of Schwalbe into ischiorectal fossa
Seiler		Posterior labial H.

TABLE 13 (*Continued*)

Eponym	Date	Description
Serafini	1917	Femoral H. posterior to femoral vessels
Spieghel	1645	Lateral, ventral H.
Teale		Prevascular femoral H.
Toldt		H. into duodenomesocolic fossa
Treitz	1857	H. into superior or inferior duodenal fossa (duodenojejunal)
Treve		Anterior retroperitoneal H.
Velpeau	1839	See Callisen-Cloquet
Von Bergmann		Intermittent hiatal H.
Waldeyer	1874	H. into mesentericoparietal fossa
Winckel		Retroperitoneal, right duodenal H.
Winslow	1824	H. through the epiploic foramen

NOTE: Where there is a single known date for the use of the eponym, it is given; otherwise, it may be assumed to be nineteenth century.

TABLE 14
Eponyms of the Inguinal Region

Eponym	Date	Description
Colles' ligament	1811	Reflected inguinal ligament
Cooper's ligament	1804, 1807	Pectineal ligament
Gimbernat's ligament	1793	Lacunar ligament
Henle's ligament		Falx inguinalis
Hesselbach's ligament	1814	Interfoveolar ligament
Polya's ligament	1912	Inferior crus of external oblique aponeurosis
Poupart's ligament	1705	Inguinal ligament
Thomson's ligament	1836	Iliopubic tract

PLATE 118
Sites of Typical and Atypical Eponymous Femoral Hernias

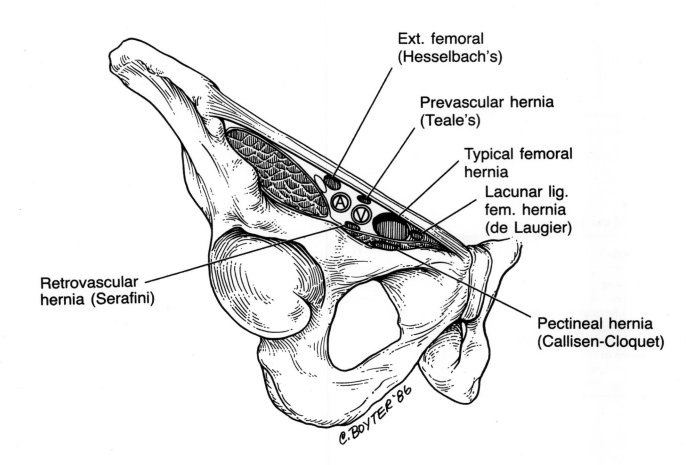

Ext. femoral
(Hesselbach's)

Prevascular hernia
(Teale's)

Typical femoral
hernia

Lacunar lig.
fem. hernia
(de Laugier)

Retrovascular
hernia (Serafini)

Pectineal hernia
(Callisen-Cloquet)